Pioneers in Neuroendocrinology

PERSPECTIVES IN NEUROENDOCRINE RESEARCH

Volume 1 • PIONEERS IN NEUROENDOCRINOLOGY
*Edited by Joseph Meites, Bernard T. Donovan,
and Samuel M. McCann • 1975*

A Continuation Order Plan is available for this series. A continuation order will bring delivery of each new volume immediately upon publication. Volumes are billed only upon actual shipment. For further information please contact the publisher.

Pioneers in
Neuroendocrinology

Edited by
Joseph Meites
Department of Physiology
Michigan State University
East Lansing, Michigan

Bernard T. Donovan
Department of Physiology
Institute of Psychiatry
London, England

and
Samuel M. McCann
Department of Physiology
Southwestern Medical School
University of Texas Health Science Center
Dallas, Texas

PLENUM PRESS • NEW YORK AND LONDON

Library of Congress Cataloging in Publication Data

Main entry under title:

Pioneers in neuroendocrinology.

(Perspectives in neuroendocrine research; v. 1)
Includes bibliographies and index.
1. Neuroendocrinology — History — Collected works. 2. Endocrinolo-
gists — Correspondence, reminiscences, etc. — Collected works. 3. Neu-
rologists — Correspondence, reminiscences, etc. — Collected works.
I. Meites, Joseph, 1913-   II. Donovan, Bernard Thomas. III.
McCann, Samuel McDonald, 1925-   [DNLM: 1. Endocrine glands
— Physiology — Personal narratives. 2. Neurophysiology — Personal nar-
ratives. W1 PE871H v. 1 / WZ112 P662]
QP356.4.P46   599'.01'88   75-19075
ISBN 0-306-34901-9

©1975 Plenum Press, New York
A Division of Plenum Publishing Corporation
227 West 17th Street, New York, N.Y. 10011

United Kingdom edition published by Plenum Press, London
A Division of Plenum Publishing Company, Ltd.
Davis House (4th Floor), 8 Scrubs Lane, Harlesden, London, NW10 6SE, England

Printed in the United States of America

Preface

In the middle and late 1960s, when it was clear that neuroendocrinology was established as a discipline in its own right, it occurred to us that auto-biographical accounts of the pioneer work in this field by the major participants would provide a highly interesting and informative account of history in the making. With the death of G. W. Harris in late 1971, and the loss thereby of an outstanding pioneer and personality in neuroendocrinology, it appeared to us to be even more urgent to undertake such a venture and collect as many stories as possible. The three of us agreed that initially we would limit our invitations to the senior investigators whose research careers lay mostly behind them, with the hope that if this venture proved successful, we could ask younger and still very active researchers in neuroendocrinology to contribute to a subsequent volume. Most of those invited to write for this book agreed to do so, but regrettably there remain some notable absentees.

The authors were requested to write a personal, and even idiosyncratic, account of the steps taken, and the motivation and drive that led them to develop their interest in the relationship between the brain and the endocrine system. They were asked to provide information on the source of their inspiration, encouragement, and financial support, and to indicate where their achievements, rewards, and disappointments lay; also to convey something of the flavor, atmosphere, and climate of opinion at the time they did their work. We have undertaken the minimum amount of editing in an effort to preserve the individual character of each pioneer.

This book deals with some of the early work on neurosecretion, neurotransmitters, releasing factors, locus and control of ADH and oxytocin secretion, neural control of the anterior pituitary, the role of the portal vessels, brain neuroanatomy and neurophysiology, effects of lesions and electrical stimulation of discrete brain areas, electrophysiological recordings and correlates, feedback mechanisms, reproductive neuroendocrinology, effects of hormones on behavior, and other aspects. There is hardly an area of modern neuroendocrinology that is not represented here by earlier investigations. We believe that the reader, be he student, teacher, or researcher, will be presented with a much livelier, broader, and more rounded picture of the development of this important branch of physiology and medicine than can

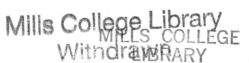

be obtained from the relatively colorless descriptions in a textbook or monograph. We hope readers will learn as much as we have from this collection, and we shall welcome comments, be they critical or otherwise.

We wish to express our appreciation to Dr. Gordon Campbell and Lindsey Grandison for help in preparing the Index, and to Carol Bradley and James Simpkins for help in proofreading the manuscripts.

Joseph Meites
Bernard T. Donovan
Samuel M. McCann

Contents

1

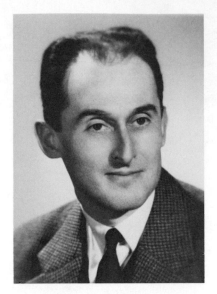

Claude Aron

Claude Aron was born on February 21, 1917, in Paris. He received an M.D. degree from the Medical School, University of Strasbourg, in 1942. He became an Assistant in Histology in 1945, Licencié dès Sciences in 1946, Maitre de Conférences in 1953, Professeur sans chaire in 1958, and Professeur titulaire in 1961 at the University of Strasbourg.

Neuroendocrine Feedbacks

CLAUDE ARON

Looking back, in an Aristotelian manner, at prime motives, I do not recall in the schoolboy I still was in 1933 any inclination for biological research, or, for that matter, the study of the relationship between the brain and the endocrine glands. On the other hand, a brief survey of my past convinces me that cerebral problems played a decisive part in the shaping of my career. These were annoying headaches that suddenly started when I was between 15 and 16 years of age and which decided my future by obliging me to leave the mathematics class as this was held to be the cause of my trouble! It was, therefore, as a philosophy student which I then became, that I enrolled in the Medical School. Of course, my belated choice of career was not strange with my family background. Neither, I think, was my rapid decision to take up biology.

But I must admit that at the outset of my medical career the problems of endocrine interrelations did not interest me greatly. Like many young people I was fascinated by biochemistry, which already wielded a vast attraction on those of us who were considering taking up research work. In my case, an additional attraction was the character of Georges Fontes, a great friend of my parents, who lectured in biochemistry at the Strasbourg Medical School. Doubtless circumstances contributed to this choice as it did not stand the test of time. Fontes died prematurely, and in wartime conditions I never came back to the laboratory of my late friend. However, at this time I had completed my theoretical scientific studies under Terroine, holder of the chair of physiology at the Science Faculty in Strasbourg, and felt more and more drawn toward physiology. I wrote, therefore, shortly before I was demobilized, in the first place to Charles Kayser, the professor of physiology at the Medical School in Strasbourg, and afterward to Alfred Schwartz, the professor of pharmacology, applying for an assistant's post in their laboratories. They were unable to grant my request. Being unfamiliar,

CLAUDE ARON ● Institute of Histology, Faculty of Medicine, University of Strasbourg, Strasbourg, France.

at that time, with the regulations governing the employment of research workers at the CNRS, I unsuccessfully applied to it for a research scholarship. This dual setback and, above all, my distaste for the Parisian hurly burly decided me to accept the post of assistant which Max Aron, who succeeded Pol Bouin, offered me at the Histology Institute at the Faculty of Medicine in Strasbourg. It is true that circumstances dictated this course for me. But it made me happy for two reasons. In the first place, it corresponded with a sincere desire to return to Alsace, and, furthermore, I fully appreciated the chance of undergoing my training as a physiologist at a school which had been the cradle of experimental morphology, and which was still a well-known center of endocrine physiology. I have never had cause to regret it from a scientific point of view. My introduction into this field thus fully satisfied my taste for research.

It is true that study of the thyroid held a more prominent place than that of the ovary in the laboratory where Max Aron had discovered thyrostimuline (TSH) and defined the morphological signs of thyroid function. But whether it was a question of ovarian biology or thyroid histophysiology, the subjects set us by Max Aron always concerned questions of correlation between endocrine glands or, what is more, study of what would now be called "feedbacks." Which, as will be seen, led as early as 1947 to my first neuroendocrinological work, and prompted me, throughout my now almost 30 years of research work, to take more interest, I must confess, in neuroendocrine feedbacks applied to the organism than in the molecular aspect of hormonal action. It is obviously fundamental to describe the mechanism whereby LH acts on the ovary or estrogens on the hypothalamic structures, but it seems to me equally important to describe the chain of events leading up to, by means of positive or negative feedbacks, the storage or "chronic" or "acute" secretion of LH during the estrous cycle. And I think in this field, to mention only that example, there is great scope for those specializing in reproduction.

But to go back to neuroendocrinology. On his return to Strasbourg Max Aron resumed experiments, using the guinea pig, which he had previously carried out on the immature female rat, and which related to the action of estrogens on follicular growth. This was the theme of my introduction to endocrinology. FSH was not measured in those days and we looked for proof of the short-term action of estradiol on the ovary of the guinea pig. To do this, the left ovary was removed, to be used as a control, from immature female guinea pigs weighing 200–220 g. One group was injected with estradiol at the time of operation and another was left untreated until the remaining ovary was removed 36 hours later. In this way, it was possible to compare the development of ovarian follicles during this period of time and find out the role attributable to estrogens in this evolution (Aron, Aron, and Marescaux, 1948). What a surprise to discover that hemicastration produced a marked stimulation of follicular activity in the controls, resulting in a hyperplastic and hypertrophic growth of the cells of the internal theca and granular membrane (Aron and Marescaux, 1948*a*). The controls became the center point of this experiment. The picture we had just exposed was never seen in the ovaries of intact animals of the same age and weight. Moreover, the administration of estrogen not only did not inhibit this phenomenon, it accentuated it. This *reactional hyperactivity* was certainly not due to hormone deficiency resulting from removal of one of the two ovaries, since the removal of the smallest ovarian fragment or the intraovarian injection of NaCl had the same effect as hemicastration (Aron and Marescaux, 1948*b*). We then thought, given the speed of the reaction, that it was a reflex starting in the ovary and relayed to the hypothalamus. We then carried out spinal cord transections between D2 and D5, either shortly before or shortly after hemicastration.

The first experiments confirmed our theory. It was not a matter arising from the effects of surgical shock, since cord section only suppressed reactional hyperactivity when it was carried out before hemi-castration (Aron, Marx, and Marescaux, 1948). It should be noted that even then we were suspicious of the complicating effects of corticosuprarenal stimulation. But it was, at the time, still a very vague idea, since nobody knew that adrenocortical progesterone was capable of stimulating the pituitary to discharge gonadotrophic hormones. Quite the reverse; if I remember correctly, H. Selye thought stress slowed down FSH production. Nevertheless, later on we noticed doubtless because cord transection was stressful, some variability in the suppressive action of this operation on reactional hyperactivity. Therefore we thought it was essential to confirm our first results, particularly as they had been greeted by an uproar at the Biological Society. Looking back at the meeting where this paper was presented, I wonder what can have so infuriated certain biologists. It must be acknowledged that they were distinctly hostile to the idea that the nervous system could intervene in the relationship between endocrine glands. To them, the compensatory hypertrophy of the surviving ovary after hemicastration, as described by Lipschutz in 1930, was the result of a purely hormonal readjustment. That the nervous system had anything to do with it was to them a heresy, even if, as early as 1927, Pines had demonstrated a rich ovarian nerve supply in many species of mammal. It was doubtless unforgivable to deprive ovarian hormones of their exclusive role as messengers.

I think the fact we persisted along this course was a sign of complete indifference. Nonetheless the fact remains that, in the following years, we went on with our experiments, and we were able to demonstrate that mesovarian sections, respecting the vascular pedicle of the ovary, had the same effect as unilateral oophorectomy, and, moreover, that novocain injected into the mesovarium prior to hemicastration suppressed the stimulatory action of this intervention (Aron, Marx, and Marescaux, 1949). This obviously confirmed the reflex nature of a phenomenon which, as we showed later, brought the pituitary into action, since cytological examination of that gland by the then available methods in the hours following hemicastration showed the presence of manifest degranulation in the gonadotrophic cells (Aron, Petrovic, Marescaux, and Isaac, 1951). And we noted that the performance of hypophysectomy shortly after hemicastration did not suppress reactional hyperactivity, whereas, of course, nothing further happened if removal of the ovary followed that of the pituitary (Aron, Aron, and Marescaux, 1952).

This research took place between 1947 and 1952, at which time we became acquainted with the exceptional work of Everett, Sawyer, and their co-workers. Moreover, we could now get Anglo-Saxon publications, such as those of Dey in 1940–41, which were unknown to us at the outset of our research; and we also bore in mind the observations of Harris in 1937, Marshall and Verney in 1936, and Haterius and Derbyshire in 1937, according to which an electrical stimulation of the hypothalamus was capable of triggering off ovulation in the rabbit. Again, we wondered why the neuroendocrine reflex we had demonstrated in the guinea pig never brought about ovulation in the female.

Obviously, we were not on forbidden ground in imagining that, under our experimental conditions, the amount of LH released was insufficient to trigger off ovulation, or again that the ovaries of the immature females on which we were working were not sensitive enough to gonadotrophic hormones to enable ovulation to occur. This being the case, it was simply necessary to extend our investigations to the mature female.

What I now wonder, 25 years later, is why we waited 15 years to do this. I can see there was one main reason at the time. In the light of our then knowledge of pituitary function in spontaneous ovulators, I found it difficult to imagine the possible significance, from a physiological standpoint, of an information system originating at the level of the ovary and solely concerned in the regulation of follicular growth. If we had observed ovulatory changes following our ovarian interventions, we could have thought of a nervous feedback system, such as growing follicles "informing" the nervous structures on their state of development.

I think, therefore, if I was rather tired of this work, it was because I was not convinced of the foundation of the arguments I have just evoked concerning the inability of the ovary to respond to hemicastration, and I finished up by considering reactional hyperactivity to be in the nature of a caricature. Does one not obtain the same result by inducing adrenocortical progesterone release at six o'clock on the morning of proestrus by means of simple ovarian traction?

I therefore thrust my definite dissatisfaction with this work to the back of my mind until one day, more than 15 years later, when I asked J. Roos and M. Roos to hemicastrate either 4- or 5-day cyclic rats, and investigate, at short term, the effects of this operation on the surviving ovary.

The fruit amply fulfilled the promise of our first flowers. Roos's observations fully confirmed our earlier results. Not only had hemicastration strongly stimulated the activity of the pituitary, but it had brought about ovulatory changes in 100% of cases in the ensuing 24 hours, when it was carried out on the morning of diestrus III in 5-day cyclic animals (Roos and Roos, 1966*a*). Yet, ablation of an ovary only exercised a mild action of this type on diestrus II of 4-day cyclic rats, and, moreover, it partially impeded the production of ovulatory changes which should occur during the night between the fourth and fifth day of 5-day cycles when it was carried out between 1600*h* and 1730*h*, on diestrus III (Roos and Roos, 1966*b*). It was tempting to compare these effects of unilateral oophorectomy with those produced by progesterone injection, administered in the morning or late afternoon of diestrus III as reported by Everett in 1948 and Zeilmaker in 1966. But I admit it was only later, on learning the results of observations made by Lorenzen, Nequin, and Schwartz in 1968, Feder, Resko, and Goy in 1968, and Resko in 1969, that we thought of associating adrenocortical progesterone with the occurrence of the ovulatory effects of hemicastration.

We knew that central nervous structures were involved in this phenomenon, since the injection of atropine prior to hemicastration had totally impeded it in an experimental series (Roos and Roos, 1966*a*). Also, in spite of the fact that this block appeared incomplete in other experiments carried out using pentobarbitone (unpublished results) we still kept to the theory that the ovulation triggered off by hemicastration was the result of a positive feedback of progesterone on hypothalamic structures. The ovarian origin of the progesterone acting in this way did not meet with our agreement.

The fact remains that, busy as we were with other experimental trials, of which more later, we did not delve deeper into this question until the adrenal cortex was suggested as being a possible factor in the control of gonadotrophic function, by reason of the progesterone secreted by it into the blood stream. We then decided to adrenalectomize 5-day cyclic rats and study the effects of hemicastration on them. I prefer to go no further. The result was unpredictable and hitherto unknown. Nature is capricious. Adrenalectomy converted all our 5-day cyclic animals into 4-day cyclics rendering our project unpractical. But this time I shall not give up the investigation of the problem. Perhaps it will be possible in the ensuing months for our laboratory to throw some light on the matter. But it will be necessary to find another experimental subject for the purpose of demonstrating that ovulation triggered off by hemicastration, in suitable hormonal conditions, is due to a discharge of extraovarian progesterone.

Perhaps it is surprising to see so much space devoted to a research project which, in spite of giving undeniable information on the neuroendocrine aspect of ovarian–pituitary interrelationships, was full of pitfalls, and resulted in findings impossible to verify completely, even in the rat, for practical reasons. It is because they seem to me to disclose the importance of psychological events in the life of a research worker. If the work on reactional hyperactivity had been well received, I would very probably, and straightaway, have been induced to take up the investigation of this problem at the level of the hypothalamus. Instead I spent several years studying ovarian function.

I know it was quite by accident I found out that vaginal stimulation was capable of eliciting follicular stimulation in the female guinea pig (Aron and Aron-Brunetiere, 1953). But this discovery was altogether the result of my professional awareness. My brother, Dr. Aron-Brunetiere, wanted to study the transmucous passage of hormones such as PMS and FSH. I suggested to him placing hormone pellets in the guinea pig's vagina. A stitch in the vaginal orifice would prevent the expulsion of the pellets. It was necessary therefore, in order to appreciate the gonadotrophic action of FSH, to eliminate any possible action due to the ligature. The experiments proved the genital area was a reflexogenic zone in the guinea pig. We later verified the same finding in the rat (Aron, Asch, and Roos, 1968; Aron, Roos, and Asch, 1968).

But this was simply an interlude, for my main work at that time was to determine the state of ovarian reactivity in the mature rat to gonadotrophic hormones at different stages in the estrous cycle. I wanted to show that even during the course of the estrous cycle, and under entirely physiological conditions, a spontaneous ovulator was capable of ovulating under the action of coitus. But first it had to be shown that, at an early stage in their development, ovarian follicles could respond to gonadotrophic stimulation by their transformation into *corpora lutea*. It was for this reason that my research into ovulation was preceded by a whole series of investigations into ovarian function. In addition, it was also necessary either to set the scene for early receptivity in the female by administering, for example, estrogen, and by doing that to ensure one did not give rise to ovarian changes, or to allow for the possibility of early receptivity in a female such as the rat, which had not been primed with hormones. I knew at that time of the 1943 work of Dempsey and Searles, that of Segal and Johnson in 1959, and particularly that of Everett in 1952. But the first, carried out on a small number of animals, did not seem convincing to me; the second failed to show any proof of induced ovulation in the rat, since the authors themselves spoke of "provoked spontaneous" ovulation, and I must admit I paid more attention to the occurrence of delayed pseudopregnancy than to that of ovulation triggered off by coitus in Everett's experiments. Moreover, in my opinion, if these investigations had conclusively proved, in the latter case, that ovulation was triggered off by sexual intercourse, it did not follow that coitus was capable of setting off LH secretion in the natural conditions normally occurring before the "critical period" of the ovarian cycle.

The work was tedious at the beginning. We set out by trial and error to find the amount of estradiol capable of producing early receptivity during the night of diestrus II to proestrus in 4-day cycles, but lacking any appreciable ovulatory action on the ovary. Luck was with us. The Wistar (WI) strain rats bred in our laboratory since 1953 lent themselves admirably to the experiment and it was soon obvious (Aron, Asch, and Asch, 1961) that in 4-day cyclic rats, primed with estradiol on the morning of diestrus I, mating could set off luteinizing or ovulatory processes; atropine cut out these phenomena just as it does at the critical period in the cycle (Aron and Asch, 1962).

All the same, I was not satisfied since our method of investigation entailed the administration of estrogen to the female. Therefore I took a stupid chance. At that time it had not been proved that the level of estrogens in the ovarian plasma rose in the late afternoon of diestrus II or diestrus III in 4- and 5-day cycles, respectively. I hoped this was the case and the hormonal level would suffice for some females to mate spontaneously at these stages of the cycle. In order to record 17 matings during the night of diestrus II to proestrus in 4-day cycles, more than 200 females were presented to the male. On the other hand, 41 out of 82 females mated during the night of diestrus III to proestrus in 5-day cycles, ovulation occurring in 75% of these cases (Asch, Roos, and Aron, 1964; Aron, Asch, and Roos, 1966) whereas in 4-day cyclic females, unprimed with estrogen, mating had no effect on ovulation (Aron, Asch, and Luxembourger, 1964; Asch, Roos, and Aron, 1964; Aron, Asch, and Roos, 1966).

I think luck was with me on two counts. In the first place, because these experiments made me a behaviorist. Secondly, because the WI strain was ideal material on which to carry out this type of experiment. In the meantime we have compared the early mating frequencies of the WI strain with those of another Wistar strain (WII) bred in our colony since 1964 and with those of Holtzman rats. Five-day cyclic females of these two latter strains only exhibit spontaneous early mating receptivity in 10–15% of cases (Aron and Chateau, 1971; Roos, Chateau, and Aron, 1971). It is true coitus brings about ovulation in both strains, but I would have perhaps thrown in my hand if I had undertaken my initial investigations on the WII strain and concluded that, compared to 4-day cyclics, there was no significant statistical increase in early mating frequency. Finally, these experiments prompted me to investigate the role of estrogens in the mechanism of stimulated ovulation in the rat, since, in 4-day cycles, an estrogen preparation was needed to produce ovulation after mating (Aron, Asch, and Luxembourger, 1964). This was the aim of the work of J. Roos (1969), which demonstrated that estradiol incited the pituitary to store FSH in the late afternoon of diestrus II and that the mating reflex only brought about ovulation if, at one and the same time, FSH and LH were secreted, as is also the case for spontaneous ovulation. Now, at 21 h to 23 h on diestrus II the pituitary level of FSH is very low. Thus early mating of a non-estradiol-primed rat cannot bring about ovulation.

I will pass over all the mechanisms of stimulated ovulation we have investigated. My intention here is to consider all the implications of a research project. This being the case it does not seem too speculative to imagine, even if recent work does not seem to favor this theory—the 1973 work of Stearnes, Winter, and Faiman, for instance—that a primate is capable of reacting to coitus in the same manner as a rat if the hormonal conditions at the time of sexual intercourse are consistent with FSH and LH secretion and if, also, there happens to be an ovarian follicle in the ovary sufficiently ripe to rupture in response to gonadotrophic hormones. I have thus always attached a greater importance to my experiments carried out on 5-day cycles, under normal conditions of cycle development, than to those conducted on 4-day cycles. This does not seem to have been the opinion of biologists interested in this question, who have always made much mention of research work done on estradiol primed rats, and never of that on 5-day cyclic rats. If my research work had been published only in French, I would have thought Anglo-Saxon readers had not read it. But from 1966 on it has appeared in English (Aron, Asch, and Roos, 1966). I expect therefore that others besides myself have put the females with the male during 5-day cycles and have been disappointed at the small proportion of early receptive females. I feel they are reassured thanks to experiments carried out on WII and Holtzman rats (Aron and Chateau, 1971; Roos, Chateau, and Aron, 1971). At present we are again carrying out trials for early receptivity in WI 5-day cyclic rats. Approximately 40% of the females are continuing to accept the male in these circumstances. I am thus greatly indebted to this strain of females who enjoy the greatest care and attention in our laboratory. This is all the more warranted since they made us interested in research into external factors affecting ovulation control and sexual behavior, as well as into estrous rhythm regulation, now a main topic in our laboratory.

But here once more we will see the part circumstances played in the setting up of a research project. If the olfactory pathways had not been involved in aggressive behavior control, we would certainly never have discovered the vital role they play in the control of estrous rhythm regulation. The rats we bulbectomized in order to determine the role of olfactory stimuli in the elaboration of early receptivity became aggressive and difficult to handle. They were housed, at that time and from 1954 on, in individual cages. Since we knew, according to Karli, that the grouping of animals counterbalanced the action of olfactory bulbectomy, from then on we housed the rats in groups whether they had been deprived of their olfactory bulbs or they were to be used as controls. It was important from then on to check all the parameters we had established, for isolated females, of cycle regularity and cycle distribution in 4- and 5-day cycles, respectively. Little was known about this subject in the rat. We knew of one experiment carried out in 1964 by Hughes, questionable on account of his methods, as he described the estrous rhythm by vaginal smears when the 5-day cyclic females were kept apart from the male, and by the occurrence of sperm in the smears when cohabitation was allowed. These experiments, therefore, did not take into account the phenomenon of early mating which we had just discovered.

Several texts had also been published dealing with a certain type of estrous synchronization in rats with nutritional deficiencies, such as the 1972 work by Cooper, Purvis, and Haynes, that of Purvis, Cooper, and Haynes, in 1971, and Cooper and Haynes in 1967. But the other observations had mainly brought negative results in this field. Did the rat differ thus to this extent from the mouse? Time has shown there was no difference and the rat is an olfactodependent type. I find it of interest here to stress a point. A research project such as this was inconceivable at the beginning on a small scale. There are phenomena which escape us because we are obliged to work on samples made up of a limited number of animals. Originally, we discovered only a 10% difference in the distribution of 4- and 5-day cycles between rats housed in groups from the time of weaning up to between 3 and 4 months of age, and those females isolated in individual cages from the age of 2.5 months. But this difference proved significant, since analysis by Cochran's combined test for 2×2 contingency tables dealt, respectively, with 1200 and 800 animals. This set our minds at rest! It is not a question of a "microphenomenon." WI Wistar rats, bulbectomized at the age of 6 weeks, at 3–4 months exhibit 70% 5-day cycles and 30% 4-day cycles. The nonoperated controls, at the same age, exhibit 70% 4-day cycles and 30% 5-day cycles (Aron, Roos, Chateau, and Roos, 1972). And WII strain rats proved very susceptible to pheromones (Aron and Chateau, 1971; Roos, Chateau, and Aron, 1973).

But I would not like to give the reader the idea that the fear of being bitten was the only determining factor in the research we are at present carrying out on the regulation of estrous rhythm and feedbacks between hormonal factors, external stimuli, and central nervous structures involved in this regulation. Logic fortunately played a part, with reference to the knowledge our team had acquired concerning ovarian response to LH at different stages of the estrous cycle (Chateau and Aron, 1970; Chateau and Roos, 1970), by process of analogy, and in pursuance of a natural interest in closely checking the estrous rhythm in females whose ventromedial nucleus we damaged, while preserving the integrity of the arcuate nucleus and anterior hypothalamus, in order to study the mechanisms of early and estrous receptivity in the rat.

All this arose from the 1969 work of Alloiteau and Acker, who, by administering an injection of LH early in the course of 4-day cycles, prolonged the cycle from 4 to 5 days. We wondered if this prolongation of the cycle was not due to luteinization of ovarian follicles, which, without the injection, would have developed to the preovulatory stage. Having succeeded in ruling out this theory (Buffler and Roser, 1972), we recalled the 24-hour delay in ovulation brought about by progesterone injected at the beginning of 4-day cycles, as Everett reported in 1948. And thus it was possible to demonstrate, in the first place, that LH prolonged the cycle by increasing ovarian progesterone secretion on the afternoon of diestrus I and the morning of diestrus II by slowing down follicular growth and by curtailing the production of estrogen in the late afternoon of diestrus II (Buffler and Roser, 1974; Roser and Aron, 1973).

As for the ventromedial nucleus, I will not dwell on it now. For us it is a symbol of the future rather than the past which I have been invited to discuss. I will therefore leave the reader to guess the next step in our experiments which disclosed to us the role it plays in regulation of the estrous cycle duration (Carrer, Asch, and Aron, 1973–74) and which are now in progress. At the time of writing I foresee the difficulties we will encounter in interpreting mechanisms of such complexity as to render it impossible for us to approach them as a whole. In actual fact, we are progressing by making abstractions from the totality of the organism, not, it must be added, without disturbing the equilibrium of the specimen whose functioning we aspire to analyze. In this aspect, moreover, I see no difference between former times and today. We altered endocrine balance in the body as much when we carried out mesovarian sections or medullary sections as now when we destroy the ventromedial nucleus or extirpate the olfactory bulbs. In this respect, nothing has changed with the use of the most modern methods of investigation. I am consequently of the opinion that prudence must be exercised in one's judgement of other peoples work and, as in the phrase from the *Cahiers de Valéry,* "Do not tend to deny what one cannot affirm." In regard to neurohormonal feedbacks, I am fairly reassured. Contrary to my experience of 26 years ago, neuroendocrinologists are no longer incensed at the mention of neuroendocrine reflexes of whatever origin.

REFERENCES

Aron, C., and R. Aron-Brunetiere (1953). Effets de la stimulation mécanique du vagin et du segment supracervical de l'utérus sur l'ovaire du Cobaye. *C. R. Acad. Sci.* **237**: 846.

Aron, M., C. Aron, and J. Marescaux (1948). Les facteurs du fonctionnement ovarien. Recherches de morphologie expérimentale sur certains facteurs intrinsèques de ce fonctionnement. *C. R. Assoc. Anat.,* 35e reunion, **53**: 10.

Aron, M., C. Aron, and J. Marescaux (1952). Influence de l'hypophysectomie sur l'hyperactivité réactionnelle de l'ovaire restant chez le Cobaye. *C. R. Acad. Sci.* **235**: 320.

Aron, C., and G. Asch (1962). Influence inhibitrice de l'atropine sur le déclenchement par le rapprochement sexuel de la ponte ovulaire chez la ratte mûre. *C. R. Acad. Sci.* **255**: 3056.

Aron, C., G. Asch, and L. Asch (1961). Déclenchement de la ponte ovulaire et de la lutéinisation par le rapprochement sexuel chez les mammifères dits à ponte spontanée. Expériences chez la ratte. *C. R. Soc. Biol.* **155**: 2173.

Aron, C., G. Asch, and M. M. Luxembourger (1964). Rôle joué par la folliculine dans le déclenchement de la ponte par le rapprochement sexuel. I. Expériences chez des rattes présentant des cycles de 4 jours. *C. R. Soc. Biol.* **158**: 182.

Aron, C., G. Asch, and J. Roos (1966). Triggering of ovulation by coitus in the rat. *Int. Rev. Cytol.* **20**: 139.

Aron, C., G. Asch, and J. Roos (1968). Données nouvelles sur l'action lutéinisante ou ovulatoire de la stimulation mécanique du vagin et du col utérin chez la ratte. *C. R. Soc. Biol.* **162**: 243.

Aron, C., and D. Chateau (1971). Presumed involvement of pheromones in mating behavior in the rat. *Horm. Behav.* **2**: 315.

Aron, C., and J. Marescaux (1948a). Nouvelles observations à propos de l'hyperactivité reactionnelle après hémicastration chez le Cobaye. *C. R. Soc. Biol.* **142**: 1554.

Aron, C., and J. Marescaux (1948b). Facteurs de l'hyperactivité réactionnelle de l'ovaire restant après hémicastration chez le Cobaye. *C. R. Soc. Biol.* **142**: 1009.

Aron, C., C. Marx, and J. Marescaux (1948). Influence de la section de la moelle épinière sur l'hyperactivité réactionnelle de l'ovaire restant après hémicastration chez le Cobaye. *C. R. Soc. Biol.* **142**: 1556.

Aron, C., C. Marx, and J. Marescaux (1949). Mécanisme de l'hyperactivité réactionnelle de l'ovaire restant après ovariectomie unilatérale chez le Cobaye. *J. Suisse Méd.* **22**: 502.

Aron, C., A. Petrovic, J. Marescaux, and J. P. Isaac (1951). Modifications histologiques de la pars distalis de la préhypophyse provoquées à court terme par l'hémicastration chez le Cobaye femelle. *C. R. Assoc. Anat.* 37e réunion, 1.

Aron, C., J. Roos, and G. Asch (1968). New facts concerning the afferent stimuli that trigger ovulation by coitus in the rat. *Neuroendocrinology* **3**: 47.

Aron, C., J. Roos, D. Chateau, and M. Roos (1972). Stimulus olfactifs et régulation de la durée du cycle ovarien chez la ratte. *Ann. Endocrinol.* **33**: 23.

Asch, G., J. Roos, and C. Aron (1964). Rôle joué par la folliculine dans le déclenchement de la ponte par le rapprochement sexuel. II. Expériences chez des rattes offrant des cycles de 5 jours. *C. R. Soc. Biol.* **158:** 838.

Buffler, G., and S. Roser (1972). New data concerning the factors involved in the lengthening of oestrous cycle duration caused by LH in the rat. *J. Interdiscip. Cycle Res.* **3:** 209.

Buffler, G., and S. Roser (1974). New data concerning the role played by progesterone in the control of follicular growth in the rat. *Acta Endocrinol.* **75:** 569.

Carrer, H., G. Asch, and C. Aron (1973–74). New facts concerning the role played by the ventromedial nucleus in the control of estrous cycle duration and sexual receptivity in the rat. *Neuroendocrinology* **13:** 129.

Chateau, D., and C. Aron (1970). Données nouvelles sur les variations de la compétence des follicules ovariques au cours du cycle oestral chez la ratte. *C. R. Assoc. Anat.* **147:** 171.

Chateau, D., and M. Roos (1970). Données qualitatives et quantitatives sur la lutéinisation expérimentale chez la ratte. *C. R. Soc. Biol.* **164:** 415.

Roos, J. (1969). Modification des cellules gonadotropes et du contenu en FSH de la glande pituitaire dans les conditions de la ponte provoquée chez la ratte. *Acta Endocrinol.* (Kbh.) **62:** 607.

Roos, J., D. Chateau, and C. Aron (1971). Comparaison de la réceptivité précoce de rattes Wistar et Holtzman au cours de cycles de 5 jours. *C. R. Soc. Biol.* **165:** 2181.

Roos, J., D. Chateau, and C. Aron (1973). Effects of olfactory bulb deprivation on estrous rhythm in the rat. *Proc. 3rd Europ. Anat. Congr.* 56. (Abstr.)

Roos, J. and M. Roos (1966b). Rôle joué par les facteurs chronologiques dans le déclenchement de phénomènes ovulatoires par l'hémiovariectomie au cours de cycles de 5 jours chez la ratte. *C. R. Soc. Biol.* **160:** 1058.

Roos, M., and J. Roos (1966a). Mise en évidence d'un déterminisme neuroendocrinien de la ponte provoquée par l'hémicastration chez la ratte. *C. R. Soc. Biol.* **160:** 647.

Roser, S., and C. Aron (1973). Modifications de l'oestradiol 17β ovarien chez les rattes traitées par LH au début du cycle de 4 jours. *C. R. Acad. Sci.* **277:** 1799.

2

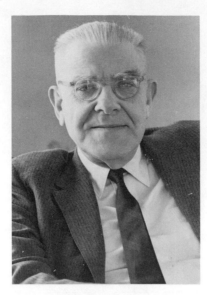

Philip Bard

Philip Bard was born on October 25, 1898 in Port Hueneme, California, the son of a former U.S. senator from California. After attending private schools in California, he enlisted in the U.S. Army Ambulance Service and served in France until his discharge in 1919. He then entered Princeton and received his A.B. in 1923 with highest honors. He received his Ph.D. from Harvard in 1927. After serving as an Assistant Professor first at Princeton and then at the Harvard Medical School, he was appointed Professor and Director of the Department of Physiology at Johns Hopkins University in 1933, a position he held until his retirement in 1964. He was Dean of the Medical Faculty from 1953 to 1957.

Dr. Bard is a member of the American Physiological Society, the Association of American Physicians, the American Neurological Association, the Association for Research in Nervous and Mental Disease, the Society for Experimental Biology and Medicine, the Society for Neuroscience, and the Harvey Society, among others.

He was a member of the editorial board of the *American Journal of Physiology* from 1939 to 1946, served as chairman of the editorial board of *Physiological Reviews* from 1950 to 1953, and has been chairman of the board of publication trustees (1959–60) and of the publication committee (1960–61) of the American Physiological Society.

He has served on many advisory committees to the government such as the Subcommittee on Shock, the Committee on Shock and Transfusions, and the Subcommittee on Motion Sickness to the Surgeons General of the Army, Navy, and Public Health Service. He has served on the physiology study section of the NIH (1947–50) and on the National Board of Medical Examiners (1935–46).

His honors include the presidency of the American Physiological Society, the Association for Research in Nervous and Mental Disease, and the Society for Experimental Biology and Medicine. He received the Jacoby Award of the American Neurological Association, the Karl Spencer Lashley Award of the American Philosophical Society, and the American College of Physicians Award for Achievement in the Science of Medicine, and he was elected to the National Academy of Sciences and the American Philosophical Society.

The Story of Some Neuroendocrinological Studies in Cats

PHILIP BARD

I must confess at the beginning of this account that whatever contributions I have made to neuroendocrinological knowledge have had their origin in hints given or chance observations made in the course of studies of central nervous mechanisms involved in the execution of emotional behavior, postural adjustments, and some other overt expressions of nervous integration. Yet, at a critical stage of my development as a physiologist, my intention was to carry on research in endocrinology. Indeed, when in 1924 I asked Dr. Walter B. Cannon to allow me to work under his direction toward the Ph.D. degree in the Division of Medical Sciences of Harvard University, I told him that my chief interest was in that area. And after nine months devoted to the courses for first year medical students I found myself engaged in a neuroendocrinological investigation.

At the time I entered the Harvard Physiological Laboratory, Dr. Cannon's chief interest was the determination of conditions which lead to activation of the sympathetic system, especially its constituent part—the adrenal medulla. He suggested to me that, since there was reason to suppose that muscular exercise is accompanied by increased sympathetic activity, it would be worthwhile to determine whether stimulation of the motor cortex evokes adrenomedullary secretion. I of course acted on his proposal and spent much time learning to prepare denervated hearts, the indicators of circulating "adrenin" then being used in the laboratory. But I soon encountered what turned out to be an insurmountable difficulty: The only anesthesia available at that time which left the motor cortex excitable was

PHILIP BARD • Department of Physiology, The Johns Hopkins University School of Medicine, Baltimore, Maryland.

light etherization, which caused such a discharge of sympathetic impulses to the adrenals that any effect of the stimulation was fully masked. Although I was forced to abandon the experiments, I later came to regard this unhappy outcome as a stroke of very good fortune, for a much more interesting problem took its place—one which proved soluble, led to significant results, formed the basis of my Ph.D. thesis, and started me on a long series of experimental studies of the central nervous system.

The neurophysiological investigation I took up was a sequel to studies that Dr. Cannon had carried out during 1924 and 1925 with Sidney Britton and Emelio Bulatao. This work had shown that, in acute experiments on cats, disconnecting the cerebral cortices from subcortical structures is followed, on emergence from etherization, by a remarkable group of activities which closely resemble the behavior of the infuriated normal animal and include widespread vigorous discharges in the sympathetic system and copious adrenomedullary secretion. Cannon termed this activity "sham rage"—"sham" because in the absence of the cerebral cortex the subjective aspects of the emotion would be absent. He suggested that I attempt to ascertain the locus of the central mechanism essential for this stereotyped form of affective behavior. This I managed to do in a long series of acute experiments by first decorticating and then transecting the brain stem at different levels and at different planes. In this way it was found that the central neural mechanism requisite for the development of sham rage (I prefer the term "quasi-rage") was located in the caudal half of the hypothalamus. This experience led to studies of a number of chronically decorticate animals in which certain neuroendocrinological observations were made. But before recounting them I would like to describe my only experimental collaboration with Dr. Cannon, for it was concerned with a possible direct neural control of an endocrine gland.

After receiving the Ph.D. degree in 1927 I remained on the Harvard physiology staff as an instructor for one year. It was at this time that Dr. Cannon proposed that I join him in testing the validity of some observations he had made in 1915 with Carl Binger and Reginald Fitz on cats with the anterior root of one phrenic nerve anastomosed to the cephalic portion of the cut cervical sympathetic trunk. The rationale of this procedure was the expectation that when regenerating phrenic motor fibers reached the superior cervical ganglion they would make synaptic connections with postganglionic neurons, including ones innervating the thyroid gland which would then be bombarded by impulses with each inspiration. Some of the animals of the initial group appeared to develop signs of hyperthyroidism, but World War I precluded a definite conclusion. Dr. Cannon and I prepared a large number of cats with phrenic-cervical sympathetic anastomoses, but throughout long survivals the animals showed no increases in resting oxygen consumption or other indications of augmented thyroid activity. We did, however, find evidence in almost all cases that the phrenic fibers had effectively innervated the superior cervical ganglion. This work was carried out long before anyone knew of TSH. Although there were strong indications, especially from the work of Philip Smith, that thyroid function is dependent on the anterior pituitary, there was still room for the supposition that it might be stimulated through a direct innervation.

Although my first two excursions into the area of neuroendocrinology were disappointing in that they led to negative results (which, by the way, were never reported), the pursuit of other problems led to a chance observation that formed the basis for much subsequent work directed toward the delimitation of the cerebral site of action of estrogen. In 1928 I went from Harvard to Princeton as an assistant professor of biology and there I developed a laboratory for experiments in mammalian physiology, including an operating room suitable for intracranial surgical procedures. Cannon had taken up his acute sham rage experiments because the chronically decorticate dog of Goltz, described in 1892, the similar animal studied by Rothmann in 1923, and the two long-surviving decorticate cats of Dusser de Barenne in 1919 had displayed rage on very slight provocation. My own interest in the cerebral mechanisms essential for angry behavior led me to attempt the preparation of chronically decorticate cats in order to study this activity at first hand and also to determine whether they are capable of displaying other kinds of emotional behavior. It turned out that my decorticates, all females, exhibited not only anger but also fear and the full, stereotyped, and rather complex estrous behavior characteristic of this species.

In 1929 at Princeton I succeeded in removing from the brain of a small, gentle, and friendly female cat all neocortex, some of the rhinencephalon, a part of the striatal complex, and the lateral portions of the thalami. The animal lived in good health for 20 months, showed anger on slight provocation and, when subjected to loud, high-pitched sounds, behaved as does a normal cat when terrified. Descriptions of her general behavior and that of three other cats lacking cortex and additional parts of the forebrain have appeared in several publications (Bard, 1934, 1939; Bard and Rioch, 1937). On her 29th decorticate day, wishing to record her temperature but noticing some rectal inflammation, I inserted a thermometer into her vagina. This immediately evoked loud growling and the assumption of a crouching posture in which, with pelvis and tail elevated, she executed rapid treading movements of the hindlegs. After removal of the thermometer she squirmed vigorously on her side and playfully rubbed cheek and occiput against the floor. This was easily recognizable as a typical and fairly full display of feline estrous behavior. Crouching and treading were at this time regularly evoked by any gentle mechanical stimulus of the vulval region and vaginal stimulation repeatedly evoked the afterreaction just described. These responses continued to be elicitable throughout an astonishingly long period, from the 29th to the 58th day, and again for a shorter time during the eighth postoperative month. It was only during these periods that vaginal smears consisted entirely of fully cornified cells and males were attracted. Unlike a normal cat in heat, she was quite indifferent to such preliminary masculine advances as vocalization and head licking. When the male grasped her neck, mounted, and executed treading movements she merely squatted and licked the floor or, if he became more violent, growled savagely and lashed her tail. But the instant he pressed against her vulval region she immediately assumed a full estrous crouch and treaded vigorously. Intromission, signaled by loud angry vocalization and followed by frantic rolling and squirming, occurred on three occasions.

At Princeton I had become much interested in the localized cortical control of certain postural and attitudinal reactions, some of which were completely absent and others very defective in the decorticate cat. The partial cortical removals and long observation periods necessary to solve this problem (Bard, 1933) occupied much of my time and it was not until I returned to Harvard in 1931 that three additional chronically decorticate cats were prepared. None of these, however, came spontaneously into estrus and I made no further studies of sexual behavior until after I went to the Johns Hopkins School of Medicine in 1933 as professor of physiology and director of the department. At that time there was not available an estrogen preparation which was effective in producing a full and sustained state of estrus, a result essential for my researches since cats enter into heat only a few times a year. Knowing that human pregnancy urine contains large amounts of estrogen of placental origin, I secured supplies of this material from the obstetrical outpatient clinic and found that about 50 ml mixed with their regular food was readily ingested by the cats and after some days induced full estrus which lasted as long as the diet was continued—in several cases for four to seven months. Fortunately it was not long before estradiol in oil became available and this was used in all subsequent experiments.

Four cats, two of them ovariectomized, were tested with estradiol before as well as after decortication, thus permitting a comparison of the postoperative with the normal responses (Bard, 1939). In each animal all neocortex had been ablated and the olfactory bulbs removed or disconnected. In one cat all rhinencephalic structures were found to have been removed, and in the others only small remnants remained. In one the striatal complex was found to be bilaterally missing. In each cat postoperative administration of estrogen evoked much the same estrual behavior as had occurred spontaneously in the first decorticate animal. In addition, crouching and treading occurred spontaneously and all four were heard to utter the "call" peculiar to feline estrus. Males were accepted on numerous occasions. Comparisons of the preoperative with the postoperative sexual activities of these females suggested that the thresholds of the reactions had been raised somewhat by the cerebral removals and that the afterreactions, although distinct and sometimes briefly frantic, lacked the vigor and nicety of execution which characterized them before operation.

Although at this stage of the work it had become quite clear that execution of the full pattern of estrual behavior is dependent on a subcortical mechanism, it remained to determine whether estrogen acts directly or indirectly on this mechanism, at least in part, by inducing marked changes in the genital tract which in turn condition or activate the "center" through afferent nervous channels. To answer this question a series of ovariectomized cats were subjected to abdominal sympathectomy and extirpation of tubes, uteri, and the proximal two-thirds of the vagina. These alterations left estrual behavior unchanged. When to them was added removal of the sacral spinal segments which rendered the remaining distal vagina, the external genitalia, and the surrounding skin areas completely anesthetic, the animals, when in estrus, rolled, rubbed themselves on the floor, crouched with pelvis raised, and treaded to the best of their abilities. They were responsive to males, cooperated when mounted, and vocalized in a provocative tone, but of course did not respond to vulval or vaginal stimulation and showed no afterreaction. When estrus was induced in two females with cord sectioned at a midthoracic level, each assumed a crouching attitude of the foreparts when a male was nearby. Often they approached a male by pulling themselves along with their forelegs, uttered typical estrual vocalizations, and rubbed their heads against him. It was concluded that afferent signals from the genitalia are not at all necessary for the development of estrous behavior in the cat (Bard, 1939).

The complex and sequential motor activity of feline estrual behavior suggests that it is dependent on a cerebral integrative mechanism. Yet, since claims of a specific action of estrogen on the isolated spinal cord had been made, Bromiley and I investigated the matter in a large number of spinal cats. Our results (Bromiley and Bard, 1940; Bard, 1940), like those obtained in spinal guinea pigs by Dempsey and Rioch (1939), showed that in these preparations the estrous condition neither causes any qualitative changes in responses obtainable from the genital region in anestrus nor unveils any not present in that state. We found this to be true also in a series of cats acutely decerebrated at a lower midbrain or a pontile level. Nine were in full behavioral estrus and 19, 10 of which had been ovariectomized, were anestrous. The reactions of all to vaginal, vulval, perineal, and anal stimuli were qualitatively the same. Of interest, however, was our finding that each responded to mechanical vaginal stimulation by a most striking collapse of the decerebrate extensor rigidity of the forelegs and a slight flexion of the hindlegs. This could not be evoked from any other part nor could it be obtained in the decerebrate male by any genital or other stimulus. In the standing animal the response imposed an attitude suggestive of the estrous crouch, but since it was entirely independent of the sexual state of the animal and since the crouch of the normal cat does not depend on vaginal stimulation, we concluded that it did not denote "the existence of a bulbospinal mechanism capable of executing the major postural adjustment of feline estrus." Again, our results were in accord with those of Dempsey and Rioch, who found that estrual guinea pigs with mesencephalic transections failed to give any response "which even remotely resembled oestrous behavior." On the other hand they obtained definite signs of the sexual behavior pattern characteristic of the species in one guinea pig and one cat, both in estrus, after an acute transection just rostral to the mammillary bodies.

Since a good many results pointed to the hypothalamus as the site of the central machinery essential for estrous behavior, I was much pleased to have the collaboration of Dr. H. W. Magoun when he spent the year 1939–1940 in the Hopkins laboratory on a Rockefeller fellowship. In Ranson's laboratory at Northwestern University Medical School he had carried out important investigations in which lesions had been made in the brain stem through electrodes positioned by the Horsley-Clarke stereotactic instrument. He at once joined me in a study of the effects of hypothalamic lesions in ovariectomized cats whose responses to estrogen had been established (Bard, 1940). Most were in full estrus at operation and all received large doses of estradiol afterward. We soon found that a subtotal but extensive destruction of the caudal half of the hypothalamus might not impair in any manner a cat's capacity to display estrous activities. Very large hypothalamic lesions, ones which caused somnolence and poikilothermia, were made in two cats. In one with the caudal supraoptic, tuberal, and mammillary areas almost completely destroyed and all known descending connections of the small remaining fragments interrupted, the only estrual actions evoked during a survival of seven weeks were some incomplete afterreactions. In the other animal a huge area of destruction began in the tuberal region and reached full size in the mammillary area where it extended from one basis pedunculi to the other. Although the anterior hypothalamus was spared, the medial forebrain bundle and the periventricular system of fibers were bilaterally interrupted, thus severing all of its known descending connections. In addition there was a triangular area of anemic softening in the upper mesencephalon which extended to the red nuclei, destroying the ventral half of the central gray, the interpeduncular area, and the adjacent portion of the medial tegmental region. During its survival of two weeks this cat, when aroused from its state of deep somnolence, repeatedly assumed a crouch and treaded in typical estrual fashion in response to light vulval stimulation, and after vaginal stimulation she engaged in a delayed but vigorous afterreaction following which she usually crouched and treaded spontaneously before lapsing into somnolence. These very positive results suggest that either hypothalamic mechanisms may not be essential for the arousal and execution of feline estrual behavior or there exist descending connections from the anterior hypothalamus not yet recognized. In view of evidence to be presented later, it is difficult to exclude the ventral diencephalon from participation in this estrogen-dependent form of emotional behavior.

The observations made with Magoun (Bard, 1940) left open the question whether estrogen may evoke feline estrous behavior by activating a central mechanism located below the hypothalamus, most probably in the mesencephalon. Shortly thereafter Martin B. Macht and I, in a study of chronically decerebrate cats (Macht and Bard, 1942), which was not fully reported until 16 years later (Bard and Macht, 1958), obtained some evidence that the mesencephalon may indeed be involved in estrous behavior. Before relating these observations it may be helpful to give a brief account of why and how we prepared and studied such animals.

Several earlier investigators had been able to keep decerebrate cats and dogs alive for periods of from 18 to 46 days, but most of these were prepared for the study of specific functions such as body temperature regulation and water balance (see Bard and Macht, 1958, for a resumé of these investigations). It appeared that none of these animals had displayed all the activities of which carnivores with brain stem truncated at a mesencephalic or pontile level are capable, and we deemed it likely that somewhat longer survivals and more general examination of responses would reveal behavior not yet observed in such preparations. Further, since the behavior of a cat with all forebrain above the hypothalamus removed (a hypothalamic cat) differs little from that of the wholly decorticate animal, such a study promised to throw light on the relative contributions of hypothalamus, mesencephalon, and rhombencephalon to the conduct of an animal lacking only cerebral cortex.

Doubtless our success in achieving survivals of 26 to 154 days (average, 54 days) in the 7 cats of the 1941–42 series and of 31 to 351 days (average, 97 days) in the 24 cats of a more recent series (Woods, Bard, and Bleier, 1966; Bard, Woods, and Bleier, 1970) was dependent on the presence in each animal of a neurally isolated island of tissue composed of hypothalamus and attached hypophysis. The necessary surgical removals were carried out by suction. After ablating all cerebral tissue situated rostral, dorsal, and lateral to the hypothalamus, a wedge or segment of brain stem was removed just caudal to the diencephalomesencephalic junction. When a high mesencephalic animal was desired, this segment was narrow rostrocaudally; in preparing a low mesencephalic cat the rostral tegmentum and tectum were included; and ablation of the entire mesencephalon produced a pontile preparation. In all cases but one under discussion, the extent and cellular integrity of the remaining brain stem were examined histologically. The hypothalamohypophyseal island, whose only connection with the rest of the body was vascular, served to maintain a normal water balance and, as will be related shortly, ensured an adequate release of TSH, ACTH, and FSH from the pars distalis of the pituitary gland.

The surgical procedures used in preparing these chronically decerebrate animals seem to be formidable, but long experience with intracranial interventions made them practical; in the last series the operative mortality was less than 10%. The postoperative hazards were greater. The chief of these is due to the fact that the mesencephalic or pontile carnivore lacks all ability to regulate its body temperature, a hypothalamic function. We soon found that hypothermia, even as low as 28°C, rarely exerts any harmful effect. But overheating to a lethal level readily developed in these animals, especially when muscular activity in the form of righting movements or locomotion added endogenous heat to that of a cage heater made necessary by the fact that at ordinary room temperatures inactive decerebrate animals become chilled. During the experiments of 1941–42 my able and conscientious collaborator, Martin Macht, then a graduate student, lived in the laboratory and spent many sleep-interrupted nights making frequent manual adjustments of cage temperatures. This dedicated effort not only saved many cat lives but also provided additional information about the animals' general behavior. Fifteen years later, when J. W. Woods and I resumed studies of chronically decerebrate cats, we had the advantage of being able to employ automatic electronic systems of control which regulated individual cage heaters and cooling fans in reference to a thermistor probe inserted in the colon or sutured in the subscapular space. Finally we achieved the luxury of regulating body temperature by signals from a telemeter implanted in the retroperitoneal region. At one stage in this technical progress we tried connecting the colonic probes in such a way that low or high temperatures signaled a downtown burglar alarm agency, which, when alerted at night or on Sundays or holidays, telephoned us at home to report impending tragedy. It proved to be a fairly effective preventive of lethal hyperthermias but was very hard on Dr. Woods, who lived about six miles nearer the laboratory than I did.

Pontile cats, unless stimulated mechanically or acoustically, tend to lie on their sides throughout their survivals. At the end of a week righting of head and foreparts could be obtained in response to a strong stimulus and later this maneuver occurred spontaneously, but locomotion in a standing position appeared to be impossible. On the other hand, the mesencephalic animals, especially those with brain stem truncated at a rostral midbrain level, began to right themselves during the first few postoperative days, soon stood up, and walked spontaneously within a week. They usually rested in a crouch on chest and belly and showed behavioral sleep and awakening.

It was in two high mesencephalic female cats that unmistakable estrous behavior was observed (Bard and Macht, 1958). Each had been bilaterally ovariectomized and, before decerebration, had responded to estrogen (estradiol benzoate in oil) by a full spontaneous display of the courtship activities (crouching, treading, vocalization) and exhibited frantic afterreactions in response to vaginal stimulation. Cat 10 was in full induced vaginal and behavioral estrus at the time of decerebration. On the second and third postoperative days, vulval stimulation caused her to assume a typical estrous crouch and to tread with pelvis elevated. On one occasion vaginal stimulation was followed by turning of the head toward the pelvis and licking. On the 11th day, when she had an anestrous smear and showed no estrous behavior, she was again given estradiol with the result that three days later genital stimulation evoked good treading in a typical crouch. Only on one occasion was vaginal stimulation followed by licking the vulva, but nothing else suggestive of a beginning afterreaction was seen. On her 14th postoperative day the other animal, cat 11, yielded a wholly anestrous vaginal smear and failed to show any estrous behavioral response. On that day and on days 17 and 18 she was given estrogen and very soon a vaginal smear consisting only of fully cornified cells was supplemented by crouching and treading with pelvis raised in response to gentle tactile stimulation of the vulval region. From the 20th to the 24th day she frequently assumed an estrous crouch spontaneously. Vaginal stimulation caused growling, the assumption of a more pronounced estrual crouch, and rapid treading. Once, on cessation of the stimulation, she lowered and rotated her head and brought one cheek in contact with the floor as if she were about to squirm on her side or roll; this was unmistakably the beginning of an afterreaction. Later, during her ninth postoperative week, cat 11 was again put into full estrus (as indicated by vaginal smears) and exhibited about the same estrual activities, but this time we failed to evoke any trace of an afterreaction.

The anatomical status of the brains of these two cats is important in any estimate of the site or sites of the effective cerebral action of estrogen. In cat 11 the truncation was rostral to the oculomotor nuclei, substantia nigra, and red nuclei. Ventrally it struck the base behind the mammillary bodies, but it cannot be said that the most rostral portion of the mesencephalon was intact, for it was the site of some mechanical damage and considerable gliosis. Unfortunately the brain of cat 10 was not sectioned and studied histologically, but careful gross inspection after fixation indicated that the level of truncation was essentially the same as in cat 11. In both cats the caudal hypothalamus, including the mammillary nuclear area, was not part of the remaining brain stem.

It remains to discuss the significance of the estrual behavior observed in the two mesencephalic cats. That behavior fell well short of the expression of sexual excitement induced in normal or even decorticate female cats by either endogenous or exogenous estrogen. The fact that it was produced by doses of estrogen much greater than those which proved effective before decerebration indicates a raised threshold, but that cannot be the sole reason for the relative paucity of expression. It seems reasonable to suppose that whatever infrahypothalamic mechanisms were activated by exogenous estrogen, they are ones incapable of integrating the complete picture of feline estrous behavior. Especially lacking was all but a hint of the afterreaction which is so conspicuous a feature in the normal cat. As already indicated, decorticate cats show a somewhat attenuated afterreaction. In the normal cat this frantic behavior may be the expression of an orgasm, for intromission is attended by loud angry cries, growling, and hissing and is frequently followed by an attack on the male. Such behavior cannot be interpreted as signs of pleasure, but the afterreaction suggests something different. All this is perhaps evidence that the feline female orgasm is dependent on the higher reaches of the central nervous system.

Obviously the evidence presented here regarding the site or sites of action of estrogen in the brain needs confirmation or correction by the results of other experimental approaches to the problem. Since the time it was obtained, several techniques other than that of exclusion of cerebral subdivisions by surgical ablation have been applied. Of these the most significant, it seems to me, is that of implanting in different parts of the brain amounts of estrogen in the solid state so minute that they do not exert any systemic effect, and the genital tract is unaffected. And yet, when properly placed, they evoked full estrous behavior in ovariectomized cats. The carefully controlled experiments carried out in this manner have recently been reviewed by Richard Michael (1973) who, with Geoffrey Harris and Patricia Scott, was a pioneer in this type of investigation. The available evidence indicates that in the cat the estrogen-sensitive central nervous mechanism whose activation results in estrous behavior is located, but not highly circumscribed, in the hypothalamus. Many extrahypothalamic sites yielded negative results, but it appears that the midbrain, including the rostral mesencephalic tegmentum, was not extensively explored. In any case it seems clear that any mesencephalic mechanism is subordinate to the hypothalamic in the management of estrous behavior just as it is in the execution of angry behavior (Bard and Macht, 1958).

Mention has been made of the fact that an isolated hypothalamohypophyseal island provides for the release of adequate amounts of antidiuretic hormone (ADH). Bard and Macht (1958) found that of their seven decerebrate cats all but one maintained a normal water balance throughout survivals of from 26 to 154 days. The exception was an animal which developed polyuria on the 14th postoperative day, but was maintained in good condition until the 35th day. Microscopic examination of sections of its island revealed that the supraoptic nuclei had undergone nearly complete degeneration. In this group of cats no quantitative studies of water balance were carried out, but the results suggested that all the hypothalamic elements—osmoreceptive, integrative, and secretomotor—necessary for regulation of ADH release were functionally intact. A similar conclusion can be drawn from the much earlier experiments of Sumwalt, Erb, and Bazett (1935).

About a year before Woods and I undertook further studies of chronically decerebrate cats with islands, Jewell and Verney (1957) had reported a delimitation of the hypothalamic osmoreceptors in the dog. This they achieved by excluding from the circulation different parts of the brain and then, weeks later, testing the animals' responses to intracarotid injections of hypertonic solutions during the course of a water diuresis. Their painstaking experiments had shown that the possible sites of the osmoreceptors are the supraoptic, suprachiasmatic, paraventricular, and ventromedial nuclei, the anterior hypothalamic area, the tuber cinereum, and the periventricular system. They showed clearly for the first time that the osmoreceptive elements are not located in the neurohypophysis. Since it had long been known that localized destruction of the supraoptic nuclei causes polyuria, the involvement of these cellular groups in the release of ADH seemed established, but it did not necessarily follow that they contain the osmoreceptors. Meanwhile a number of investigators,[*] employing the method of recording the electrical activity of neural units in the hypothalamus, had found cells in or near the supraoptic nuclei which are responsive to changes in blood osmolarity. But since osmotic stimuli evoke increased electrical activity in such remote regions as the medulla oblongata and olfactory bulbs,[*] these hypothalamic responses constitute nothing better than circumstantial evidence. More significant was the demonstration by Chandler Brooks and his several colleagues (see Brooks and Koizumi, 1965) that unit electrical activity in the supraoptic and paraventricular nuclei can be related

---

[*] See references on Woods, Bard, and Bleier (1966).

to impulse discharge in the fine fibers of the hypophyseal stalk and to the induced release of ADH and oxytocin. But none of these studies had demonstrated that the responding units are the osmoreceptors of Verney.

Over forty years ago I suggested (Bard, 1933) that the permanent abolition of a given cerebral function by a specific ablation does not afford proof of localization. I insisted that the function in question can be regarded as strictly localized only when it has been determined how much cerebral tissue can be removed without disturbing that function. In the case of the osmoreceptors, Woods and I, with the anatomical cooperation of Ruth Bleier (Woods, Bard, and Bleier, 1966), were able to apply this criterion with fair success to the localization of the hypothalamic osmoreceptors. This was accomplished by fashioning islands of different sizes and dimensions in a series of 19 decerebrate cats which survived from 28 to 346 days (average, 110 days). During their survival periods, 18 regulated their water balance under basal conditions and under conditions of water loading and water deprivation. One animal developed diabetes insipidus on its 25th day and examination of its island yielded information of considerable interest. In contrast, diabetes insipidus developed immediately in each of 28 cats which survived removal of the hypothalamus as well as the rest of the forebrain for periods of 28 to 112 days (average, 55 days). In them the pituitary gland was left in situ (with severed stalk), neurally isolated except for a possible sympathetic innervation. The pars neuralis of course degenerated, but the arterial blood supply and venous drainage sustained the glandular portions. These animals, which may be termed isolated pituitary preparations, were maintained by Pitressin therapy. One, when Pitressin was withheld for several days, excreted 1,700 ml of urine in one 24-hour period. It is notable that after withdrawal of exogenous ADH, withholding all food and water failed to reduce urinary output and the animals became dehydrated and hypernatremic; they survived only if rehydrated by intravenous fluids.

The water balance of the island cats was compared to that of eight animals in which, weeks before, the spinal cord had been sectioned between the sixth and eighth cervical segments. With their intact brains they served as good controls since they resembled the decerebrates in four respects: (1) Being essentially poikilothermic they were kept under the same thermal conditions; (2) they were fed the same food thinned with water to pass easily through a stomach tube; (3) their motor activity was about the same; and (4) their bladders, as were those of the island cats, were emptied manually without evoking sensory or affective responses which might affect the release of ADH. With the same water intake, the urine output and specific gravity were essentially the same in the two groups. In both, over periods as long as 50 days, body weight did not change appreciably and serum electrolytes, total solids, and total nitrogen remained within normal limits—evidence that the animals were in water balance.

To determine the responsiveness of the osmoreceptor-ADH system, the cats were subjected to water deprivation and water loading and, in many cases, to antidiuretic stimuli. To these the island cats reacted in a normal fashion with respect to urine output and specific gravity. After the onset of a water diuresis, stimuli known to increase release of ADH were applied. Intravenous injections of nicotine hydrogen tartrate were used in some cases, but reliance was placed chiefly on intravenous injections of hypertonic solutions of NaCl. Intracarotid injections, which were used by Jewell and Verney (1957), are not practical in cats since the internal carotid arteries are not patent in the majority of these animals. It was found that by the intravenous route 5–10 ml of a 2.9% NaCl solution or 2.0 mg of the nicotine compound quickly and markedly reduced urine flow from a diuresis level of about 1.0 ml to less than 0.1 ml per minute with corresponding increase in specific gravity. All cases in which recovery of the previously high rate of urine production failed to occur were considered inconclusive.

Tabulation of the anatomical findings in each of the 19 island cats indicated that only the anterior portion of the hypothalamus is required for a normal output of ADH and for its suppression and augmentation by physiological and pharmacological stimuli. One cat which, throughout its survival of 34 days, showed a normal water balance and responded normally to dehydration and water loading, had a hypothalamic remnant consisting of only the dorsal chiasmatic, suprachiasmatic, and anterior hypothalamic nuclei and fractions of other nuclei—one-fourth of the anterior supraoptic, one-half of the tuberal supraoptic, one-third each of the anterior paraventricular and anterior periventricular, one-fourth of the infundibular together with one-half of the anterior hypothalamic area, and one-fourth each of the lateral hypothalamic areas and the area of the tuber cinereum. The smallest remnant was found in the animal which developed diabetes insipidus 25 days after operation. Here the only cell groups remaining were the dorsal suprachiasmatic nucleus, about one-fourth of the tuberal component of the supraoptic nuclei, and some cells in a narrow strip consisting of about a fourth of the area of the tuber cinereum. There was marked cell loss throughout the remnant, and the cytoplasm of most of the large cells seen at the site of the tuberal supraoptic nuclei appeared to be replaced by large vacuoles. Although this animal was not tested by antidiuretic agents, it maintained water balance and excreted hypertonic urine for 24 days after the very small island was surgically fashioned. It is not unlikely that during this period the neurons essential for ADH release were undergoing transneuronal degeneration secondary to the almost complete deafferentation effected in this series of experiments and that at a crucial stage in this process hormone production, transportation, and release ceased. In any case, it appears that in the cat the neurohypophysis need be connected with only a very small island of anterior hypothalamus in order to maintain water balance and to respond to diuretic and antidiuretic stimuli. The conclusion was drawn that the elements essential for this are within an area which "must contain, at the most, the dorsal chiasmatic and suprachiasmatic nuclei, about half of the supraoptic nuclei, the rostral tip of the infundibular nucleus, the most ventral portion of the anterior periventricular nucleus, and the most ventral portions of the anterior and tuberal hypothalamic areas" (Woods, Bard, and Bleier, 1966). Jewell and Verney adopted the working hypothesis that the osmoreceptors lie in or very close to the supraoptic nuclei and our results are in accord with this supposition, for every cat that maintained fluid balance presented a hypothalamic remnant in which one-third or more of these cellular groups were present.

Although we succeeded in reducing further than did Jewell and Verney the confines of the cerebral region within which regulation of ADH release can be managed in normal fashion, there remains the question whether the essential neurons serve as both receptors and effectors. It is of course possible that the osmoreceptive function resides in cells which project to the effector neurons. While both ascending and descending neural traffic does affect the output of ADH in the normal animal, our experimental results show that after exclusion of all extrahypothalamic neural input the basal secretion of the hormone continues and can be modified by the osmolarity of blood flowing through a small anterior hypothalamic remnant. Further, no change in the sensitivity of the osmoreceptors was detected during long survivals. These facts suggest that the neurons in control of ADH release may be unique in that their basic excitability and impulse firing are independent of afferent bombardment. Certainly tonic excitation from extrahypothalamic sources is in no way requisite for their normal secretomotor activity. Finally, it is interesting to speculate whether this characteristic was evolved to provide a high degree of security for the phylogenetically ancient mechanism that developed for the production of hypertonic urine.

Dr. James W. Woods returned to the Johns Hopkins department of physiology in 1957 after a fellowship spent in Geoffrey Harris's laboratory at the Maudsley Hospital, where his interest in endocrinology had been further stimulated. It was just at this time that I was getting back into investigative work after four physiologically sterile years spent as dean of the medical faculty. Woods had become especially interested in the pituitary and thyroid glands and I had long wanted to take up again the studies of chronically decerebrate cats with islands, an endeavor which had been interrupted by World War II. We joined forces with the idea that it would be interesting to examine the output of TSH by the hypothalamohypophyseal islands (the ADH studies just described came later). This we determined by measuring the rate of disappearance of neck radioactivity following a tracer dose of I^{131}, a technique which had been recently described by Brown-Grant, von Euler, Harris, and Reichlin (1954). Very soon we established that under basal conditions the amount of isotope accumulated by the thyroid and its rate of release from the gland were essentially the same in six decerebrate island cats as in nine normal animals (Woods and Bard, 1960). Also we found that the responses to injection of thyroxin or exogenous TSH were not qualitatively different in the two groups. Thus it appeared that in the island cats the feedback inhibition of TSH secretion by thyroxin and the sensitivity of the thyroid to that tropic hormone were within the normal range.

In our studies we soon observed that when the wholly poikilothermic island animals (Bard, Woods, and Bleier, 1970) became even mildly hypothermic there was complete inhibition of thyroid secretion (Woods and Bard, 1960). In nine tests on six cats carried out between the 31st and 108th postoperative days, reduction of core temperature to 35.5°C or below caused cessation of thyroid activity as indicated by a complete flattening of the release curve. This inhibition was due to an effect on the island, not to any decreased sensitivity of the thyroid, for the response to a standard test injection of exogenous TSH was always somewhat greater during hypothermia than when core temperature was at a normal level—an interesting but unexplained phenomenon. It is most significant that the same results were obtained in three experiments on a cat whose brain was intact but whose spinal cord had been sectioned at the level of the eighth cervical segment. Since cutaneous vasoconstriction and piloerection could not occur and shivering was possible only in muscles innervated by cervical and cranial nerves, she was almost but not quite as deficient as the decerebrates in maintaining body temperature in the face of a cool environment.

The inhibitory effect of hypothermia on thyroid secretion in the island cats and in the low cervical spinal cat stands in marked contrast to the well-established increase engendered in normal animals by exposure to cold, a response which we found readily detectible by the radioisotope method we employed. Woods and I were unable to offer any certain explanation of the inhibition, but we did rule out as a cause any elevation of the thyroid threshold to TSH. Although the total body cooling involved the hypothalamus, this is an unlikely causative factor in view of the evidence, obtained since our experiments were done, that local hypothalamic cooling increases TSH release in the intact animal (Andersson, Ekman, Gale, and Sundsten, 1963; Andersson, Brook, and Ekman, 1965). Woods and I suggested that a potent factor might be an increased feedback action of circulating thyroid hormones, for it is reasonable to suppose that in hypothermia there is a lessened tissue utilization of them. Still, the fact that in the intact animal hypothalamic cooling increases thyroid activity raises the question why this does not occur in the cat with an isolated island or in the low cervical spinal cat. One could summon good neurophysiological reasons for suggesting that the total absence of afferent hypothalamic input from peripheral thermoreceptors in the former and a great reduction of such input in the latter accentuated the inhibitory effect of a raised blood level of the thyroid hormones.

I regret that we did not explore in depth the capacity of the islands to provide other tropic hormones of the pars distalis. It may be noted, however, that in our long surviving animals the adrenal cortices were found to be histologically normal and that well-developed follicles were present in the ovaries of several, indications that ACTH and FSH as well as TSH were being released.

In reviewing my excursions into the field of neuroendocrinology, I see that my own limitations have restricted the extent to which they might have been expanded. Having no special training or experience in the methods, especially the biochemical ones, which have so greatly advanced endocrinology during the period of my scientific career, I was unable to follow a number of promising lines of attack. I was, however, fortunate in having collaborators who provided essential neuroanatomical knowledge, skills, and ideas or devised techniques that made my own contributions, mainly surgical and observational, significant. Whatever this work may signify, I have had many months of pleasure and satisfaction in carrying it out.

REFERENCES

Andersson, B., A. H. Brook, and L. Ekman (1965). Further studies of the thyroidal response to local cooling of the "heat loss center." *Acta Physiol. Scand.* **63:** 186.

Andersson, B., L. Ekman, C. C. Gale, and J. W. Sundsten (1963). Control of thyrotrophic hormone (TSH) secretion by the "heat loss center." *Acta Physiol. Scand.* **59:** 12.

Bard, P. (1933). Studies on the cerebral cortex. I. Localized control of placing and hopping reactions in the cat and their normal management by small cortical remnants. *Arch. Neurol. and Psychiatry* **30:** 40.

Bard, P. (1934). On emotional expression after decortication with some remarks on certain theoretical views: Part II. *Psychol. Rev.* **41:** 424.

Bard, P. (1939). Central nervous mechanisms for emotional behavior patterns in animals. *Res. Publ. Assoc. Res. Nerv. Ment. Dis.* **19:** 190.

Bard, P. (1940). The hypothalamus and sexual behavior. *Res. Publ. Assoc. Res. Nerv. Ment. Dis.* **20:** 551.

Bard, P., and M. B. Macht (1958). The behavior of chronically decerebrate cats. *Ciba Foundation Symposium on Neurological Basis of Behavior,* p. 55. Little, Brown and Co., Boston.

Bard, P., and D. McK. Rioch (1937). A study of four cats deprived of neocortex and additional portions of the forebrain. *Bull. Johns Hopkins Hosp.* **60**: 73.

Bard, P., J. W. Woods, and R. Bleier (1970). The effects of cooling, heating, and pyrogen on chronically decerebrate cats, *Comm. Behav. Biol. Part* A. **5**: 31.

Bromiley, R. B., and P. Bard (1940). A study of the effect of estrin on the responses to genital stimulation shown by decapitate and decerebrate female cats. *Am. J. Physiol.* **129**: 318.

Brooks, C. McC., and K. Koizumi (1965). Control of neurons in the supraoptic and paraventricular nuclei. Page 18 *in* D. R. Cross and A. K. McIntyre, eds. *Studies in Physiology Presented to John C. Eccles.* Springer-Verlag, New York.

Brown-Grant, K., C. von Euler, G. W. Harris, and S. Reichlin (1954). The measurement and experimental modification of thyroid activity in the rabbit. *J. Physiol.* **126**: 1.

Dempsey, E. W., and D. McK. Rioch (1939). The localization in the brain stem of the oestrous responses of the female guinea pig, *J. Neurophysiol.* **2**: 9.

Jewell, P. A., and E. B. Verney (1957). An experimental attempt to determine the site of the neurohypophysial osmoreceptors in the dog. *Philos. Trans. R. Soc.* (London), Ser. B. **232**: 197.

Macht, M. B., and P. Bard (1942). Studies on decerebrate cats in the chronic state. *Fed. Proc.* **1**: 55.

Michael, R. P. (1973). The effects of hormones on sexual behavior in female cat and rhesus monkey. Pages 187-221 *in Handbook of Physiology, Section 7: Endocrinology,* vol. 2, part 1, chap. 10. American Physiological Society, Washington, D. C.

Sumwalt, M., W. H. Erb, and H. C. Bazett (1935). The water and chloride excretion of decerebrate cats. *Am. J. Physiol.* **112**: 386.

Woods, J. W., and P. Bard (1960). Thyroid activity during hypothermia produced without the use of drugs. *Bull. Johns Hopkins Hosp.* **107**: 163.

Woods, J. W., P. Bard, and R. Bleier (1966). Functional capacity of the deafferented hypothalamus: Water balance and responses to osmotic stimuli in the decerebrate cat and rat. *J. Neurophysiol.* **29**: 571.

3

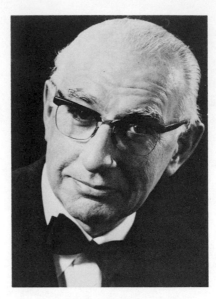

Wolfgang Bargmann

Wolfgang Bargmann was born in 1906 in Nuremberg, Bavaria. He received a liberal education at the humanistic Lessing Gymnasium in Frankfurt-am-Main and began his medical studies at the University of Frankfurt, where his teachers were Albrecht Bethe, Gustav Embden, Franz Volhard, Franz Weidenreich, and Karl Zeiger. Additional semesters were spent at the Universities of Munich, Vienna, and Berlin. His doctoral thesis at the University of Frankfurt dealt with the histology of the kidney glomerulus.

He became an Instructor in the Department of Anatomy at the University of Frankfurt, and it was there that he made the acquaintance of Ernst Scharrer, whose investigations on neurosecretion influenced him many years later to begin studies in this field. He became a *Privatdozent* in 1935 at the University of Zürich, where he served for several years and during which time he made several sojourns to the Stazione Zoologica in Naples. In 1938 he was appointed a Prosector in Leipzig. He was a military doctor for one year during World War II.

In 1942 he took charge of the laboratories for histology and embryology at the University of Königsberg in East Prussia, where he remained until his escape in 1945. After spending some months in Göttingen, he took over the chair of anatomy at Kiel University in 1946, and he remained there to build up the Anatomical Institute. The years at Kiel were devoted not only to research and teaching, but also to the reconstitution of scientific life in West Germany. Much of his time also has been devoted to editing Zeitschrift für Zellforschung (now Cell and Tissue Research) together with Berta Scharrer, Donald Farner, and Andreas Oksche, and also to the editorship of v. Möllendorff's *Handbuch der mikrokopischen Anatomie des Menschen.*

Dr. Bargmann enjoys travel in foreign lands, and reading history, fiction, and history of art. Some of his own publications have dealt with historical topics, including a contribution to *History of the World,* edited by Golo Mann. He became a Professor Emeritus in March, 1974.

A Marvelous Region

WOLFGANG BARGMANN

More than 20 years ago, the distinguished neuroanatomist and neuropathologist, Hugo Spatz, asked me at the end of a controversial discussion on hypothalamic neurosecretion, "Isn't the hypothalamus a marvelous region? Don't you think so?" My affirmative reply was one of the few points of mutual agreement, as far as the function of the hypothalamic-neurohypophyseal system was concerned. How and when did I become acquainted with this neuronal system in the diencephalon of vertebrates, since recognized as the source of the so-called posterior lobe hormones?

When I was a young assistant in the department of anatomy in Frankfurt/Main (1933–34), I had my first contacts with Ernst and Berta Scharrer, both having arrived from Munich, where Ernst had performed his pioneer investigations on secretory nerve cells in the brain. In Frankfurt, Ernst Scharrer was head of a modest but renowned laboratory housed in the Institute of Pathology, the neurological institute bearing the name of its founder, Ludwig Edinger. I remember still its homely atmosphere and Edinger's famous portrait, painted by Lovis Corinth, that hung on the wall above an old-fashioned sofa. It was there that Ernst Scharrer demonstrated to me his brilliant microscopical preparations, showing granular and dropletlike inclusions within the perikarya of certain diencephalic nerve cells, which he interpreted as *Drüsen-Nervenzellen*, their function still being enigmatic at the time.

Approximately one year later, our paths diverged. The Scharrers went to the United States in 1937, and I came via Freiburg/Breisgau (1934) to Zürich, Switzerland (1935) to work in the anatomy department headed by my teacher, Wilhelm v. Möllendorff. He asked me to write some review articles on endocrine organs (except the hypophysis) to be published in *Handbuch der mikroskopischen Anatomie des Menschen* (Springer-Verlag),

WOLFGANG BARGMANN ● Anatomical Institute, University of Kiel, 23 Kiel, West Germany.

despite my sparse experience in this field. This was my first approach to the morphological aspects of internal secretion.

I followed the endocrine line later on, when I was appointed as prosector in Leipzig (1938) and as professor of anatomy in Königsberg/East Prussia (1942). It was in Königsberg (today Kaliningrad) that I began histological investigations on the neurohypophysis, but without getting remarkable results. Such research, doomed to be interrupted in view of an imminent catastrophe, ceased altogether in autumn 1944.

After having examined the last medical students in January 1945, I escaped from Königsberg just at the beginning of its siege by the Russian army, joined my family in Bavaria, and responded some months later to a call from the Medical Faculty in Göttingen. My final refuge was almost totally bombed Kiel in northern Germany, where I started a new career as full professor of anatomy in February 1946, under primitive living conditions, but happily facing the new tasks and aspects of life in security and freedom.

It was not until spring 1948 that I was able to begin again with research work. Having published some histological papers on the pancreatic islands, I became interested de novo in this subject and stimulated one of my students, Werner Creutzfeldt (today professor of medicine, Göttingen University) to reproduce the alloxan diabetes experiments performed during the war in England by Dunn and co-workers, and to reinvestigate the islet necrosis with Gomori's 1941 chromalum-hematoxylin-phloxin staining method. At the same time another student of mine, Walter Hild (today professor of anatomy, Galveston, Texas), asked me for a theme for an M.D. thesis just at the moment when I had become stimulated by the problems of neurosecretion in vertebrates. It was inevitable that he would participate in this research, investigating the brain of lower vertebrates, while my attention was primarily directed toward the hypothalamic-hypophyseal system in mammals.

The origins of this activity were rather complex: The memories of the past (Frankfurt), the disappointing histological investigations of the neurohypophysis (Königsberg), and last but not least, one of the first letters I received after the war from the outside world. In it Ernst Scharrer mentioned that his work on neurosecretion had made progress, but that one of the questions still open was whether and how the diencephalic *Drüsen-Nervenzellen* were related to the unmyelinated nerve terminals in the posterior lobe of the hypophysis. Additionally, I felt myself challenged by the negative attitude of many of my colleagues as far as the phenomenon of neurosecretion was concerned. I cannot forget, for example, the somewhat sarcastic question of Hans Gerhard Creutzfeldt (Jacob–Creutzfeldt disease; father of my student W. Creutzfeldt) that he asked me during a stroll in the evening after a faculty meeting: "Do you really believe in neurosecretion? These *Drüsen-Nervenzellen* are certainly nothing more than degenerating neurons." Well, I had still stored in my memory the images of Ernst Scharrer's preparations that, according to my impression, were far from representing pathological events.

The problem was how to find a new methodological approach to the characterization of these glandular nerve cells. My reasoning was simple: Scharrer's observations suggested the existence of secretory, possibly endocrine cell groups in the brain. It was known that the cells of endocrine glands may be differentiated by various staining methods. One distinguishes, for example, the A- and B-cells in the islets of Langerhans by their different affinities for chromalum-hematoxylin and phloxin, and the various cell types of the anterior lobe of the hypophysis by means of many differential staining procedures.

As a consequence of this unsophisticated consideration, I asked my technician, Miss K. Jacob, to stain a first series of slides from a dog's brain according to Gomori's technique with chromalum-hematoxylin-phloxin, already introduced by W. Creutzfeldt in his alloxan diabetes studies. When I took the first look through the microscope—the slides still being wet—I was lucky enough to perceive at once a selectively stained neuronal system, extending uninterruptedly from the nuclei supraopticus and paraventricularis to the neural lobe of the hypophysis. This finding was soon confirmed for other mammals, and I wrote instantly and with enthusiasm the paper, *Über die neurosekretorische Verknüpfung von Hypothalamus und Neurohypophyse,* that was published in 1949. Fortunately enough, being at that time the sole editor of this journal, I had none of the barriers to overcome that might have been erected by members of an editorial board more or less prejudiced (as far as neurosecretion was concerned).

The article just mentioned is obviously the reason for my having been invited by the editors of the present volume to write this sketch. It seems therefore justified to repeat briefly its essential results:

1. The nerve cells of the supraoptic and paraventricular nuclei (in lower vertebrates, the preoptic nucleus) form a neurosecretory pathway, containing selectively stainable material. The network of terminals of this via neurosecretoria, which surround the blood capillaries in the neurohypophysis, is particularly rich in neurosecretory substance. The so-called Herring bodies, for a long time misinterpreted as isolated colloidal particles, are in reality circumscribed swellings of hypothalamic axons, filled with neurosecretion (string of pearl fibers).

2. The cytological aspect of the via neurosecretoria was interpreted to

indicate transport of neurosecretory material. This transport begins
in their perikarya and ends in the neurohypophysis. From a
considerable number of these perivascular nerve terminals in the
neural lobe neurosecretory substance is released.

3. The hypothesis was put forward that the magnocellular neurosecretory hypothalamic system releases into the bloodstream antidiuretic
hormone, elaborated in the perikarya.

4. The question was raised whether the visualized neurosecretory material within the neurons was a carrier substance of hormone or the
hormone itself.

5. Relationships between neurosecretory fibers and the pars intermedia
of the hypophysis were indicated.

These observations and hypotheses proved to be very stimulating, and a
happy period of light microscopic and experimental research work began in
the Kiel Institute for Anatomy, which was then lodged in a former factory
and only modestly equipped. Since the production of electron microscopes
was not allowed in Germany after the war, we were for some years confined
to light microscopy. At any rate, our institute would not have been prepared
to undertake expensive studies; the financial outlay for our pilot studies ran
to no more than approximately 100 U.S. dollars. Rather late in 1956, my
co-worker, the physicist Dr. Anne-Marie Knoop, was able to organize our
first laboratory for electron microscopy.

The results published in 1949 gave rise to a sequence of new investigations, carried out by my co-workers and myself. The transport hypothesis
was substantiated by hypophyseal stalk sections performed by Hild in 1951.
Ortmann, in 1951–52, and Kratzsch, also in 1951–52, demonstrated a relationship between water metabolism and amount of neurosecretory material.
Hild and his friend G. Zetler (now professor of pharmacology, Lübeck)
gave evidence in 1953 that extracts exert antidiuretic, vasopressor, and
oxytocic activity only when prepared from those parts of the hypothalamus
that contain the stainable secretory products of the supraoptic and paraventricular neurons.

During the postwar period in which the studies I mentioned were carried out, it was still difficult for German research workers to make personal
contact with the outside world and to have discussions with scientists on the
international level. My first experience of this kind, a lecture given in Oxford by invitation of Professor Glees, was soon followed by a gratefully
welcomed three-month travel grant from the Rockefeller Foundation, that
generously gave me the opportunity to visit many colleagues and institutions
in the United States (1950). I demonstrated my slides to Dr. Gomori,
among others, who was very astonished by the unexpected side effect of his

staining method, and to Dr. Bodian, who at the time was interested in the peculiarities of the opossum neurohypophysis. The outstanding event was of course to meet again after so many years with Ernst and Berta Scharrer, who were at that time living in Denver, Colorado. I remember vividly a lecture I gave in less than literate English and the long discussion I had afterward with the audience. Ernst Scharrer proposed that we write a joint paper. It appeared in *American Scientist* (1951) and summarized the main results of his and my efforts and the studies of my co-workers and formulated the concept of a hypothalamic-neurohypophyseal system, consisting of sites of hormone production (hypothalamic nuclei), transport (axons), and storage and release (neural lobe). As may be easily understood, we found it very gratifying that this concept was finally generally accepted. Neurosecretion in vertebrates was no longer considered to be conjecture or a matter of faith.

Denver was also the place where we first discussed how to arrange international symposia on this topic, nowadays one of the roots of neuroendocrinology. The sixth meeting of the "family of neurosecretionists" was carefully organized in 1973 by Sir Francis Knowles in London, under the auspices of the Royal Society.

One day after having returned from the United States (1950), I was elected *Rector magnificus* of my university and became considerably involved in administration and representation affairs. Nevertheless, I was keen on not losing contact with the laboratory and with my co-workers.

A variety of topics have been examined in the course of time: e.g., lactation and the neurosecretory system, its ultrastructure, the innervation of the intermediate lobe by peptidergic and adrenergic endings, the contact between neurosecretory terminals and the capillary loops in the median eminence, and the problem of exocytosis in the neural lobe. Electron microscopic research work on the median eminence is still going on in our institute (Br. Krisch). Valuable contributions towards the knowledge of the neuroendocrine system have also been made by foreign guests I had the pleasure to welcome in our laboratory—among them Malandra (Italy), Rodeck (Düsseldorf), Sloper (London), Sano (Kyoto), Lederis (Bristol), and Hartmann (United States).

Looking back, I find it instructive to ponder how useful light microscopic observations and their functional interpretation may be as a basis for the development of new concepts. I am still impressed by the explosion of literature that followed the first postwar publications on the histology of classical neurosecretory cells. This expansion includes increasingly the large field of hypophysiotropic ("releasing" and "release inhibiting") hormones.

Since I became involved in neuroendocrinology as an anatomist, one might ask about my motives and my approach to morphology as a lifetime task. When I was still a schoolboy I felt myself attracted by form and structure of living organisms, admiring their esthetics and mysteries. But how was I to get access to these structures? In order to cover the expenses for a simple microscope, petrol-heated thermostat, microtome, etc., I wrote meagerly paying articles for magazines and changed my bedroom—somewhat to the family's dismay—into a laboratory. Having finished the gymnasium, I studied—instead of zoology—medicine because it promised to yield more information on the human organism than does zoology.

At the university, I was so fortunate as to enjoy the guidance of such excellent anatomists as Karl Zeiger, Franz Weidenreich, and Hans Bluntschli. While still a medical student, I published my first papers in Z. Zellforsch., the editor of which I became two decades later. I also remained in touch with morphology as intimately as possible during my clinical years in Vienna, Munich, and Berlin, and I was delighted to obtain after the final examination the position of an assistant in institutes of anatomy, first in Frankfurt, later in Freiburg/Breisgau. At that time anatomy began more and more to adopt dynamic aspects and to devote itself to the interrelationships between structure and function, v. Möllendorff being one of the prominent representatives of this new line. The spirit in his institutes in Freiburg and Zürich met my basic inclinations.

The study of endocrine organs that I had begun in Freiburg made me familiar with structures, the development and pattern of which change strikingly under the influence of internal and external factors —a fascinating example of functional morphology. This is one of the reasons why research work on endocrine organs prevails among other investigations of mine. The incentives, some of them accidental, that led to my preferential involvement in problems of neurosecretion and neuroendocrinology have been already mentioned. In retrospect, I regret that I neglected in younger years to learn the methods of biochemistry and pharmacology. Without this sin of omission my contributions to neuroendocrinology might have been more successful than my exploration of a "marvelous region" actually was.

REFERENCES

Bargmann, W. (1949). Über die neurosekretorische Verknüpfung von Hypothalamus und Neurohypophyse. Z. Zellforsch. 34: 610.

Bargmann, W. (1953). Uber das Zwischenhirn-Hypophysensystem von Fischen. Z. Zellforsch. 38: 275.

Bargmann, W. (1954). Die endokrine Funktion neurosekretorischer Zellen bei Wirbeltieren. Pubbl. Stn. Zool. Napoli 24 (Suppl.): 11.

Bargmann, W. (1954). *Das Zwischenhirn-Hypophysensystem*. Springer-Verlag, Berlin/ Göttingen/Heidelberg.

Bargmann, W. (1955). Weitere Untersuchungen am neurosekretorischen Zwischenhirn-Hypophysensystem. *Z. Zellforsch.* **2**: 247.

Bargmann, W. (1956). Relationship between neurohypophysial structure and function. *Colston Papers VIII*, 11–22. Butterworths Scientific Publ., London.

Bargmann, W. (1960–61). Neurosekretorische Nervenfasern und Adenohypophyse. Anat. Anz. **109**:(Ergänzungsband): 260.

Bargmann, W. (1966). Neurosecretion. *Intern. Rev. Cytol.* **19**: 183.

Bargmann, W. (1967). Über neuroendokrine Zwischenhirnsysteme. Freiburger Universitätsreden, N.F. Heft 42. H.F. Schulz Verlag, Freiburg/Br.

Bargmann, W. (1967). Gehirn and Hypophyse. Schleiden-Vorlesung. *Nova acta Leopold., N.F. 181*, vol. **341**: 3.

Bargmann, W. (1968). Neurohypophysis. Structure and Function. Pages 1–39 *in* Eichler, Farah, Herken, and Welch, eds. *Handbuch d. experim. Pharmakol.* vol. 23. Springer-Verlag, Berlin/Heidelberg/New York.

Bargmann, W. (1969). Das neurosekretorische Zwischenhirn-Hypophysensystem und seine synaptischen Verknüpfungen. *J. Neuro-Visc. Relat. Suppl.* IX: 64.

Bargmann, W., and B. v. Gaudecker (1969). Über die Ultrastruktur neurosekretorischer Elementargranula. *Z. Zellforsch.* **96**: 495.

Bargmann, W., and W. Hild (1949). Über die Morphologie der neurosekretorischen Verknüpfung von Hypothalamus und Neurohypophyse. *Acta Anat.* **8**: 264.

Bargmann, W., W. Hild, R. Ortmann, and T. H. Schiebler (1950). Morphologische und experimentelle Untersuchungen über das hypothalamisch-hypophysäre System. *Acta Neuroveg.* **1**: 233.

Bargmann, W., and A. Knoop (1957). Elektronenmikroskopische Beobachtungen an der Neurohypophyse. *Z. Zellforsch.* **46**: 242.

Bargmann, W., A. Knoop, and A. Thiel (1957). Elektronenmikroskopische Studie an der Neurohypophyse von Tropidonotus natrix (mit Berücksichtigung der Pars intermedia). *Z. Zellforsch.* **47**: 114.

Bargmann, W., E. Lindner, and K. H. Andres (1967). Über Synapsen an endokrinen Epithelzellen und die Definition sekretorischer Neurone. Untersuchungen am Zwischenlappen der Katzenhypophyse. *Z. Zellforsch.* **77**: 282.

Bargmann, W., and E. Scharrer (1951). The site of origin of the hormones of the posterior pituitary. *Am. Sci.* **39**: 255.

4

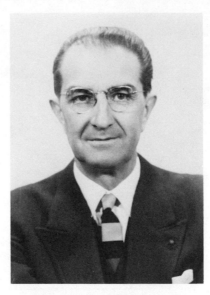

J. Benoit

J. Benoit was born in Nancy (Meurthe et Moselle), France, on February 26, 1896. He passed the university entrance examination in 1913. In 1914 he joined the French army. He was wounded and became a prisoner of war, and was freed in January 1919. In May 1919 he began work in the Histology Laboratory of the Strasbourg Medical Faculty, whose director was Prof. Pol Bouin. He became a Doctor of Medicine in 1925 and a Doctor of Science in 1929. He was an Assistant Professor of the Faculty of Medicine in 1930, and a Fellow of the Rockefeller Foundation for one year in 1936–37 at Yale University in the Department of Anatomy under Prof. E. Allen. He became Titular Professor of Histology and Embryology at the Faculty of Medicine and Pharmacy at the University of Algiers in 1939, Professor of Embryology at the Strasbourg Medical Faculty in 1946, and Professor of Histophysiology at the Collège de France, Paris, from 1952 to 1966.

He is a member of the National Academy of Medicine, corresponding member of the Royal Academy of Belgium, and founder and president of the National Committee of Coordination for Vertebrate Neuroendocrinology (1963) and of the Society of Experimental Neuroendocrinology (1971). His honors include Commander of the Academic Palms (1967) and Commander of the Legion of Honor (1970).

My Research in Neuroendocrinology: Study of the Photo-Sexual Reflex in the Domestic Duck

J. BENOIT

INTRODUCTION

Attracted at the age of 9 years by the marvels and variety of living organisms and their structure, I undertook, as a young self-made histologist, microscopic studies of vegetable and animal tissues, and obtained at the age of 16 years, a silver-gilt medal at a competition organized by the French Photographic Society where I had shown color photographs of histological sections. On this occasion in 1912. I was privileged to meet Prof. Pol Bouin, who held the chair of histology at the Nancy Medical Faculty. His exceptional personality and scientific and human value impressed me and I decided to join his team. The Great War of 1914, during which I served, delayed my project and it was only in 1919, after a long captivity, that I was able to join Professor Bouin at Strasbourg, where he had just been appointed. An eminent specialist of the genital glands and secondary sexual characteristics, he advised me to work on male birds. Several French and German biologists considered that the testes did not contain any trace of the interstitial cells which, according to Professor Bouin and his friend and colleague Prof. Paul Ancel, was the source of male hormone responsible for the development of the secondary sexual characteristics. For this reason, I became rapidly familiar with the histophysiological study of the gonads and of the sexual characteristics of the cock and, a little later, the domestic duck.

J. BENOIT ● Laboratory of Histophysiology, Collège de France, Paris, France.

During the long vacation in 1933 I read a report by T. H. Bissonnette (1931) concerning strong stimulation of the testes of the starling by artificial light. This article was of great interest to me and I resolved that I would attempt to determine the mechanism of this phenomenon. Between this cosmic factor of light and the genital glands, there were numerous intermediate steps which had to be discovered: a photoreceptor, the eye perhaps, which probably commanded a chain of nervous impulses, then a hormonal mechanism. This immediately raised a neuroendocrine problem in a laboratory where the endocrine sex glands were the main object of study.

I chose for my experiments the domestic duck. Its annual testicular sex cycle is very marked. This bird is large, resistant to infection, and easy to manipulate. Its large beak would permit one, after attaching the animal to a work bench, to immobilize its head and carry out certain operations. I believed, in fact, that light might act on the eye and that operations and exposure to light at various points on the head would perhaps be necessary to solve the problem.

DEVELOPMENT OF RESEARCH

Before undertaking these operations, I applied the bold reasoning which I had learned during the mathematics course at the secondary school and which consisted of "supposing that the problem has already been solved." I attached colored glasses to my ducks! I had glasses made with an oval shape, colored red, yellow, green, and blue, and each glass was inserted within a metal ring, attached by a hinge to another ring of the same shape.

The latter was stitched to the skin of the duck, in front of his eyes. Twenty-one ducks were thus supplied with colored glasses and let loose outside the laboratory, in December 1933, for several weeks. The duck is not a particularly clean animal; it was necessary to open the glasses every day and clean them. In spite of the low light intensity during winter at Strasbourg, the testes underwent definite growth with red and yellow spectacles but little growth or none with green or blue spectacles. But these glasses were far from monochromatic and the animals did not all receive the same amount of light energy. Thus, I did not consider these results worthy of publication. I reported them 10 years later however, but as a footnote and after acquiring precise results by strict technical procedures, thanks to the collaboration of a physicist, Dr. L. Ott, in a publication of the Yale Journal of Biology and Medicine in 1944.

This first and picturesque experiment was no doubt evidence for my theory concerning the role of the eye, but it was in this form, simply a guess.

Putting off until later a routine study of the action of colored light using recognized optical techniques, I attempted to draw up a few basic facts for my future experiments. Here are briefly the main results:

a. Prepubertal Peking or Rouen ducklings, aged from 3 to 5 months, submitted to 15 hours daily of white light, may present after 3 weeks, *strong testicular growth:* 60 to 80 times in terms of weight. *It is definitely the light,* and not the waking condition nor the increased food nor the increased movement which provokes testicular growth (Benoit, 1934).

b. *Dividing up* the daily dose of light into small repeated doses favors the development of the gonads (Benoit, 1936).*

c. The *anterior pituitary* is essential for the phenomenon of light stimulation of the gonads. Its removal prevents growth of the testes before puberty and testes already stimulated by light return to the resting condition. When implanted in the female mouse before puberty, stored hormone is released (Benoit, 1936). A cytological study of its gonadotropic cells reveals its activation (Benoit, 1937; Tixier-Vidal, Herlant, and Benoit, 1962).

Light thus exerts a *powerful and specific effect* on the development of the gonads in the duck before puberty. The anterior pituitary plays an essential role in this phenomenon.

Once these facts were determined, I sought the region of the body on which light rays exerted their action. Ducks before puberty had their feathers partly removed, and their heads covered by an opaque headdress.

---

* This modest finding, which emerged during an experiment which I carried out at the Algiers Medical Faculty, where I was professor of histology and embryology from 1938 to 1946, almost led me and my assistant, Jean Clavert, before a court-martial on a charge of high treason! These were the facts: W. U. Gardner, working with Prof. E. Allen, of Yale University, had kindly informed me of his research on the osteogenic effect of estrogen in the chick, which Zondek reported in 1937, and the mouse cited by Gardner and Pfeiffer in 1938. I undertook with Jean Clavert a study on the female duck of the mechanism of this action. Several ducks were placed in an open air hen run in the court of the Medical Faculty and submitted, during the night, to stimulation of their ovaries by intermittent flashes of light, which proved more economic and more efficacious than continuous light stimulation. Unfortunately, we started our experiment the night preceding J-Day (November 8, 1944) when the American troops arrived in Algiers! We had thus involuntarily alerted the civil defence of the Medical Faculty area and, the following morning, when J. Clavert went along to his laboratory, he was arrested by the area chief who said to him, "There are here some traitors who throughout the night sent light signals to the American planes which were flying over the town before their disembarkment. We have not been able to determine the origin, but we are carrying out investigations and will take the necessary steps." Fortunately for Clavert and myself, and above all for Algeria, the Allied disembarkment succeeded within a few hours. In the evening, in the joy of the success, everything was forgotten. We almost went to prison, or worse; our ducks betrayed us by playing the opposite role to the famous Capitole ducks!

Others were enclosed in opaque sacks, with small openings at the level of the eyes. Light stimulation of all these animals showed that *only the eye region* intervened in gonad stimulation (Benoit, 1934). I then showed that neither division of the optic nerves nor removal of both eyes prevented intense light from strongly stimulating testicular growth: Thus, I concluded that *deep retro-orbital organs* (for the orbits were completely emptied of their contents) were *light sensitive and produced stimulation of the gonads* (Benoit, 1935b,c).

I first believed, by shedding light on the pituitary region (using a quartz rod introduced within the orbit and across its bony wall up to the level of the pituitary), that light could stimulate this organ directly. But the light also reached the hypothalamus at the level of the median eminence. Light stimulation above the pituitary, using the quartz rod towards the upper border of the optic chiasma in the region of the supraoptic and paraventricular nuclei, convinced me that direct light stimulation of the hypothalamus strongly stimulated the gonads (Benoit, 1938b).*

The hypothalamus was thus the deep photoreceptor intervening during light stimulation of the ocular window.

I was able to show later, by shedding light on other regions of the duck brain, that only the rhinencephalon stimulated the development of the gonads in the same way as the hypothalamus, to which it is linked by nervous pathways (Benoit and Kehl, 1939).

It was thus demonstrated that light acting at the *level of the eyes* passed through an essential relay, the hypothalamus, which controlled the following stages of the light sexual reflex, stimulating the anterior pituitary by a mechanism to be discovered later.

But did the eye therefore have no role? Experiments on the eye alone, surrounded by an opaque cup made of metal, rubber, or paraffin blackened with india ink, in ducks firmly fixed to the work bench, and after division of the optic nerve in some cases, showed that the eye intervened positively in gonad stimulation and behaved truly as a *superficial photoreceptor*. The retro-ocular light stimulation of the eye, partially surrounded by a glass strip bent in the form of a spoon and through which light was passed through the cut edge, also produced definite development of the testes.

A more convincing experiment consisted of placing at gradually increasing distances from a feeble source of light (25 w) two series of ducks, one normal, the other having undergone division of the optic nerve on the light-stimulated side. Testicular growth, from zero to a maximum, at about 40 cm from the lamp, was definitely stronger in intact animals. In the latter, both photoreceptors, the superficial (retina) and deep (hypothalamic) recep-

---

* In 1911, K. von Frisch illuminated the top of the head of minnows (*Phoxinus laevis*) and obtained, by stimulation of the mesencephalon, a pigmentary response of the fishes. That is, I think, the first evidence for stimulation of hypothalamic centers by lighting.

tors, had been brought into play. The operated series, on the other hand, only responded by hypothalamic stimulation. This experiment showed *the role of the eye,* thus probably the role of the retina.

The *eye* represents a *superficial photoreceptor,* which stimulates the hypothalamus, the deep photoreceptor.

But which rays are the most active? And how do they penetrate as far as the hypothalamus?

To determine the active wavelength, I used successively as sources of light, car headlights, ordinary electric light bulbs, and a mercury lamp. As filters, I used gelatin filters or colored glasses, then interference filters, which were only found on the market after 1948, as far as I know. My technical advisor was, first, Prof. Fred Vlès, a very competent physicist who, unfortunately, during the Second World War, was sent to a German concentration camp and died of exhaustion and asphyxia in a cattle wagon of the train which was taking him into captivity! Later, at Yale University, where I was able to work for one year as a Rockefeller Fellow, the optical physicist L. Ott, and, finally, in Paris, at the Collège de France, the physicists of the Pasteur Laboratory of the Radium Institute, B. Muel and D. Lavalette, advised me.

Our first experiments, carried out with colored nonmonochromatic filters, gave strong responses in the red, feeble responses with yellow light, and nil responses in the indigo blue part of the spectrum. But with the mercury lamp, rays were isolated in the indigo, green, and yellow bands. Even using strong light energy, these three rays were totally inactive. As for the other part of the visible spectrum, the interference filters used with an ordinary electric light bulb demonstrated strong stimulant effect of *orange and, above all, red rays.* Ultraviolet and infrared were both totally inactive. The *photo-sexual retina,* insensitive to yellow light, is thus different from the visual retina, which has maximum sensitivity to yellow light. It has an *autonomic nervous function,* quite different from the visual function (Benoit, 1936, 1970; Benoit and Ott, 1944; Benoit, Da Lage, Muel, Kordon, and Assenmacher, 1966).

As far as the hypothalamus is concerned, when stimulated directly by the quartz rod, it is insensitive to ultraviolet and to infrared light, but is *very sensitive to indigo, green, yellow, and red light.* The hypothalamus was 100 times *more sensitive than the retina* to white light (Benoit, Walter, and Assenmacher, 1950).

The photo-sexual retina is thus only sensitive to orange and red light. The hypothalamus, when stimulated directly, is sensitive to light rays between indigo and red. When stimulated directly by white light, the hypothalamus is more light sensitive than the retina in influencing gonadotropic secretion.

Considering the *penetration* by light rays of various wavelengths of tissues situated in front of the hypothalamus, a photoelectric method shows that this penetration is all the greater when the wave length is greater. The coefficient of transmission was found to be equal to $\frac{1}{66}$ for red light of 745 nm and $\frac{1}{1260}$ only for indigo light (435 nm): i.e., a ratio of 20 of 1 (Benoit, Tauc, and Assenmacher, 1954).

Ducks exposed to white light, even when powerful, respond only to orange and red rays for (1) the retina is insensitive to indigo and yellow light rays and (2) the transmission of blue, green, and yellow rays is too low for them to reach the hypothalamus across the tissues of the socket.

An essential problem remains to be solved: *By what mechanism does the hypothalamus,* stimulated through surrounding tissue or indirectly by the retina, *stimulate the activity of the anterior lobe of the pituitary* and the secretion of gonadotropic hormone?

I tackled this problem in close collaboration with a young medical student who had astonished me at the embryology examination by his knowledge and critical faculties and the clearness of his exposition—Ivan Assenmacher, at present professor of comparative physiology at the Montpellier University of Sciences and Techniques. We undertook together the histophysiological study of the pituitary of the duck, and were able to discover in 1950 a certain number of new facts:

The anterior lobe of the pituitary receives all its blood supply through portal veins which, grouped together in a bundle situated 2 mm in front of the purely nervous stalk, extended from the median eminence to the pituitary hilum, and drained the blood from a rich capillary network covering the median eminence which is supplied by arterioles derived from the internal carotid arteries (Benoit and Assenmacher, 1950, 1951) (see Figure 1).

We were able to detect the presence, at the surface of the median eminence, of numerous nerve fibers mainly derived from the magnocellular hypothalamic nuclei containing numerous *neurosecretory granules* (Benoit and Assenmacher, 1953). In my opinion, there are few cases where the morphology of certain structures suggests as clearly what may be their physiology and function. These structures suggested to us possible surgical operations. These operations consisted, as indicated in Figure 2, of division of the median eminence (Benoit and Assenmacher, 1952), the portal veins (Assenmacher and Benoit, 1953), and the pituitary stalk (Benoit and Assenmacher, 1953), and the destruction of the magnocellular nuclei (Assenmacher, 1957). The testicular response suggested that *mediators* triggering off anterior pituitary activity *must be secreted by the magnocellular nuclei and are linked to neurosecretion by these nuclei.* These chemical mediators must pass through the capillaries which cover the median eminence, and through the portal veins, to reach the anterior lobe of the pituitary, in which they stimulate gonadotropic activity.

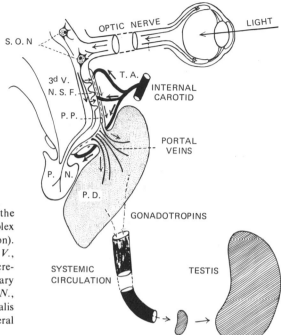

FIGURE 1. Vascularization of the hypothalamohypophyseal complex of the duck (sagittal section). *S.O.N.*, supra optic nucleus; $3^d V.$, third ventricle; *N.S.F.*, neurosecretory fibers; *P.P.*, primary capillary plexus of the portal system; *P.N.*, pars nervosa and *P.D.*, pars distalis of the hypophysis; *T.A.*, tuberal artery.

Thus we were able to confirm the neurohumoral theory of Green and Harris (1947) with more evidence than in mammals, where the portal veins and the nerve fibers between the hypothalamus and the pituitary are mixed together within a single pituitary stalk, and where selective division of the portal veins or the nerve fibers is anatomically impossible.

All this illustrates the strong gonadostimulant effect of visible light in the duck. But *internal factors* also intervene. By removing ducks from the action of light, by placing them in total darkness, or removing daily fluctuations by constant continuous light, I observed with Assenmacher and Brard (1955), among other things, that ducks placed together have synchronous testicular function. Only social factors, or group factors, may explain this phenomenon. Although they are still in progress, our experiments suggest that *tactile factors* may be responsible.

However, apart from the question of light, one problem intrigued us: Are ducks sensitive to sound and liable to respond by an *audiosexual reflex* to noises, sounds, or music—like cows, where it has been found that music increases their daily milk output?

The problem was attractive. We studied it by placing male ducks before puberty in a totally dark room, with a radio which produced for several weeks all kinds of noises and sounds, including news bulletins, songs

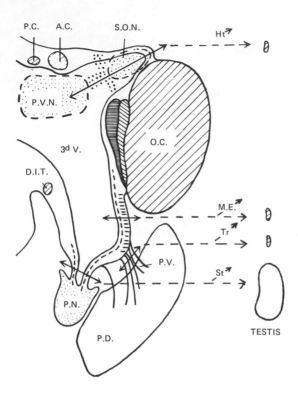

FIGURE 2. Four types of lesions in the hypothalamo-hypophyseal complex of the duck—their actions on the development of the testes of immature drakes submitted to the light (see Assenmacher, 1958). *P.C.*, palleal commissure; *A.C.* anterior commissure; *S.O.N.*, supra optic nucleus; *P.V.N.*, paraventricular nucleus; $3^d V.$, third ventricle; *O.C.*, optic chiasma; *D.I.T.*, decussation of the infundibular tract; *P.N.*, pars nervosa; *P.D.*, pars distalis; *P.V.*, portal veins. To the right, from top to bottom: lesion in the anterior hypothalamus; section of the median eminence; section of the portotuberal tract; section of the hypothalamic stalk.

by Maurice Chevalier, Edith Piaf, or Charles Trenet, jazz music, and classical music. Would ducks respond by growth of the testes on hearing the works of Bach, Debussy, Britten, Gershwin, or Stravinsky? The answer was no. After several weeks, the testes of our ducks remained indifferent to this musical and sound treatment. Wishing to control the experiment more closely, Assenmacher verified the function of the radio and its programs. One day he came along smiling, "Sir, the radio is giving out cooking recipes including full details on how to prepare the delicious dish, called 'duck with an orange sauce.' Should we continue the experiment?" With great amusement, we stopped the experiment, without concluding that there was not in the duck any audiosexual neuroendocrine reflex. We continued, moreover, the search for a reflex of this type in the laboratory of René Guy Busnel, director of the acoustic physiology laboratory at the National Institute for Agricultural Research. Mr. Busnel recorded, on a taperecorder, the cries of ducks during sexual activity and played back these cries to drakes before puberty placed in a dark room. No positive result was obtained with this experiment, which was abandoned.

This is a summary of the main results which I obtained, both alone and with several co-workers, studying the neuroendocrine mechanism of the photo-sexual reflex of the duck. The main aspects of this mechanism are thus established. However, we still do not know the sensitivity curves to various visible rays of the retina alone and of the hypothalamus alone, nor do we know the precise nature of the photoreceptor cells of the autonomic retina, nor of the hypothalamic photoreceptor cells.* And last but not least, we have no knowledge of the chemical processes which occur in the retina and in the hypothalamic centers under the influence of light.

RELATED MATTERS

To respond to the wish expressed by the Editors, I will now briefly describe other aspects of the problem which I have studied and the favorable or unfavorable circumstances during which my research was carried out.

Firstly, what are the *original results* of the research which I have carried out, first alone, then with my co-workers? Let's examine the main results of Rowan and Bissonnette, who were the first to study the action of light in birds.

Rowan had demonstrated in 1925 that light stimulation causes development of the testes of the junco. But in his opinion, light acted simply by prolonging the period of awakeness and thus increasing general activity and movements in the bird (1928). Bissonnette demonstrated in the starling that light exerts a specific effect on testicular activity (1931*a*). But, according to this author, light acted directly on the testes across the skin and muscles (1931*b*) and perhaps also on the skin of the bird's foot (1932). In 1938, this author observed in the ferret that the gonads underwent involution after removal of the pituitary, even in the presence of light. Also in the ferret, Bissonnette showed in 1938, by division of the optic nerves, that the eye was a photoreceptor necessary for gonad stimulation. Let us note that in his publication in 1933 on the possible role of the eye and pituitary in the ferret, Bissonnette wrote these prophetic words: "It appears probable that the light rays, of the long-wave variety, react upon some part of the head of the ferret and, through that receptor, upon the anterior lobe, to stimulate it to increased secretion or liberation into the blood stream of the hormone which causes increased gonadal activity. A neurohumoral effect of this sort, described by H. Parker, is suggested." It is curious to note that the ideas of Bissonnette are more true for birds than for mammals.

---

* Bons and Assenmacher (1973) have recently demonstrated the existence of retinal fibers which pass, in the duck, from the anterior central hypothalamic region to the region above the optic chiasma.

My personal contribution, aided by that of my co-workers, in the study of the light-sexual reflex in the duck, consisted of showing in the bird the roles of the eyes, the hypothalamus, the pituitary, and the histophysiological peculiarities of the hypothalamopituitary complex: its blood supply, its nerve supply, and the neurosecretory links between the anterior lobe of the pituitary and the median eminence. Four operations carried out on this complex permitted us to conclude that, stimulated by the eye and, across tissues, by penetrating light rays, the hypothalamus stimulates the anterior lobe of the pituitary by a neurohumoral mechanism proposed in 1947 by Green and Harris. This, we believe, is a basic problem in neuroendocrinology, where the duck has permitted us to demonstrate the main details.

The bibliographic references at the end of this report will permit one to follow the dates of the successive results, detailed in the text, which we have obtained. They also permit one to appreciate the great help given to us by our co-workers, and we would like to express here how grateful we are to them.*

Have I been encouraged in my research? Definitely yes. The atmosphere of the Histology Laboratory at the Strasbourg Medical Faculty, where I entered as an assistant in 1919, was excellent under the stimulating and paternal direction of Professor Bouin. His second in command was Dr. Max Aron, and I also met there Robert Courrier, who was an assistant like me. Marc Klein, Gaston Mayer, Robert and Claude Aron—then other younger workers came and joined our group, which formed a large family.

The universal renown of Professor Bouin, after the end of the great World War, led to a visit of a delegation from the Rockefeller Foundation, which, after noting his dynamic nature and that of his young pupils, proposed to finance a histology institute in Strasbourg, for one-half of its cost if the other half could be obtained from the French state. I was thus able, in our new institute, to continue my research under excellent conditions, using laboratories adapted to my research program.

But I also have a second debt toward the Rockefeller Foundation. I received, in 1936, an annual visit of one of its representatives, Dr. W. E. Tisdale. Without asking me to give him further experimental results, he offered to let me stay for a year in the United States as a Rockefeller Fellow, in the laboratory of Prof. Edgar Allen (Department of Anatomy of the Yale University Medical school). I accepted enthusiastically and I left with my wife for New Haven, where we passed a very agreeable and fruitful year with Professor Allen, who was so hospitable and generous toward young research workers that some called him "The Peach." Our relations with his

---

* I am also grateful to the technical collaborators who contributed to the realization of our experiences: Mmes. E. Laplante and A. Statian; Mr. and Mrs. A. Lyleire; Misses S. Bayon and A. Stäubli; MM. A. Collinet, R. Combes, P. Moechler, and M. Morgen.

sympathetic co-workers were very friendly and we were able to carry out various research projects, including those of which I spoke earlier in collaboration with Dr. L. Ott, physicist.

As far as concerns the *financial help* which I obtained in Strasbourg for my research, I must admit that my numerous ducks proved very expensive. While encouraging me in my work, my chief attracted my attention to the limited funds available. My animals obviously cost more than the toads and frogs of Max Aron or the bats and sticklebacks of Robert Courrier. One day, Professor Bouin said to me, "Benoit, you're going to make us broke!" This remark led me to save a little money by selling at half price the control animals which had undergone the minimum of operations. One day I invited a friend to taste an appetizing three-month-old duckling, which before operation had suddenly died after inhaling a few breaths of ether. My friend did not compliment me on this duckling, which he found uneatable, and I had to agree with him. Once in the United States I renewed this attempt, offering a laboratory boy a duck killed five days after ether anesthesia. I hoped that the ether, which is very volatile, would by then have left the animal's tissues. Unfortunately, although ether is very volatile in air, it persists for a long time in the adipose tissue of animals that have inhaled it, and the boy did not appreciate this preparation of the duck. I did not continue my trials to determine what lapse of time is necessary for duck flesh to become entirely purified. I am now resigned: "ether duck" has justifiably a poor reputation as a dish.

I have already noted that Monsieur Bouin had limited funds available for research in his unit. The only funds at that time were obtained from the Faculty of Medicine. Later, other grants were made, coming from the National Council of Scientific Research (CNRS). I am very grateful to this organization for its generosity to me. Later, they did even more, for in 1957 they created a CNRS Photobiology Laboratory at Gif-sur-Ivette which included in a large area numerous enclosures where I was able to raise and experiment on a considerable number of ducks.

There also I carried out with several co-workers, including the Reverend Father Pierre Leroy, experiments to attempt to modify certain hereditary characteristics of the duck by interracial exchange of DNA. These experiments gave us great satisfaction, but they also attracted a good deal of criticism and deception from colleagues who were irritated by the revolutionary aspect of the results which we obtained. However, after us, several authors obtained—mutatis mutandis—similar results to ours in insects, birds, and mammals. But this is another story.

To young research workers who sometimes hesitate to engage themselves totally in scientific research, I would like to end by saying how much thirst for knowledge and the pursuit of truth in this unlimited field of the origin of life are, or are becoming, absolutely fascinating. The phenomena that nature offers for our study are so extraordinary and remain so mysterious that they attract us irresistibly. We never cease to marvel at them, they constantly give us new joy, even if we do not fully understand them.

These are the reflections that are inspired by many years that I have devoted to one of the mysteries of "Donald Duck." With my co-workers I have penetrated the first mysteries of this neuroendocrinological problem but, fortunately, there are still many unknowns.

CONCLUSION

The duck has proved to be a particularly favorable animal for the study of a neuroendocrine problem concerned with reproduction. We were able to show that light stimulates two photoreceptors—one superficial: the retina, the other deep: the hypothalamus—to which one must add the rhinencephalon. Under normal conditions, in daylight or artificial light, the duck only responds to orange and red light rays. This is evident at the level of the retina, because the latter is not sensitive to other parts of the visible spectrum, and at the level of the hypothalamus also, because the latter, although sensitive to the whole of the spectrum, only receives orange and red rays, for the others are absorbed by the tissues.

Stimulated indirectly by the retinal fibers or directly by red and orange rays, across the tissues, the magnocellular hypothalamic nuclei produce chemical substances linked to neurosecretion, which reach the superficial part of the median eminence and the capillary network which covers the latter so that, via the portal veins, they reach the gonadotropic cells of the anterior lobe of the pituitary. This is a typical example which illustrates the neurohumoral theory of Green and Harris.

REFERENCES

Assenmacher, I. (1957). Répercussions de lésions hypothalamiques sur le conditionnement génital du Canard domestique. *C. R. Acad. Sci.* **245**: 210.

Assenmacher, I. (1958). Recherches sur le contrôle hypothalamique de la fonction gonadotrope préhypophysaire chez le Canard. *Arch. Anat. Microsc. et Morphol. Exp.* **47**: 447.

Assenmacher, I., and J. Benoit (1953). Répercussions de la section du tractus porto-tubéral hypophysaire sur la gonado-stimulation par la lumière chez le Canard domestique. *C. R. Acad. Sci.* **236**: 2002.

Benoit, J. (1934). Activation sexuelle obtenue chez le Canard par l'éclairement artificiel pendant la période de repos génital. *C. R. Acad. Sci.* **199**: 1671.

Benoit, J. (1935a). Rôle de l'hypophyse dans l'action stimulante de la lumière sur le développement testiculaire chez le Canard (avec démonstrations). *C. R. Soc. Biol.* **118**: 672.

Benoit, J. (1935b). Stimulation par la lumière artificielle du développement testiculaire chez des Canards aveuglés par section du nerf optique (avec démonstrations). *C. R. Soc. Biol.* **120**: 133.

Benoit, J. (1935c). Stimulation par la lumière artificielle du développement testiculaire chez des Canards aveuglés par enucléation des globes oculaires (avec démonstrations). *C. R. Soc. Biol.* **120**: 136.

Benoit, J. (1936). Facteurs externes et internes de l'activité sexuelle I. Stimulation par la lumière de l'activité sexuelle chez le Canard et la Cane domestiques. *Bull. Biol. Fr. Belg.* **70**: 487.

Benoit, J. (1937). Facteurs externes et internes de l'activité sexuelle II. Étude du mécanisme de la stimulation par la lumière de l'activité testiculaire chez le Canard domestique. Rôle de l'hypophyse. *Bull. Biol. Fr. Belg.* **71**: 394.

Benoit, J. (1938a). Action de lumières de différentes longueurs d'onde sur la gonadostimulation chez le Canard mâle impubère. *C. R. Soc. Biol.* **127**: 906.

Benoit, J. (1938b). Rôle des yeux et de la voie nerveuse oculo-hypophysaire dans la gonadostimulation par la lumière artificielle chez le Canard domestique. *C. R. Soc. Biol.* **129**: 231.

Benoit, J. (1961). Opto-sexual reflex in the duck: Physiological and histological aspects. Ferris Lecture, Yale J. Biol. Med. **34**: 97.

Benoit, J. (1964a). The structural components of the hypothalamo-hypophyseal pathway, with particular reference to photostimulation of the gonads in birds. *Ann. N.Y. Acad. Sci.* **117**: 204.

Benoit, J. (1964b). The role of the eye and of the hypothalamus in the photostimulation of gonads in the duck. *Ann. N.Y. Acad. Sci.* **117**: 23.

Benoit, J. (1970). Étude de l'action des radiations visibles de différentes longueurs d'onde sur la gonadostimulation et de leur pénétration transcranienne chez les Oiseaux et les Mammifères. *Colloque International du CNRS sur la Photorégulation de la Reproduction chez les Oiseaux et les Mammifères*, Montpellier, ed. CNRS N° 172.

Benoit, J., and I. Assenmacher (1950). Quelques données relatives à la vascularisation de l'hypophyse du Canard domestique. *Bull. Biol. Appl.* **27**: 182.

Benoit, J., and I. Assenmacher (1951). Étude préliminaire de la vascularisation de l'appareil hypophysaire du Canard domestique. *Arch. Anat. Microsc. et Morphol. Exp.* **40**: 27.

Benoit, J., and I. Assenmacher (1952). Influence de lésions hautes et basses de l'infundibulum sur la gonadostimulation chez le Canard domestique. *C. R. Acad. Sci.* **235**: 1547.

Benoit, J., and I. Assenmacher (1953). Rapport entre la stimulation sexuelle préhypophysaire et la neurosécrétion chez l'Oiseau. *Arch. Anat. Microsc. et Morphol. Exp.* **42**: 334.

Benoit, J., and I. Assenmacher (1954). Sensibilité comparée des récepteurs superficiel et profond dans le réflexe opto-sexuel chez le Canard. *C. R. Acad. Sci.* **239**: 105.

Benoit, J., and I. Assenmacher (1955). Le contrôle hypothalamique de l'activité préhypophysaire gonadotrope. *J. Physiol.* **47**: 427.

Benoit, J., and I. Assenmacher (1957). Photorécepteurs rétiniens et encéphaliques impliqués dans la gonadostimulation par les radiations visibles chez le Canard domestique. *Minerva Med.* **24**: 13.

Benoit, J., and I. Assenmacher (1958). The control by visible radiations of the gonadotropic activity of the duck hypophysis. *Recent Prog. Horm. Res.* **15**: 143.

Benoit, J., I. Assenmacher, and E. Brard (1955). Evolution testiculaire du Canard domestique maintenu à l'obscurité totale pendant une longue durée. *C. R. Acad. Sci.* **241**: 251.

Benoit, J., I. Assenmacher, and S. Manuel (1953). Pénétration, variable selon la longueur d'onde, des radiations visibles jusqu'à l'hypothalamus et au rhinencéphale, à travers la région orbitaire chez le Canard. *C. R. Acad. Sc.* **235**: 1695.

Benoit, J., I. Assenmacher, and F. X. Walter (1953). Dissociation experimentale des rôles des récepteurs superficiel et profond dans la gonadostimulation hypophysaire par la lumière chez le Canard. *C. R. Soc. Biol.* **147**: 186.

Benoit, J., C. Da Lage, B. Muel, C. Kordon, and I. Assenmacher. (1966). Localisation dans le spectre visible de la zone de sensibilité rétinienne maximale aux radiations lumineuses impliquées dans la gonadostimulation chez le Canard Pékin impubère. *C. R. Acad. Sci.* **263**: 62.

Benoit, J., and R. Kehl (1939). Nouvelles recherches sur les voies nerveuses photoréceptrices et hypophyso-stimulantes chez le Canard domestique. *C. R. Soc. Biol.* **131**: 89.

Benoit, J., and L. Ott (1944). External and internal factors in sexual activity. Effect of irradiation with different wave-lengths on the mechanisms of photostimulation of the hypophysis and on testicular growth in the immature duck. *Yale J. Biol. Med.* **17**: 27.

Benoit, J., L. Tauc, and I. Assenmacher (1954). Mésure photo-électrique de la pénétration transorbitaire des radiations visibles jusqu'au cerveau, chez le Canard domestique. *C. R. Acad. Sci.* **239**: 451.

Benoit, J., F. X. Walter, and I. Assenmacher (1950). Nouvelles recherches relatives à l'action de lumières de différentes longuers d'onde sur la gonadostimulation du Canard mâle impubère. *C. R. Soc. Biol.* **144**: 1206.

Bissonnette, T. H. (1931a). Studies on the sexual cycle in Birds. IV. Experimental modification of the sexual cycle in male of the European Starling (*Sturnus vulgaris*) by changes in the daily period of illumination and of muscular work. *J. Exp. Zool.* **58**: 281.

Bissonnette, T. H. (1931b). Studies on the sexual cycle in Birds. V. Effects of light of different intensities upon the testis activity of the European Starling (*Sturnus vulgaris*.) *Physiol. Zool.* **4**: 542.

5

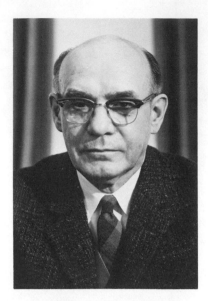

Chandler McC(uskey) Brooks

Chandler Brooks was born in Waverly, West Virginia, on December 18, 1905. He attended public schools in Weston, West Virginia, and later in Everett, Massachusetts, before enrolling at Oberlin College where he received the A.B. in Zoology in 1928. He entered graduate school and received the Ph.D. in Biology from Princeton University in 1931. He then joined the Department of Physiology at Harvard as a National Research Council Fellow from 1931 to 1933. He moved to Johns Hopkins School of Medicine as Instructor in Physiology in 1933 and rose to the rank of associate professor. In 1948 he was appointed Professor and Chairman of the Departments of Physiology and Pharmacology at Long Island College of Medicine and continued to hold these positions when this school became the State University of New York. From 1956 to 1972 he continued to serve as Chairman of Physiology and became Dean of the Graduate School of Downstate Medical Center. He was Acting President and Dean of Medicine at the Downstate Medical Center from 1969 to 1971, and has been Distinguished Professor of Physiology since 1971. He has held visiting professorships in Montevideo, Uruguay, Recifi, Brazil, Tokyo and Kobe, Japan, and in Aberdeen, Scotland.

He is a member of many societies, which include the Academy of Neurology, the American College of Cardiology, the American Heart Association, the American Physiological Society, the American Society for Pharmacology and Experimental Therapeutics, the Association for Research in Nervous and Mental Diseases, the Harvey Society, the International Brain Research Organization, the Society for Experimental Biology and Medicine, the Endocrine Society, the Royal Society of Medicine and the National Academy of Sciences.

He has served on the editorial boards of *Circulation Research,* 1956–61, the *Journal of Neurophysiology*, from 1961 to 1965, and *Physiological Reviews* from 1962 to 1965. He was chairman of the editorial board of *Proceedings of the Society of Experimental Biology and Medicine,* 1960–65. He has also served on the editorial board of the *Journal of Electrocardiography*, the *Federation of American Societies for Experimental Biology,* and *Brain Behavior and Evolution.*

He has received a number of awards, including citations from the Japanese Physiological Society, Tokyo University, and the U.S.P.H.S. He was president of the Harvey Society from 1965 to 1966 and Honorary D.Sc. Berea College, Kentucky, 1970.

Development of the Convergent Themes of Neuroendocrinology

CHANDLER McC. BROOKS

INTRODUCTION TO NEUROENDOCRINOLOGY

It is an honor to be included among those considered to have contributed to the development of neuroendocrinology. Although I have always thought of myself as a physiologist interested in the control and integration of body functions, I am pleased to be also a neuroendocrinologist. During my time I have had many interests and at least some of them represent the major themes which have resulted in the establishment of this new discipline. A discussion of the history of neuroendocrinology requires some description of these contributory interests responsible for its development and a definition of neuroendocrinology.

The study of the innervation and neural control of endocrine glands is as old as endocrinology (Rolleston, 1936; Brooks, Gilbert, Levey, and Curtis, 1962), but neuroendocrinology has become a recognized autonomous discipline only during the last 30 to 40 years. I consider the unique feature of modern neuroendocrinology to be the study of hormone production by neurons and the control of the endocrine system by humoral agents formulated by and released from the brain into the blood stream. However, if this discipline is considered to include all studies of the "relationship between the brain and endocrine system," then there are at least two major contributory interests.

One of these fundamental themes is the study of the autonomic nervous system's influence on endocrine gland functions. The second is the study of hormone effects on the brain and nervous system itself. Certainly I have never strayed very far nor for very long from one or another of these three

CHANDLER McC. BROOKS. • Distinguished Professor of the State University of New York and Department of Physiology, Downstate Medical Center, Brooklyn, New York.

channels of interests which neuroendocrinology comprises. I can remember very clearly many of the developments in these fields which have occurred in my time.

One is not often fully conscious of the significance of movements in which he participates and I can claim no early consciousness of the development of neuroendocrinology until the early 1940s. I do not know when or by whom the term *neuroendocrinology* was first used. A book by that title was published in 1946 by Roussy and Mosinger but I am sure that many of the basic concepts of this subject had developed before that time. I personally cannot remember when I was not interested, professionally and nonprofessionally, in the neuroendocrine control of behavior.

My father, in addition to being a Presbyterian minister, was a naturalist whose chief interest was ornithology. The first paper I ever wrote was on the behavior of birds and it was published in a journal called the *Ornotogist*. As a child living in Weston, West Virginia, I collected moths, studied their life histories, and observed metamorphosis. One of my first books was *The Moth Book* by W. J. Holland (1908).

This exposure to natural phenomena tended to terminate when we moved to the city of Boston in 1916, but this was more than compensated for by associations with some of Boston's famous naturalists and acquaintances with men like George H. Parker of Harvard (Parker, 1948). I was no longer able to collect the giant moths but I retained my interest and was much impressed when I was told of the discovery of a *pupation hormone* (Kopeć, 1917). Because of my father's instructions and my own experience as a boy on my grandfather's farm in West Virginia, I knew something of the peculiar factors influencing egg laying and brooding in birds. I also was aware that food, light, and changing seasons determined pelt color and plumage, affected reproductive activity, and established cycles of behavior. Long before I entered Oberlin College in 1924 and began to study zoology and ecology and long before I read the intriguing papers of Hammond 1925, 1951; Marshall 1936, 1937; and Parkes 1930, 1961, which described reversal of breeding seasons in some but not all species of mammals and birds when they were transferred from one hemisphere to the other, I knew something about this concern of the neuroendocrinologists. The point I wish to make is that when in 1933 Philip Bard invited me to go to the Johns Hopkins with him and told me that he had a grant for studying "sex and the central nervous system," I was interested and took pleasure in finding the literature in which the effects of light were described and in which other mysterious phenomena suggesting hypothalamic or neural control of endocrines were mentioned.

In 1928 I obtained a fellowship to study biology at Princeton and it was there that the two other themes of interest which led me to neuroendocrinology developed. I took a course in comparative histology with Ulric Dahlgren, who had described (Dahlgren, 1914) cells in the nervous system of the skate which appear to produce and store secretory materials. He told me of the work done on the tissue in 1919–22 by Speidel (Speidel, 1922). I cannot remember whether he spoke of the presence of similar secretory cells in other parts of the nervous system, but I was prepared for description of other such cells in the nervous system by Scharrer (1933). I also participated in the 1940 Symposium on the Hypothalamus organized by the Association for Research in Nervous and Mental Disease when the Scharrers presented one of their major papers on the secretory cells within the hypothalamus (Scharrer and Scharrer, 1940) but I do not wish to imply that I understood their significance. My focus, like that of the Russians who missed the discovery of secretin (see Brooks, Gilbert, Levey, and Curtis, 1962, p. 27), was on control by reflexes and impulses transmitted by neurons. I do think I should point out here that this early work by the Scharrers was on the SON and PVN, not on cells which produce the releasing factors. Nevertheless, this started the work which became a major contribution to the founding of neuroendocrinology: the demonstration that ADH and oxytocin are produced by neurons.

At Princeton I had two other experiences related to my interest in humoral and neural control of functions. The first was with Edwin Grant Conklin, one of that great group of cytologists and experimental embryologists to which E. B. Wilson and Thomas Hunt Morgan belonged. Morgan was at Woods Hole in the summer of 1929 when I went there as Conklin's assistant, but he had become a geneticist by then. Conklin set some three problems, which I failed to resolve. The major one was to find the mechanism of sex determination and reversal in crepidula (*Crepidula fornicata*—"slipper shell"). The basic observation was that when a female crepidula lives on a rock and a little veliger comes along and settles down by her it becomes a male. If the female then disappears, the male turns into a female. My problem was to see what happens when one puts two males on a rock together; which becomes a female and why? I could not get two males to stay on the same rock together and discovered nothing. I did not even confirm the original observation but I did read a bit of literature on sex determination and reversal. I also acquired some appreciation of the fact that there are modulator compounds produced by the body which can be humorally transported and which act at a distance. Probably the greatest consequence of that experience was that it cooled my enthusiasm for the mysteries of the invertebrate world. I became and have remained a mammalian physiologist. I have, however, always retained a great respect for that generation of biologists to which Conklin belonged.

The other experience at Princeton to which I have referred was that of meeting Philip Bard. I became his student and he suggested, as a project I might undertake, an analysis of the mechanism of *reflex hyperglycemia*. Consequently I studied the functions and the control of the autonomic system, most particularly its role in the release of *epinephrine* from the adrenal medulla and glucose from storage reservoirs (liver and muscle glycogen) during stress or when afferent nerves were stimulated. This question of the neural involvement in blood sugar level control had its origin in Claude Bernard's observation that an injury to the floor of the fourth ventricle produced a transient hyperglycemia (piqûre diabetes). It had been rather well demonstrated that the sympathoadrenal complex was responsible, but there remained the question of hypothalamic involvement. Unquestionably stimulation of and reflex activation of hypothalamic centers could raise blood sugar. My analysis of the situation and my contributions were published (Brooks, 1931) and since then many have worked on the central control of adrenal and autonomic activity (see Harrison, 1964). At that time there were even those who felt sensors and centers in the hypothalamus regulated, through the vagus nerve, insulin output from the pancreas and blood sugar mobilizing hormones from the adrenal medulla through the sympathetic system. This concept was soon thereafter rejected, but it is of interest that in 1974 it seems to be agreed that the vagi innervate the islets of Langerhans and can influence insulin secretion (Watari, 1973). It is also held now that there are glucoreceptors in the hypothalamus which can sense blood sugar levels and initiate appropriate reactions (Bray, 1974; Panksepp, 1974). Releasing factors also can affect insulin output directly, it is now claimed (Endocrine Society Papers—Meeting of June, 1974).

But to return to reminiscences, I can say that by 1929 I had acquired a variety of interests which led me eventually into the realm of neuroendocrinological research. I had begun to study the function of the hypothalamus and control of the autonomic nervous system. I was interested in those "stimuli" which initiate neuroendocrine reactions.

THE AUTONOMIC SYSTEM AS AN INTEGRATOR OF BODY FUNCTIONS

In the 1920s and 1930s the possibility that the autonomic system might control endocrine functions was a living issue. Autonomic nerves were known to cause secretory activity in salivary glands, stomach, adrenal medulla, and possibly the islets of Langerhans. Cannon had obtained some strange results from the thyroid gland, a seeming hyperthyroidism, following cross suturing of the phrenic and cervical sympathetics in cats (Cannon,

Binger, and Fitz, 1914–15). Despite many attempts, this work could not be repeated, but since that time others have found evidence of sympathetic action on the thyroid (see Brooks, Koizumi, and Pinkston, 1974). Much of this early work on the relationship between the autonomic nervous system and the endocrines was reviewed by Roussy and Mosinger in their *Neuroendocrinologie* (1946) and in a *Bibliographia Neurovegetativa* (Fenz, 1953). However, all this suggestive evidence soon came to be regarded as insignificant as knowledge of the hypothalamic-hypophyseal control developed. The importance of this change to me was that something which seemed promising, a study of the autonomic control of endocrine function, was turning out to be unrewarding. Today, however, the question again arises. It is claimed that the pineal gland is controlled through a sympathetic innervation; my associates and I are working on this problem now, in 1974. I believe that restudy of the autonomic system's influence on other endocrines could be quite warranted.

In 1931 I left Princeton and went to Walter B. Cannon's department at Harvard with Philip Bard. There I temporarily gave up my concern for autonomic system control of the endocrines. Instead I concentrated on the central control of the autonomic system and most specifically on autonomic activity and reflexes in chronic spinal animals. At Harvard, Philip Bard continued his study of the behavior of chronically decorticate, hemidecerebrate, and other types of "brain-reduced" animals. I worked with him in the study of the hopping-and-placing reactions. The pertinence of all this to neuroendocrinology is that brain-reduced animals showed relatively normal endocrine functions and sexual behavior. They also maintained those body states requiring autonomic and endocrine cooperation. We concluded that many, if not all, neuroendocrine reactions could be carried on at very basal levels.

I met a great many people at Harvard who were interested in the autonomic system, the central nervous system, somatosympathetic reactions to stress, emotional response, and the endocrine system. The *Journal of Endocrinology* was being edited from there by R. G. Hoskins and Milton O. Lee. I really felt that the scientific world was alive and, despite the depression, there was excitement; better still, there was local as well as international good will among scientists. It seemed a period of great hope and progress.

In the early thirties the major concentration of interest in Cannon's laboratory was, of course, on humoral transmission of the nerve impulse. The story of the discovery of *sympathin* by Cannon and his associates is well known. They found both excitatory and inhibitory actions of sympathetic nerve transmitters which they endeavored to explain as due to a *sympathin E* and *I*. The presence of receptors in effector tissues was recognized. I was involved in none of this directly although I did use denervation-sensitized organs (nictitating membrane and heart) to assay the transmitter and adrenal medulla hormone release in spinal reflex actions. While speaking of autonomic control at the spinal level, it is pertinent to mention that I became interested in temperature regulation and response to cold stress. This introduced me to the study of hypothalamic-hypophyseal-thyroid responses to cold, a subject which was investigated in Cannon's laboratory by U. U. Uotila some years later (1939) at a time when I was working on neuroendocrine control systems. A hypothalamic influence on the thyroid by way of the hypophysis was recognized.

But to return to the matter of chemical transmission of the nerve impulse, it can be said that the production and release of chemical transmitters by nerves is, in one sense, neuroendocrinology. It was reasoned also that if neurons can formulate catecholamines and cholinergic compounds, they might well manufacture other materials. We have at present, in 1974, the complex problem of humoral transmission and production of modulators, activators, and inhibitors in the central nervous system, particularly in the hypothalamus. It is my impression that such study began with Marta Vogt (1954) in Dale and Feldberg's laboratory while people were still arguing about peripheral chemical transmission (Wurtmann, 1970; Yagi and Yoshida, 1973). I knew Sir Henry Dale and Otto Loewi before and after they had received the Nobel Prize for discovery of chemical transmission. They well deserved all honors received, but we who had worked with him were disappointed that Cannon's contributions were not similarly recognized (Brooks, Koizumi, and Pinkston, 1974).

It happened that I had another contact with the chemical transmission story. In 1946–47, when Eccles was mounting the last resistance to the nerve transmitter theories, I was working with him in Dunedin, New Zealand. By 1949 this resistance was ended. The point I wish to make is that the period of discovery of chemical transmission of nerve impulses was very exciting. The atmosphere of the time resembled that of the era in neuroendocrinology during which the releasing factors were discovered.

STUDIES OF THE HYPOTHALAMIC–HYPOPHYSEAL SYSTEM

My most direct participation in the development of neuroendocrinology began when I went to the Hopkins in 1933. As stated previously, Philip Bard had a grant to support our research if it dealt with sex and the nervous system. I chose as my problems ovulation in the rabbit and the production of pseudopregnancy in the rat. Later I tried to unravel the complexities of experimentally produced adiposogenital dystrophy in the monkey and rat.

Ovulation and pseudopregnancy appeared to be due to secretion of hormones from the anterior lobe of the hypophysis due to specific stimuli. I thought the stimuli might be transmitted neurally to the anterior lobe through sympathetic nerves or from the hypothalamus by way of the stalk.

To make a long story short, I was interested in the role of the cortex and higher centers as well as that of the hypothalamus and peripheral stimuli which produce ovulation or pseudopregnancy. It soon became apparent that coitus was not necessary; sexual activity and excitement was enough. Convulsant drugs and electric shock were also effective. Neocortex was essential to maternal behavior and initiation of sexual activity but not to ovulation or production of pseudopregnancy; neither was the sympathetic system. Section of the pituitary stalk, however, abolished coitus-produced ovulation in the rabbit and pseudopregnancy in the rat. When chemical stimuli were used, section of the stalk within an hour after their application blocked ovulation (Brooks, Beadenkopf, and Bojar, 1940). It did seem to me that by severing the stalk an essential connection between hypothalamus and the anterior lobe had been interrupted. I studied the blood supply and I knew that there was a portal system which might be damaged by the operation. I did see lesions in the hypophysis but injections of the circulation showed what appeared to be an adequate blood supply. Furthermore when these "isolated" pituitaries were assayed for ovulation-producing action, they were found to contain several times the required amount of hormone.

The major problem of course, was whether the anterior lobe of the hypophysis was innervated from the stalk. The literature contained some claims that the anterior lobe received innervation from the hypothalamus but it was not very convincing. I therefore began with the advice of Isidore Gersh of the anatomy department to restudy the situation. For quite a few years one of our pictures of nerve fibers to anterior and posterior lobe of the hypophysis was published in Howell's *Textbook of Physiology* when edited by John Fulton (now the Ruch and Patton, 1965). In the species I studied (rat, cat, rabbit, and monkey) the pars neuralis and pars intermedia received a rich innervation from the stalk. A considerable number of fibers also crossed into the anterior lobe. These fibers were not present after stalk transection and I even observed them in process of degeneration. There were two problems: First, the fibers were relatively few in number and I did not know, nor do I know now, how many fibers are required to produce secretion from a gland. Second, although many friends and visitors such as E. C. Hoff, who had written papers dealing with neuron fiber staining, saw my preparations and said they were nerves, other neurohistologists just flatly claimed none existed. I was convinced that at least a meager innervation exists and others have confirmed this, but I felt rather insecure.

I finally concluded and stated that physiological evidence strongly suggested that either "nerve impulses or some other excitatory agent" pass between the hypothalamus and the anterior lobe to evoke liberation of ovulation-producing hormones. I did state in a paper submitted July 23, 1937 (Brooks, 1938, p.174): "The reason that these experiments cannot be considered absolute proof of the nervous activation of the gland is that stalk section interrupts or injures the hypothalamicohypophysial portal system. Conceivably this system could carry some specific chemical excitant from brain to pituitary under normal conditions but could not do so following stalk section." That is as close as I ever got to the concept of "releasing" factors. I felt I had gone about as far as I could without additional techniques. Also, other observations were attracting my attention. I had concluded that in order to prove the involvement of nerves I would have to record action potentials from them. Opportunity to learn that technique did not arise until 1946–47, but I was then diverted from this specific project for many years. Several of the papers I published during this era are listed and their titles show what was done (Brooks, 1931–46).

Numerous other individuals had become interested and were working in this field when I was. Most prominent among them was Geoffrey Harris. I met Goeffrey first in Zurich during the International Physiological Congress of 1938. He was a very friendly, strong, determined young man and I always admired him greatly. We had performed similar experiments for several years, but he went on beyond the point where I stopped to make his magnificent studies of the portal system and its role in conducting neuroendocrine secretions from the hypothalamus to the pars anterior of the hypophysis. The book he published in 1955 is a classic (Harris, 1955).

There were many others with whom I was well acquainted in those early years and with whom I corresponded. There were young men besides Gersh and Harris and my own students with whom I worked and talked: J. E. Markee, H. D. Haterius, J. Derbyshire, H. B. Friedgood, E. W. Dempsey, and others. There were also men of an older generation, too, besides Bard and Cannon: P. E. Smith, J. C. Hinsey, G. W. Corner, C. G. Hartman, and Oscar Riddle. I remember one warm evening in Odessa on the Black Sea in 1935—Oscar Riddle, my wife, and I walked out of a Russian banquet to get some air. We tried to count the steps from the palace down to the sea. We tried it three times and got three different answers.

I also met Bernardo A. Houssay and for some reason he adopted me as one of his students, among whom were Oscar Orias, Braun-Menendez, Foglia, Covian. They and their children and their students have been my friends for life.

While endeavoring to cut the stalk and produce hypothalamic lesions which would block ovulation and pseudopregnancy or interfere with the menstrual cycles of the macaque, I inadvertently produced diabetes insipidus and obesity. This work was done chiefly on rats and monkeys. I worked with Isidore Gersh on diabetes insipidus (Gersh, 1940). We studied the transient and then the following permanent diabetes and its course (Gersh and Brooks, 1941). Gersh developed a technique for staining materials which were evidently transported from the hypothalamus to the posterior lobe. This substance accumulated in the median eminence above a stalk section and we felt it was or contained the material secreted. I am not sure that he ever got much credit for that discovery nor was our demonstration of nerve fibers and terminals accepted by the neurohistologists (Brooks and Gersh, 1941). Strangely enough, this is merely an academic speculation to me now, but when one is young there is always hope of doing something important; one feels disappointment when no one is impressed. That is probably true now as well as in the days when neuroendocrinology was young.

One of the accomplishments of this project was that it brought me into contact with that magnificent group which had been assembled by Ranson at Northwestern. Their book on diabetes insipidus (Fisher, Ingram, and Ranson, 1938) was studied as carefully by me as was the book by Long and Evans (1922) on the estrous cycle of the rat. It was Hetherington at Northwestern who showed me how to make lesions in the ventromedial nuclei of the rat. Other members of the group were well known to me for years, but the two with whom I have maintained closest contact are H. W. Magoun and W. R. Ingram. I really think the revival of the use of the Horsley-Clarke apparatus for studies of hypothalamic and basal structure functions advanced the study of neuro endocrinology very significantly. The studies I conducted with the use of this instrument also convinced me that one should relate activity in the supraoptic and paraventricular neurons and their axons with the release of secretions from the pars neuralis. I did not do this, however, for some 20 years or until the 1960s.

My next interest was in obesity. I suppose there was a sort of contest between Northwestern, Yale (John Brobeck), and me at the Hopkins as to who could produce the fattest monkey and the fattest rat. The adiposogenital dystrophy which I produced in my monkeys resembled that occurring in man and was originally thought to be an endocrine disorder. The group at Northwestern quickly demonstrated that obesity could be produced in the hypophysectomized rat and that obesity could be produced independent of reproductive system disorders or diabetes insipidus. I never did completely publish the work I did on the monkey. Frankly speaking, I was intimidated or inhibited by the neurohistology. In those days one worked pretty much alone; he had to do it all. I was able to identify all nuclei destroyed but I could not or I was unwilling to try to identify all tracts severed and the possible indirect consequences of that relative to the nuclear lesions. I should have ignored the ideal and made the best analysis within my power. Idealism and humility are good but one should never be deterred by the criticism of others who may feel you are not qualified to invade their fields. I eventually learned this, but that is another story.

While studying obesity, I worked some with Curt Richter, whom I consider to be a very great scholar; he was interested in the food selection made by rats following obesity-producing lesions. I was not able to help him much and I think the job never got done. I also worked with a young pediatrician by the name of E. M. Bridge. We found that during the dynamic phase of obesity in the monkey as well as in the rat (Brooks and Bridge, 1944; Brooks, 1946) a test meal drove the RQ way above unity. Because of this and considerable other work I did on obesity, I developed a desire to study the metabolism of obesity more carefully and to examine the accompanying endocrine disorders, but I felt inadequately prepared. It was time for me to receive some additional training if I intended to pursue my interests in neuroendocrinology.

In 1945 I was granted a John Simon Guggenheim fellowship by nomination of Isidore Gersh and due to approval gained in an interview with Henry Allen Moe. I have had the honor of Dr. Moe's friendship since that day. I had intended to study with Dr. Houssay but Peron put him in prison and he wrote advising me not to come to Argentina. When I finally did visit him it was in 1952, but I went as a cardiologist and not an endocrinologist.

My other opportunity was to join J. C. Eccles in New Zealand and learn the techniques of action potential recording. This I did, arriving in Dunedin during the summer of 1946. Eccles quickly informed me it would be impractical to try to record from fibers of the pituitary stalk or nuclei of the hypothalamus; I should join him in his research. This I did and I found him to be a kind and patient instructor and a very stimulating scholar and I have continued to work in neurophysiology throughout the years since that time. I was with him when he began his analysis of central inhibitory processes for which he eventually received a Nobel Prize.

This divergence finally broke my associations with Geoffrey Harris and others working in the fields of neuroendocrinology. When I returned to the United States and moved to Brooklyn in 1948 as chairman of physiology and of pharmacology at the Long Island College of Medicine, I had no time to immediately pick up old interests. I had to start research in this school and I choose to do it initially in cardiac and neurophysiology. I used the techniques of neurophysiology in the study of the heart, and when in 1949 the technique for recording intracellularly, by using the Ling-Gerard micropipette was developed, we used it first on the heart cell. However, I soon revived my interest in the autonomic system but I was not able to return to neuroendocrinology until 1961 (see Kao, Koizumi, and Vassalle, 1971). When I did so we used the methods developed for studies of the motoneuron and the heart cell.

RETURN TO NEUROENDOCRINOLOGY

During the winter of 1961 some of my associates and I returned to the study of hypothalamic nuclei and the liberation of hormones therefrom. We were able to monitor the activity of units within and close to the supraoptic nucleus and to record potentials from axons of the pituitary stalk (Brooks, Ushiyama, and Lange, 1962; Suda, Koizumi, and Brooks, 1963). That was only 12 years ago and can hardly be regarded as ancient history. But for the record, I should like to say that we have since then done intracellular as well as extracellular recording from units of the supraoptic and paraventricular nuclei; we have studied their osmosensitivity, their reactions to other stimuli and various chemical agents; we have made quantitative assays of ADH and oxytocin output, relating this to the activity recorded from the neurons of the SON and PVN; we have recorded reciprocal action between the ventromedian nuclei and lateral hypothalamic areas while subjecting the units of these regions to activating influences. To a degree an objective of the early 1940s has been attained. The work has been interesting but Dr. Koizumi and I, or at least I, have felt we were completing an old story rather than working in new territory.

There is, however, always something new to try. It is obvious that one cell of the SON and PVN cannot secrete enough hormone to effect a reaction. Therefore there must be a mass action and this raises the question: What is going on within the hypothalamic nuclei and what intercellular reactions occur? At the present time my associates and I are studying the interaction between units of these nuclei and determining the effects of their axonal collaterals (Koizumi, Ishikawa, and Brooks, 1973). We are doing other things which relate to neuroendocrinology using the techniques of neurophysiology.

During the last three or four years I have also endeavored to assist other associates in conducting some studies of the maturation of the hypothalamicohypophyseal reactions to stress. We have found that thyroid and adrenal reactions to cold exposure require some 12 to 16 days to mature in rats but we are just beginning this approach to neuroendocrinology. I think this is a good problem.

Finally, I and my associates have also returned to studies of the autonomic system and how it integrates visceral, somatic, and endocrine functions to meet specific behavioral needs. We are reinvestigating how this system may affect the functions of the endocrines.

There is modern history as well as ancient. The world seems quite different to me now. Very major advances have been made by new groups and I have not participated in what was probably the principal one—the isolation and identification of releasing factors. It is a different, larger, and more difficult world. During the period when neuroendocrinology began we worked pretty much alone. Now, it seems, magnificent team operations determine the pace of advancement. A man alone cannot compete. There is much to be said, however, for giving a brilliant man a team of capable technicians and associates but it does create obvious problems which we never encountered 30 years ago. I might also say we were not encumbered by wealth and its disturbing influences but had we had money, we might have done more—I personally doubt it.

Much is also the same; in my return to neuroendocrinology I have found some old and some new associates. Relative to our studies of the SON and PVN we can mention our friends H. Heller at Bristol, Barry A. Cross, a student of Geoffrey Harris, and his student Richard Dyball, both now in Babraham; we know J. D. Vincent of France, Horatio Ferreyra of Cordoba in the Argentine, Hiroshi Yamashita of Japan, and many others who have worked with us or visited us here in Brooklyn. Another group shares our interests in the autonomic system and its integrative function: Charles Downman of London, Horst Seller of Munich, Robert Schmitt of Kiel, Akio Sato in Japan, as well as our students, one of whom, Mary Schmitt, was primarily responsible for our new studies of the circadian and other rhythms of activity in hypothalamic neurons (Schmitt, 1973).

THE SIGNIFICANCE OF NEUROENDOCRINOLOGY AND THE ROLE IT HAS PLAYED IN THE DEVELOPMENT OF PHYSIOLOGICAL SCIENCE

Those who have lived for some time have the advantage of perspective. One purpose of a consideration of history is to estimate the effects of discoveries, to consider the consequences of the development of new disciplines. It seems appropriate to try to define what neuroendocrinology has accomplished.

Neuroendocrinology is a bridge in addition to being a well-organized discipline. It has united neuroscience and endocrinology. It has an even greater integrating influence in that it has shown how the releasing factors and the hormones produced by the hypothalamus regulate growth, metabolism, and water and salt balance, as well as specific endocrine gland activities. It is known that there are interactions within the hypothalamus important to the control of all body states and systems functions. One cannot study neuroendocrinology without dealing with the body as a whole. This is a good counterbalance to our usual reductionist approach and philosophy.

Neuroendocrinology has developed in parallel with other fields and also as a consequence of progress made, for example, in endocrinology, neuroanatomy, and neurophysiology.

It is rather obvious that there are surges of interest and accomplishment in science and to a degree neuroendocrinology is the "new" field of the middle third of this century. Dominant thought in neuroendocrinology resembles that of endocrinology rather than physiology. Thus it is reasonable to consider it a third phase in the development of endocrinological thought.

In my opinion, the first phase of endocrinology was concerned with the identification of the glands and the determination of their function by ablation and replacement procedures. This era was practically completed before my time, but I did witness the advent of hypophysectomies and the analysis of the cause of death following removal of the adrenals. Study of the effects of thymectomies and pineal gland removals are relatively recent. Phases overlap and work in any field continues despite new developments; no approach is completely abandoned.

The second phase of endocrinology was that robust period during which hormones were extracted from tons of tissues, purified, analyzed, and synthesized. One could say it began in 1899 with the isolation of epinephrine by Abel, or in 1902 with Bayliss' and Starling's discovery of secretin and use of the term *hormone* (Brooks, Gilbert, Levey, and Curtis, 1962). My closest contacts with this age of endocrinology were at Princeton when W. W. Swingle and J. Pfiffner were in a contest with Hartman, Rogoff, and others relative to isolation of the adrenal cortical hormones. I was also at a scientific meeting, in 1929 I believe, which was interrupted by a telegram announcing that Doisy had analyzed estrone. I was impressed but rather intimidated by those enthusiasms and contests.

The third great surge in endocrinology came with the concept and then the identification and analysis of the releasing factors. That is neuroendocrinology. The exquisite techniques which have been developed in this field make those of the older eras seem crude indeed. I think, however, that the neurophysiologists and those who have studied water balance, temperature regulation, and even metabolism would like some credit for the advent of neuroendocrinology. This third era, if we can call it that, will be in existence for some time to come.

There are many interesting problems remaining for the neuroendocrinologists. In addition to questions such as which structures or cells produce the releasing factors, how are they synthesized, and how do they act on their target cells, we need to know what controls their release. There are cold- and heat-sensitive receptors in the hypothalamus which conceivably could initiate release or inhibition of release of TRF; there are hormonal feedbacks and chemical changes in the blood or tissue surroundings which might trigger the release of other secretion-producing factors. A glance at the titles of articles in recent issues of *Neuroendocrinology* gives one assurance that a traditional interest of the neuroendocrinologist—the effect on the endocrine system of exposure of animals to light—will continue (Krieger and Allen, 1974; Smith and Davidson, 1974). One also sees frequent reference to the clearly defined circadian rhythms in discharge of some of the releasing hormones (Jacoby, Sassin, Greenstein, and Weitzman, 1974). The cause of these fluctuations in hormonal discharge is not known and neither do we understand the origins of circadian variations in the firing rates and responsiveness of some hypothalamic neurons (Schmitt, 1973). These problems will attract attention in the future and we can predict that still other related types of research interest also will develop as time passes. The dominant interests of neuroendocrinologists will change, as will those who deal with the relationship of brain and the endocrine complex, but one perceives no sign that this field is approaching depletion.

When one tries to compare meetings attended in one's youth with meetings held by the endocrinologists and neuroendocrinologists today, some interesting paradoxes become apparent. The young men now are extremely well trained; their technical competence is impressive; the meticulousness of their work in comparison with that done 50 or even 25-years ago is amazing. I perceive that the theme "control" is as strong as "action"; certainly neuroendocrinologists are in a position of dominance. However, I see difficulty ahead for any who think matters are reaching a solution. Neuroendocrinology seems to be in the same kind of trouble as is the field of "digestive system endocrinology" and "central humoral transmission." There is evidence that some of the releasing factors, once thought to be specific entities, are the same or at least have overlapping actions. The catecholamines and related compounds, at least in high doses, have similar effects in some instances. The releasing factors or hormones seem to be produced or are found in all parts of the brain and cord. The releasing factors have widespread effects, modifying secretory activities in the pancreatic islet tissues as well as in the hypophysis. What appeared to be a neat chapter drawing to a close has opened up again and one wonders just where these compounds fit into the functional picture. This is not a defeat; it can be a new excitement, but it does suggest need for a greater caution and modesty. In the early days the concept of director compounds—releasing factors—developed. Evidence indicated they were essential to the release of specific hypophysial hormones when appropriate stimuli were received. Now the problem is not the presence of these messengers; they are known. The problem is that of how they function. One could say that masses of facts are available but complete understanding seems ever harder to attain.

Despite our problems and the elusiveness of understanding, we are indeed a fortunate people, free to go as far as we can, free to diverge but also to return when we have acquired new skills, new ideas, and new opportunities. We are helped by the progress of many others. In each adventure there is excitement and the certainty of finding new knowledge and new friends. Although it may seem now more than in the pioneering days of neuroendocrinology that one needs much money and a big team to accomplish anything at all, there is still a place for the one man and the idea produced by one man's or one woman's mind.

REFERENCES

Bissonnette, T. H. (1938). Influence of light upon pituitary activity. *Res. Publ. Assoc. Res. Nerv. Ment. Dis.* **17**: 361.

Bray, G. A. (1974). Endocrine factors in the control of food intake. *Fed. Proc.* **33**: 1140.

Brooks, C. McC. (1931). A delimitation of the central nervous mechanism involved in reflex hyperglycemia. *Am. J. Physiol.* **99**:64.

Brooks, C. McC. (1935). The role of the cerebral cortex in the sexual activities of the rabbit. *Sechenov Physiol J. USSR.* **21**(5).

Brooks, C. McC. (1935). Studies on the neural basis of ovulation in the rabbit. *Am. J. Physiol.* **113**(1).

Brooks, C. McC. (1937). The role of the cerebral cortex and of various sense organs in the excitation and execution of mating activity in the rabbit. *Am. J. Physiol.* **120**: 544.

Brooks, C. McC. (1938). A study of the mechanism whereby coitus excites ovulation-producing activity of the rabbit's pituitary. *Am. J. Physiol.* **121**: 157.

Brooks, C. McC. (1938). The effect of transection of the pituitary stalk on the FSH and LH content of the rabbit's pituitary. *Proc. Am. Physiol. Soc.* **123**:25.

Brooks, C. McC. (1938). The reproductive functions of male and female rabbits after transection of the pituitary stalk and ablation of the cervical sympathetic nerve supply. *Proc. XII International Physiol. Congress.*, Zurich.

Brooks, C. McC. (1946). A study of the respiratory quotient in experimental hypothalamic obesity. *Am. J. Physiol.* **147**: 727.

Brooks, C. McC., W. G. Beadenkopf, and S. Bojar (1940). A study of the mechanism whereby copper acetate and certain drugs produce ovulation in the rabbit. *Endocrinology* **27**:878.

Brooks, C. McC., and E. M. Bridge (1944). Changes in the respiratory quotient associated with development of experimentally produced obesity in the monkey (*Macaca mulatta*). *Endocrinology* **35**: 208.

Brooks, C. McC., and I. Gersh (1941). Innervation of the hypophysis of the rabbit and rat. *Endocrinology* **28**: 1.

Brooks, C. McC., J. L. Gilbert, H. A. Levey, and D. R. Curtis (1962). *Humors, Hormones and Neurosecretions: The Origins and Development of Man's Present Knowledge of the Humoral Control of Body Function.* State University of New York Press, Albany.

Brooks, C. McC., K. Koizumi, and J. O. Pinkston (1974). *The Life and Contributions of Walter Bradford Cannon, 1871–1945, His Influence on the Development of Physiology.* State University of New York Press, Albany.

Brooks, C. McC., and E. Lambert (1939). The effect of hypophysial stalk transection on the gonadotropic functions of the rabbit's hypophysis. *Am. J. Physiol.* **128:** 57.

Brooks, C. McC., and S. W. Page (1938). The occurrence of coitus-induced ovulation in the adrenalectomized rabbit. *Endocrinology* **22:** 613.

Brooks, C. McC., I. Suda, and K. Koizumi (1962). Unit activity in supraoptic area of hypothalamus. *Proc. XXII International Congress of Physiological Sciences,* Leiden. 1138.

Brooks, C. McC., J. Ushiyama, and G. Lange (1962). Reactions of neurons in or near the supraoptic nuclei. *Am. J. Physiol.* **202:**487.

Cannon, W. B., C. A. L. Binger, and R. Fitz (1914–15). Experimental hyperthyroidism. *Am. J. Physiol.* **36:** 363.

Dahlgren, U. (1914). The electric motor nerve centers in the skate (*Rajaidae*). *Science* **40:** 862.

Fisher, C., W. R. Ingram, and S. W. Ranson, (1938). *Diabetes insipidus and the neurohormonal control of water balance.* Edwards Bros., Ann Arbor.

Gersh, I. (1940). Water Metabolism: Endocrine Factors. pages 430–448 *in The Hypothalamus* J. F. Fulton, S. W. Ranson, and A. M. Frantz eds. Res. Publ. Assoc. Res. Nerv. Ment. Dis. Williams & Wilkins Co., Baltimore.

Gersh, I., and C. McC. Brooks (1938). Pericellular nerve fiber terminations in the pars nervosa and pars distalis of the rat's pituitary. *Anat. Rec.* **70:** (4) Suppl. No. 3.

Gersh, I., and C. McC. Brooks (1941). Correlation of physiological and cytological changes in the neurohypophysis of rats with experimental diabetes insipidus. *Endocrinology* **28:** 6.

Hammond, J. (1925). Reproduction in the Rabbit. London.

Hammond, J. (1951). Control by light of reproduction in ferrets and mink. *Nature* **167:** 150.

Harris, G. W. (1955). Neural Control of the Pituitary Gland. Edward Arnold, Ltd., London.

Harrison, T. S. (1964). Adrenal medulla and its regulation. *Physiol. Rev.* **44:** 161.

Hartman, C. G. (1939). Pages 630–719 *in* Allen's *Sex and Internal Secretions.* Williams & Wilkins, Baltimore.

Holland, W. J. (1908). *The Moth Book.* Doubleday, Page & Co., New York.

Jacoby, J. H., J. F. Sassin, M. Greenstein, and E. D. Weitzman (1974). Patterns of spontaneous cortical and growth hormone secretion in Rhesus monkeys during the sleep-waking cycle. *Neuroendocrinology* **14:** 165.

Kao, F. F., K. Koizumi, and M. Vassalle, eds. (1971). *Research in Physiology, A Liber Memorialis in Honor of Professor Chandler McCuskey Brooks.* Aulo Gaggi, Publisher, Bologna.

Koizumi, K., T. Ishikawa, and C. McC. Brooks (1973). The existence of facilitatory axon collaterals in neurosecretory cells of the hypothalamus. *Brain Res.* **63:** 408.

Kopeć, S. (1917). Experiments on metamorphosis of insects. *Bull. Acad. Sci.* Cracovie, Classe Sci. Math. Nat. Ser. **B:** 57.

Krieger, D. T., and W. Allen (1974). Effect of ocular enucleation and altered lighting regimens of various ages on adrenal and gonadal weight and mean plasma corticosteroid levels in the rat. *Endocr. Res. Commun.* **1:** 19.

Long, J. A., and H. M. Evans (1922). The estrous cycle in the rat and its associated phenomena. *Memoirs of the University of California.* Vol. 6.

Marshall, F. H. A. (1936). Sexual periodicity and the causes which determine it. *Philos. Trans., Ser. B* **226:** 423.

Marshall, F. H. A. (1937). On changeover in oestrous cycle in animals after transference across equator, with further observations on incidence of breeding seasons and factors controlling sexual periodicity. *Proc. R. Soc. London, Ser. B* **122**: 413.

Panksepp, J. (1974). Hypothalamic regulation of energy balance and feeding behavior. *Fed. Proc.* **33**:(5): 1150.

Parker, G. H. (1948). *Animal Color Changes and their Neurohumors*. Cambridge Univ. Press, Cambridge, England.

Parkes, A. S. (1961). Chapter on cycles and seasonal variations *in* Marshall's *Physiology of Reproduction*, vol. 1, part 2. Longmans, Green and Co., London.

Parkes, A. S., and A. R. Fee (1930). Studies on ovulation; effect of vaginal anaesthesia on ovulation in the rabbit. *J. Physiol.* **70**: 385.

Rolleston, H. D. (1936). *The Endocrine Organs in Health and Disease with an Historical Review*. Oxford Univ. Press, London.

Roussey, G., and M. Mosinger (1946). *Traité de Neuro-endocrinologie*, Masson et Cie., Paris.

Roussey, G., and M. Mosinger (1953). Bibliographia neurovegetativa Fenz, Egon, Springer, Wein, XVIII, 343p.

Ruch, T. C., and H. D. Patton (1965). *Physiology and Biophysics*, 19th ed. W. B. Saunders Co., Philadelphia.

Scharrer, E. (1933). Über neurokrine organe der wierbeltiere. Verh. Dtsch. Zool. Ges., *Zool. Anz.* **6**: 217.

Scharrer, E., and B. Scharrer (1940). Secretory cells within the hypothalamus. *Res. Publ. Assoc. Res. Nerv. Ment. Dis.* **20**: 170.

Schmitt, M. (1973). Circadian rhythmicity in responses of cells in the lateral hypothalamus. *Am. J. Physiol.* **25**: 1096.

Smith, E. R., and J. M. Davidson (1974). Luteinizing hormone releasing factor in rats exposed to constant light: Effects of mating. *Neuroendocrinology* **14**: 129.

Speidel, C. C. (1922). Further comparative studies in other fishes of cells that are homologous to the large irregular glandular cells in the spinal cord of the skate. *J. Comp. Neurol.* **34**: 303.

Suda, I., K. Koizumi, and C. McC. Brooks (1963). Study of unitary activity in the supraoptic nucleus of the hypothalamus. *Jpn. J. Physiol.* **13**: 374.

Uotila, U. U. (1939). On the role of the pituitary stalk in the regulation of the anterior pituitary with special reference to the thyrotropic hormone. *Endocrinology* **25**: 605.

Vogt, M. (1954). The concentration of sympathin in different parts of the central nervous system under normal conditions and after the administration of drugs. *J. Physiol.* **123**: 451.

Watari, N. (1973). K. Yagi and S. Yoshida, eds. *Innervation of Pancreatic Islet Cells in Neuroendocrine Control*. Halsted Press Book, John Wiley & Sons, New York.

Wurtmann, R. J. (1970). Brain catecholamines and the control of secretion from the anterior pituitary gland. *In* J. Meites, ed., *Hypophysiotropic Hormones of the Hypothalamus: Assay and Chemistry*. Williams & Wilkins, Baltimore.

Yagi, K., and S. Yoshida (1973). *Neuroendocrine Control*. John Wiley & Sons, New York.

6

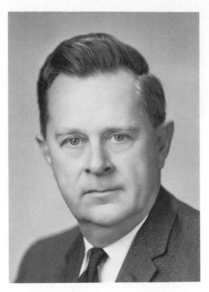

Edward W(heeler) Dempsey

Edward W. Dempsey was born on May 15, 1911, in Buxton, Iowa. He received his A.B. degree from Marietta College in 1932 and entered graduate school at Brown University where he received his Sc.M. in 1934 and his Ph.D. in 1937. He obtained a National Research Council fellowship to work in the Department of Anatomy at Harvard in 1937 and was appointed Instructor in Physiology there in 1938. In 1946 he was appointed Associate Professor of Anatomy. In 1950 he left Harvard to become Professor and Chairman of the Department of Anatomy at Washington University School of Medicine in St. Louis, a position which he held until 1966. He also served as Assistant to the Dean at Washington University from 1956 to 1958 and was Dean from 1958 to 1964. He was appointed Special Assistant to the Secretary of Health, Education and Welfare in 1964 and then assumed the chairmanship of the Department of Anatomy at the College of Physicians and Surgeons of Columbia University in 1966, a position which he held until 1974. He was a Professor of Anatomy at the school until his death in January 1975.

Dr. Dempsey was a member of many societies, including the American Association of Anatomists, American Physiological Society, Society for Experimental Biology and Medicine, the Histochemical Society, the Electronmicroscopy Society of America, the Endocrine Society, the American Academy of Neurology, the Anatomical Society of Great Britain and Ireland, and the American Neurological Association.

He served as editor of *Endocrinology* from 1944 to 1952 and on the editorial boards of the *Proceedings of the Society of Experimental Biology and Medicine,* the *Journal of the National Cancer Institute,* the *Journal of Histochemistry and Cytochemistry, Experimental Neurology,* and the *American Journal of Anatomy.* He also served as advisory editor of the *International Review of Cytology* from 1957 to 1960.

At the national level, he was on the Morphology and Genetics Study Section from 1952 to 1956 and served on the Anatomical Sciences Training Committee of NIH from 1956 to 1960. He was also on the Medical Committee of the National Science Foundation and served as its chairman in 1953.

During his career he received many honors. He was Treasurer of the Histochemical Society from 1950 to 1954 and President of the American Association of Anatomists in 1961 and was elected to the American Academy of Arts and Sciences.

Wanderings in Neuroendocrinology

EDWARD W. DEMPSEY

"Looking back," Nat King Cole once sang, "there's one mistake I'd never make again." I can accept no such limitation. Many mistakes I have made, many more I would make, and many I would probably make again. It would have been pleasant had I realized sooner how my own observations were pointing toward neuroendocrine mechanisms. I regret that the quantitative importance of the hypophyseal portal blood supply did not occur to me until Harris's elegant surgical procedures made it abundantly clear. And I am sorry that distractions deflected me only too often from the mainstream of neuroendocrine research.

The invitation to contribute this account of a personal relationship to neuroendocrinology emphasized that autobiographical and anecdotal statements were requested—not a review of the developing field. I shall respond to this request unabashedly. In many instances credit and acknowledgement to others will be scanty or absent. Also (memory being faulty) errors, mistakes, and misinterpretations will conveniently be forgotten. Nonetheless, I shall try to recall something of the people and ideas that dominated the field at particular times and that made it so exciting. This period now extends over more than four decades.

My first scientific work began in 1932 under the direction of the late Dr. William C. Young of Brown University. It concerned estrous behavior. In female guinea pigs, we were able to show that estrus has a circadian rhythm—it begins most often in the middle of the night and its diurnal rhythmicity becomes random in animals maintained in darkness. Endocrinologically, it can be induced concomitantly with ovulation by suitably timed injections of gonadotropic hormones and in ovariectomized animals by progesterone following priming with estrogens. Taken together, these facts indicated that light influences the rhythm of the pituitary and ovary, which in turn controls behavioral phenomena. Neural factors were strongly indicated—one mediating the effect of light on the hypophysis and another responding to the sex steroids to effect the behavioral manifestations of estrus.

My introduction to controversy came early. At the meeting of the American Association of Anatomists at Duke University in, I believe, 1935, I presented my first scientific paper. It concerned the role of progesterone in inducing estrous behavior. In discussion of my presentation, George Corner, chairman of the session, led off by pointing out that estrus in the sow preceded ovulation and that the luteal hormone had, therefore, not yet been produced. This was followed in turn by similar critical remarks by Edgar Allen, Philip Smith, Herbert Evans, and F. L. Hisaw. In defense against this formidable group, I offered the rebuttal that I had presented experiments and observations, repeatedly and easily verified, whereas their objections were on grounds of theory and not facts. When the next paper was called, I left the room to walk off my agitation. In the hallway two men accosted me to ask questions about my paper. They got from me a rather uninhibited opinion about the fairness and quality of the discussion. I have always been grateful for their forbearance, as it turned out that my intemperate remarks were made to George Wislocki and Franklin Snyder, both of whom were to play important roles in my future. Years later, when I was editor of *Endocrinology,* I asked Dr. Corner to read a paper for me. Together with his editorial comments, he sent me a note recalling his criticism and apologizing both for having been wrong and for having been unduly harsh to a young investigator presenting his first paper. I have always tried to remember these two episodes —when tempted to criticize hastily or to avoid a position because it was controversial.

At this point, deficiencies in my background and training had become seriously apparent. Although reasonably well informed about reproductive physiology and competent in histology and cytology, I had had no experience in neuroanatomy and neurophysiology, and it seemed abundantly clear that I must either remove these deficiencies or find other research interests. Fortunately for me, Dr. Young suggested that I approach Dr. Wislocki, then chairman of the Department of Anatomy at Harvard Medical School. Dr. Wislocki, as indicated above, had earlier expressed interest in my research. Together with Dr. David Rioch, the neuroanatomist of the department, they suggested that I apply for a National Research Council fellowship to work under their direction. There, I might learn something about neuroanatomy and also attempt to locate the centers and pathways which mediate the estrous reflexes. Largely due to the support of these three—Drs. Young, Wislocki, and Rioch—I was awarded the fellowship for the year 1937–38.

As it must have happened to many others, this and the following post-doctorate years influenced enormously everything I have done since. These years occurred toward the end of the great depression, during which academic positions were scarce and competition keen. I was thrown into intimate contact with contemporaries who were able indeed and who were to become noteworthy figures in American medicine. To name a few: Robert Gross, one of the pioneers in heart surgery; Stanley Bennett, who influenced histochemistry at a decisive time and later became successively professor of anatomy at Seattle, dean of medicine at Chicago and now professor of anatomy at North Carolina; Oliver Lowry, whose micromethods ushered in an era of cytochemistry and cell biology; E. B. Astwood, whose development of antithyroid drugs extended our knowledge of thyroid physiology and the clinical management of thyrotoxicosis; and Robert Morison, whose ability in neurophysiology was matched only by his wisdom in later guiding the medical affairs of the Rockefeller Foundation and, still later, of Cornell University.

My need to learn something about the nervous system was abundantly satisfied. Dr. Rioch and Dr. Arturo Rosenblueth, of the Physiology Department, collaborated that year in teaching a summer course in neuroanatomy and neurophysiology. The didactic portion consisted of the lectures normally given to medical students but the laboratory part was much more advanced and up to date, since with a small class it was possible to use equipment ordinarily available only for research. This course, and my association in it with Rioch, Rosenblueth, and Morison, and through them with Drs. Walter B. Cannon, Hallowell Davis, and Alexander Forbes, provided me with both information and sponsorship sufficient to gain entrance into neurological circles.

A third, somewhat interlocking, group which influenced me greatly was a supper club interested in the philosophy of science. At its regular meetings, each of its members in turn provided scientific entertainment for the evening in the form of an account of his current interests. This was a broadly representative group—Norbert Wiener, mathematician from the Massachusetts Institute of Technology; Smith Stevens, experimental psychologist from Harvard; Baird Hastings, biochemist of Harvard Medical School; and several others. At one of these meetings, Rosenblueth described how the cerebellum smooths out the motor activities of the corticospinal system, and mentioned that the nerve impulse is an all-or-nothing phenomenon. At this point Wiener became tremendously excited—indeed agitated—and marched up and down the room developing the idea that digital feedbacks could regulate servomechanisms. This idea developed rapidly during the war years and became the basis of an entire science of control mechanisms, later collectively described by Wiener under the name *cybernetics*. At another meeting, Smith Stevens proposed the idea of a *Handbook of Experimental Psychology*. The resulting volume markedly influenced the development of experimental methods in psychology; it also forced me to think through the concept of the steady state and to apply it to the higher intellectual and sociological functions of the body and the body politic, in addition to its more commonly understood physiological aspects.

These were the years that psychosomatic medicine was a great vogue. The journal of that name was relatively new; Freudian concepts were prevalent among psychiatric circles in Boston; Bard and Rioch's classical work on the behavior of cats deprived of neocortex had just appeared; and, above all, Cannon's work on the sympathetic nervous system and adrenal medulla had recently provided clinicians with physiological mechanisms linking emotional or environmental stress to pathological responses. Bernard's statement describing the constancy of the internal environment had been substantiated and developed into Cannon's concept of homeostasis. The time was ripe for Selye to extend this idea still further to include the endocrine events collectively described as the *alarm reaction*. It was also ripe for our own investigations of the histophysiology and histochemistry of the endocrine system.

A final aspect of my development during these prewar years at Harvard was the serendipity of circumstance. Academic appointments were rare in those depression days. On the advice of Wislocki, I had applied for a renewal of my fellowship, and in due course it was awarded. However, during the first year, Rioch was offered and accepted a professorship of neuropsychiatry at Washington University in St. Louis. He invited me to go with him. Concurrently, to fill his slot in neuroanatomy, Wislocki offered the position to Robert Morison, who then was a member of the Department of Physiology. His acceptance left Dr. Cannon with an open position. Since he was to retire in a few years, he was amenable to Wislocki's suggestion that I might join the physiology department for three years, at the end of which time scheduled retirements would provide an opportunity for me to return to anatomy. Thus, I resigned my fellowship, declined Rioch's flattering offer, and became an instructor in physiology. There, to my consternation, I was put in charge of the course. It is a truism that the most effective way to learn is to teach. I learned, and rapidly. In the process, I introduced into the course a formalized sequence of lectures and laboratory exercises on endocrinology, a subject which previously had received only casual attention.

These, then, were the people, concepts, and forces which influenced me during my formative years. They occupied my energy and they challenged my thoughts. They led to the demonstration that progesterone blocks the processes causing ovulation. They led also to fruitless efforts to find electrical changes in the nervous system after treatment with sex steroids. The crude methods then at our disposal caused me to seek further experience with electrophysiological procedures with Rosenblueth. These later initiated a series of studies with Robert and Benigna Morison, in which we demonstrated that anatomical pathways in the brain can be traced by the electrical activity recorded through probe electrodes, and that the corticothalamic systems so investigated can be shown to control the electroencephalographic events heralding sleep and awakening, attention reactions, and other behavioral attributes.

Such excursions into experimental neuroanatomy and neurophysiology confirmed my growing suspicions that, although fine things in their own right, the methods of these disciplines alone would hardly solve the problems of environmental influences on endocrine activity. To tackle these problems, it seemed apparent that other and different experimental questions must be asked. Are external and internal environmental changes mediated by the same mechanisms? Can morphological procedures be devised which are more sensitive than the then current criteria involving weight of target organs or the height of glandular epithelia? Is it possible that blood-borne substances modify the activity of specific nervous pathways by reaching them more expeditiously or by being fixed more firmly by them, thus acting to increase or decrease excitatory levels? These questions, modified and reshaped according to the rapidly developing technologies of morphological science, underlie most of the investigations undertaken by me, alone or together with students and associates during the last three decades.

Maintenance of rats in a constantly illuminated environment leads to a state of steady estrus with large follicles but no corpora lutea in the ovaries. In this state, female rats will mate with normal or sterile males, becoming pregnant with the former and pseudopregnant with the latter. Ovulation, therefore, is induced in such animals by copulation, as is the case normally in the rabbit. Also like the rabbit, ovulation can be induced in these animals by the injection of chorionic gonadotrophin. We concluded, therefore, that the hypophysis can be stimulated by neural events associated with sexual activity or by the hormonal stimulus of gonadotropin. In either case, the final common pathway from the hypophysis to the ovary appeared to be the same. Since we had previously found that section of the pituitary stalk did not interrupt follicular growth or ovulation in spontaneously ovulating species, these experiments pointed strongly toward a neuroendocrine factor produced by nervous stimuli and circulating to the hypophysis via the blood stream. We now know, of course, that this factor is the LH releasing hormone of the hypothalamus.

Somewhat similar results were obtained in experiments designed to elucidate hypophyseal-thyroid relationships. Rats maintained in cold environments have active thyroid glands, judged by the cell-height index of their follicular epithelia. Conversely, hot environments depress thyroid function as judged by the same criteria. Similar, but more delicate, control of the thyroid can be shown by determining the amount of thyroxin necessary to prevent the thyroid hypertrophy induced by antithyroid drugs. In rats kept in the cold, this quantity of thyroxin is many times that required in animals kept in hot environments (Dempsey and Astwood, 1943). Thus, it appears that heat—a nervous stimulus—depresses the hypophysial thyrotrophin just as it is suppressed by an excess of thyroxin. As is the case with the ovary, the final common pathway seems to be the same. However, in this case the results were equivocal in that section of the pituitary stalk depressed or inhibited the effect of cold on the thyroid, leading to the then current interpretation that thyrotrophic stimulation of the hypophysis was induced by nerves. Had we studied more carefully damage to the pituitary blood supply caused by the stalk section, we would probably have seen that the suppressed effect of cold was partial and not complete, and that these experiments, like those with light and the ovary, also pointed toward a neuroendocrine thyrotropin releasing factor. But we did not, and hindsight is always perfect.

These somewhat equivocal results, together with our success in demonstrating the increased precision of thyroxin assay using properly prepared animals, led to a long diversion from the line of investigation outlined earlier. At this time, histochemical methods were being developed which promised more delicate means of evaluation than had previously been possible. Moreover, many of these methods yielded results which could be correlated with known metabolic events. Consequently, we embarked on what became a long search for staining and enzymatic methods which could be interpreted chemically. These procedures were many and various. They included the characterization of lipids by their solubilities, their affinities for nonpolar dyes, their content of phosphorus and of carbonyl groups, and their physical nature as determined by polarization and fluorescence microscopy. They involved also the physical-chemical behavior of proteins whereby the strength of their ionizable groups could be determined. Carbohydrates, too, could be characterized by their acidic groups and by their conversion to aldehydes identifiable by the Schiff or silver reduction reagents. Enzymes, particularly phosphatases and lipases, were localized by modifications of Gomori's basic methods. All of these and various other procedures, putatively identifying substances such as calcium and iron, were applied to endocrine glands and their target organs in various degrees of stimulation and suppression. These physiological states were sometimes produced by environmental stimuli such as light, heat, and cold and sometimes by naturally occurring rhythms such as the estrous cycle, seasonal activities, or pregnancy.

A review of our work on the histochemistry of endocrine and target organs is beyond the scope of this account. Nevertheless, a few instances should be mentioned since they indicate the greater precision obtainable with histochemical as opposed to conventional staining, and since in some instances conclusions made many years ago are only now being confirmed with methods more elegant, accurate, and precise.

Basophilic staining of the hypophysis and chorionic trophoblast was shown to be abolished by prior digestion with ribonuclease (Dempsey and Wislocki, 1945). This localization of ribonucleic acid antedated by many years the identification of ribosomes and of rough endoplasmic reticulum in these locations.

Alkaline phosphatase reactions indicated dramatic depression of this enzyme's activity in many organs of hypophysectomized as compared to normal rats. This was true in thyroids, the adrenal fasciculata (but not glomerulosa), gonads, and their target organs. Interestingly, the phosphatase reaction of the parathyroid glands is depressed after hypophysectomy but it is unchanged in the pancreatic islets (Dempsey, 1948).

Iron, as detected by the Turnbull blue reaction, is present throughout the trophoblast in early human placentas, but becomes concentrated at the base of the syncytium as pregnancy advances (Dempsey and Wislocki, 1944). Iron can also be demonstrated by this method in the paraplacental chorionic cells of the cat's brown border (Wislocki and Dempsey, 1946). Calcium was also detected provisionally in placentas by modified von Kossa reactions. These reactions are of current interest since recent electron microscopic studies have revealed small dense bodies corresponding to the location of the Turnbull blue reactions in placentas from early and late stages of pregnancy (Dempsey and Luse, 1971). Still more recently, energy dispersive X-ray analysis has positively identified these elements in placentas of primates and carnivores (Dempsey, 1975).

The development of histochemical methods such as those mentioned above led directly to explorations of the blood-brain barrier, in the hope that more detailed knowledge of its structure would lead to improved concepts concerning the origin of neuroendocrine factors and of the locations in which hormones could leave the blood stream to reach the nervous tissues.

The idea of a hematoencephalic barrier came from the observations of Goldmann (1913), who found that chronic administration of acid colloidal dyes such as trypan blue stains most of the tissues of the body but not the nervous system. Later, more detailed search indicated that there were certain exceptions to this generalization. A group of neural organs now often described as circumventricular stain with varying degrees of intensity when trypan blue is administered intravitally. These organs include the area postrema, choroid plexuses, intercolumnar tubercle, pineal body, supraoptic recess, neurohypophysis, and the infundibulum. These same organs are blackened when silver nitrate is administered chronically in rat's drinking water (Wislocki and Leduc, 1952).

With the identification of the neurohypophyseal hormones, with the determination that blood flows from the infundibulum toward the hypophysis in the hypophyseal portal system (Wislocki, 1938), and with our later improvements in histological methods, it became important to investigate the circumventricular organs in greater detail. Various histochemical studies were carried out (Wislocki and Dempsey, 1948a; 1948b; Wislocki and Leduc, 1952).

The decade of the forties was scientifically productive—more so than any other period of my life. However, it introduced a number of distractions which accumulated with time and which were to restrict seriously the investigations I should pursue in the future. An invitation to serve on the endocrinology panel of the Committee on Growth led to further participation in the advisory groups of granting agencies—the Study Section on Morphology and Genetics of the National Institutes of Health, the advisory committee of the National Multiple Sclerosis Society, the Committee of Consultants on Medical Research of the United States Senate, the National Advisory Health Council, the President's Commission on Heart Disease, Cancer and Stroke, and the National Advisory Council of the Institute of General Medical Sciences. The activities of these committees required a great deal of travel and the study of research and research support, but they were time consuming. Similarly, editorial activities on various journals (*Endocrinology, Proceedings of the Society of Experimental Biology and Medicine, Journal of Histochemistry and Cytochemistry, Experimental Neurology,* and the *American Journal of Anatomy*) have broadened my horizons, but each has been a chronophage. Finally, administrative responsibilities, as acting chairman of the Department of Anatomy (1946–48) at Harvard, chairman of anatomy at the Washington University School of Medicine at St. Louis (1950–66), dean of the School of Medicine, Washington University (1958–64), Special Assistant for Health and Medical Affairs to the Secretary of Health Education and Welfare (1964–66), and chairman of the Department of Anatomy, the College of Physicians and Surgeons of Columbia University (1966–74) all have consumed time and energy. Nevertheless, during these years I have been able to continue some work of my own but more importantly to attract and encourage a number of people whose work was directly or collaterally related to neuroendocrinology. Among them, but by no means exhausting the list, were Sarah Luse, Paul Lacy, Jack Davies, Allen Enders, Duncan Chiquoine, Bryce Munger, and, as visitors to the laboratory, E. C. Amoroso, A. G. Weddell, Jeffrey Lever, and Alan Muir.

I can, and have, justified diversions from research by arguing that these administrative efforts created opportunities for others, just as opportunities had earlier been created for me. Nevertheless, in the interim many indeed have been the advances made by others without my being able to participate in the excitement of their discoveries. I may explain, but not excuse, therefore, the sporadic record of whatever contributions I have been able to make.

At about the time I left Harvard to go to St. Louis, sectioning, embedding, and fixing methods for electron microscopy had progressed to a point that ultrastructural observations could be made reliably in histophysiological investigations. In 1955, Dempsey and Wislocki reported that silver nitrate administrated chronically to rats led to electron-dense deposits in the basement membranes of the capillary vessels located in the circumventricular organs and also in a second layer constituting a pial investment. Between these two basement membranes, a perivascular connective tissue sheath characterized these organs, whereas in the nervous tissue proper the glial processes touched directly the single basement membrane surrounding the capillary endothelium. Thus, the circumventricular organs all share a common property—a perivascular connective tissue sheath unique to these neural structures.

More recent investigations have established that a portal circulation exists in the area postrema (Roth and Yamomoto, 1968) and probably in all of the circumventricular organs (Duvernoy and Koritké, 1965). Thus, the microcirculatory pattern, like the perivascular sheath, is similar in all of these organs, two of which (the neurohypophysis and the pineal body) certainly are neuroendocrine glands.

Electron microscopy of the intercolumnar tubercle (Dempsey, 1968) and area postrema (Dempsey, 1973) has revealed still other details similar to those of the neurohypophysis and pineal body. In all four of these organs, nerve axons penetrate the pial membrane and end in bulbous protrusions located in the perivascular sheath. These enlarged endings, like those constituting the Herring bodies of the neurohypophysis, contain dense-cored vesicles of various sizes. Also, although the relationships have not been worked out in satisfactory detail, tanycyte processes extending into the ventricle are associated with the infundibular system. Similar nerve cells with processes approaching the ventricular fluids are to be found in the regions of both the intercolumnar tubercle and the area postrema. All of these details, taken together, demonstrate that the circumventricular organs are constructed on a morphologically similar pattern, and that at least two of them have neuroendocrine functions. It remains for future investigations to establish what, if any, neuroendocrine properties characterize the remainder of this enigmatic group of structures which, as Tilney (1938) has shown have a long evolutionary history.

A final remark may be added. From 1966 to 1974, I have been chairman of the Department of Anatomy at Columbia University. During these past eight years it has been possible again to construct a laboratory equipped to carry out work in the forefront of morphology. The addition of scanning electron microscopy and of energy dispersive X-ray analysis to the armamentarium of anatomy has already permitted important advances and promises many more. With current instruments it is possible to identify positively any element of atomic number greater than 10, in a volume of tissue as small as one-tenth micron in cubic dimension and in quantities approaching 20,000 atoms. This qualitative, quantitative, and spatial precision, which is now obtainable, places histochemistry on an entirely new plane. Application of these exciting new procedures to endocrine events has already begun. We have been able to localize iron in the small dark granules of syncytial trophoblast (vide supra). Sulfur and phosphorus have been measured in individual spermatozoa (Dempsey, Jarvis, and Purkerson, 1974). We are currently investigating the microcirculation of endocrine organs by using the resolution and magnification possible with scanning electron microscopes as applied to ultrastructurally accurate casts of the vessels in various organs (Lee, Purkerson, Agate, and Dempsey, 1972). We have been able recently to localize iron in hemoglobin and sulfur in the membranes of individual erythrocytes. As these methods are developed further and utilized more widely, they will throw light on new investigative territories which, one hopes, will illuminate not only neuroendocrinology but all of morphology as well.

REFERENCES

Dempsey, E. W. (1937). Follicular growth rate and ovulation after various experimental procedures in the guinea pig. *Am. J. Physiol.* **120:** 126.

Dempsey, E. W. (1948). The chemical cytology of endocrine glands. *Recent Prog. Horm. Res.* **3:** 127.

Dempsey, E. W. (1951). Homeostasis. Pages 209–235 In S. S. Stevens, ed. *Handbook of Experimental Psychology,* John Wiley and Sons, New York.

Dempsey, E. W. (1968). Fine-structure of the rat's intercolumnar tubercle and its adjacent ependyma and choroid plexus, with especial reference to the appearance of its sinusoidal vessels in experimental argyria. *Exp. Neurol..* **22:** 568.

Dempsey, E. W. (1973). Neural and vascular ultrastructure of the area postrema in the rat. *J. Comp. Neurol.* **150:** 177.

Dempsey, E. W. (1975). Ultrastructural and x-ray analysis after electron excitation of primate placentas, with remarks on the transport of iron and calcium. *Am. J. Anat.,* in press.

Dempsey, E. W., and E. B. Astwood (1943). Determination of the rate of thyroid hormone secretion at various environmental temperatures. *Endocrinology* **32:** 509.

Dempsey, E. W., J. U. M. Jarvis, and M. L. Purkerson (1974). The location of sulfur in spermatozoa by energy dispersive X-ray analysis and scanning electron microscopy. Pages 631–637 in *Scanning Electron Microscopy/1974* (Part 3). IIT Research Institute, Chicago.

Dempsey, E. W., and S. A. Luse (1971). Regional specializations in the syncytial trophoblast of early human placentas. *J. Anat.* **108:**545.

Dempsey, E. W., and H. F. Searles (1943). Environmental modification of certain endocrine phenomena. *Endocrinology* **32:** 119.

Dempsey, E. W., and G. B. Wislocki (1944). Observations on some histochemical reactions in the human placenta, with special reference to the significance of the lipoids, glycogen and iron. *Endocrinology,* **35:** 409.

Dempsey, E. W., and G. B. Wislocki (1945). Histochemical reactions associated with basophilia and acidophilia in the placenta and pituitary gland. *Am. J. Anat.* **76:**277.

Dempsey, E. W., and G. B. Wislocki (1955). An electron microscopic study of the blood brain barrier in the rat, employing silver nitrate as a vital stain. *J. Biophys. and Biochem. Cytol.* **1:** 245.

Duvernoy, H., and J. G. Koritké (1965). Contribution a l'étude de l'angioarchitectonie des organes circumventriculaires. *Arch. Biol.* **75:** 849.

Goldmann, E. E. (1913). Vitalfärbung am Zentralnervensystem. K. Academie de Wissenschaften, Berlin. 9.

Lee, M. L., M. L. Purkerson, F. J., Jr. Agate, and E. W. Dempsey (1972). Ultrastructural changes in renal glomeruli of rats during experimentally induced hypertension and uremia. *Am. J. Anat.* **135:** 191.

Roth, G. I., and W. S. Yamomoto (1968). The microcirculation of the area postrema in the rat. *J. Comp. Neurol.* **133:** 329.

Tilney, F. (1938). The glands of the brain with special reference to the pituitary gland. In *The Pituitary Gland. Proc. Assoc. Res. Nerv. Ment. Dis.,* **17:** 1.

Wislocki, G. B. (1938). The vascular supply of the hypophysis cerebri of the Rhesus monkey and man. In *The Pituitary Gland. Proc. Assoc. Res. Nerv. Ment. Dis.* **17:** 48.

Wislocki, G. B., and E. W. Dempsey (1946). Histochemical reactions in the placenta of the cat. *Am. J. Anat.* **78:** 1.

Wislocki, G. B., and E. W. Dempsey (1948a). The chemical histology and cytology of the pineal body and neurohypophysis. *Endocrinology* **42:** 56.

Wislocki, G. B., and E. W. Dempsey (1948b). The chemical cytology of the choroid plexus and blood brain barrier of the Rhesus monkey (*Macaca mulatta*). *J. Comp. Neurol.* **88:** 319.

Wislocki, G. B., and E. H. Leduc (1952). Vital staining of the hematoencephalic barrier by silver nitrate and trypan blue, and cytological comparisons of the neurohypophysis, pineal organ, area postrema, intercolumnar tubercle and supraoptic crest. *J. Comp. Neurol.* **96:** 371.

7

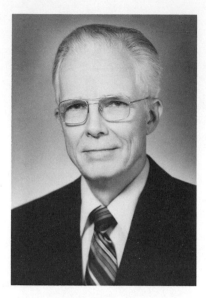

John W. Everett

John W. Everett was born on March 5, 1906, in Ovid, Michigan. He was educated in the public schools of Big Rapids, Michigan, and received an A. B. degree from Olivet College, Olivet, Michigan, in 1928. He received a Ph.D. from Yale University Graduate School, Department of Zoology, in 1932. He served as a Graduate Assistant in Zoology from 1928 to 1930 and 1931 to 1932, and was an Instructor in Biology at Goucher College from 1930 to 1931. In 1932 he accepted a position as Instructor in Anatomy at Duke University School of Medicine, Durham, North Carolina, where he has remained, and became a Professor in 1950. He served as a Visiting Professor of Anatomy at the University of California at Los Angeles in 1952, and at the University of Tennessee in 1954.

Dr. Everett is a member of many societies, including the American Association of Anatomists, American Physiological Society, American Institute of Biological Sciences, The Endocrine Society, Society for Experimental Biology and Medicine, Biological Stain Committee, American Association for the Advancement of Science, New York Academy of Science, International Brain Research Organization, Sigma Xi, Society for the Study of Reproduction, and the International Society of Neuroendocrinology. He has served on the editorial boards of *Endocrinology* (1953–1956, 1959–1975) and *Neuroendocrinology* (1966–1973), was associate editor of *Anatomical Record* from 1957 to 1963, section editor of *Biological Abstracts* from 1956 to 1971, and associate editor of *Biology of Reproduction* from 1968 to 1969.

His honors include presentation of the annual lecture, Neuroendocrine Dinner Discussion Group, Federation of American Societies for Experimental Biology, 1968; Third Annual Carl G. Hartman Lectureship Award of the Society for the Study of Reproduction, 1971; the First Annual Kathleen M. Osborn Memorial Lecture, University of Kansas Medical Center, 1971; the Fred Conrad Koch Award of the Endocrine Society, 1973; jointly with Dr. Charles H. Sawyer; president of the American Association of Anatomists, 1973–74.

His major research interests have been centered on the physiology of reproduction, particularly on the hypothalamopituitary-ovarian system.

Contributions to the Substructure of Neuroendocrinology

JOHN W. EVERETT

At the 56th annual meeting of the American Association of Anatomists, two adjacent exhibits were the demonstration by F. L. Dey (1940) describing the follicular ovaries of guinea pigs resulting from anterior hypothalamic lesions and my demonstration (Everett, 1940a) concerned with spontaneous and light-induced persistent estrus in rats. I doubt that either of us recognized that we were concerned with closely interrelated phenomena.

How I came to be involved with persistent estrus is one of those accidents of time and place that so often determine the trend of events in one's personal affairs. In 1932 I had brought with me from J. S. Nicholas' colony at Yale several rats with which to establish a colony of inbred stock, later designated as the DA strain. It happened that these animals of mixed ancestry had acquired a trait leading to early female infertility. In virgin females and in breeders not immediately returned to the male after littering or lactation, there was an early onset of persistent estrus. These characteristics became acute problems around 1936–37 after several generations of inbreeding. There were also seasonal influences, with a marked decline in fertility during the winter months. In an attempt to compensate, I left the colony lights burning continually for nine days in late December 1938. Promptly nearly every cycling rat in the colony began to show persistent estrus, which in most cases was replaced by cyclic estrus once the light–dark rhythm was restored. During the previous year two independent reports had described similar induction of persistent estrus by continuous illumination

JOHN W. EVERETT ● Department of Anatomy, Duke University School of Medicine, Durham, North Carolina.

(Browman, 1937; Hemmingsen and Krarup, 1937). In the DA rats, the onset of the condition was exceedingly rapid in even young animals.

There was an obvious challenge in these various peculiarities. I felt that if persistent estrus could be prevented or if estrous cycles could be restored to rats that had already become persistent-estrous, much would be learned about normal reproductive physiology. Since lighting was clearly involved, rats were studied in parallel under conditions in which the daily exposure to light was regulated at either 9.5 hours or 14.5 hours, the approximate lengths of the solar days in this latitude at the winter and summer solstices, respectively. Details of that study were recently described elsewhere (Everett, 1970). From comparison with other strains and from hybridization experiments the conclusion was reached that the persistent estrus trait is governed by hereditary factors relating both to the age of the animal and to the length of daily illumination. One important observation was that in rats that had become persistent-estrous during the longer days, estrous cycles (with renewed corpus luteum formation) returned after a few weeks' exposure to the shorter days. Here was clear evidence that persistent estrus was not a permanent condition and could be counteracted.

Various hormonal treatments were instituted. Administration of a crude pituitary extract demonstrated that the persistent follicles could be luteinized. Estradiol benzoate in comparatively massive doses failed to induce luteinization and resulted in only a short anestrus several days later. In retrospect, the very fact that these animals failed to luteinize in response to their own estrogen was a foretoken of that result. Progesterone treatment then suggested itself, for the very reason that luteal tissue was conspicuously absent in persistent-estrous rats. I have the impression that Dr. George Corner may have encouraged me to try progesterone. I am sure that we discussed the general problem at one time. Phillips (1937) had shown that small daily dosages of progesterone (< 1.0 mg) would not interfere with the normal estrous cycle of rats. My initial trials with progesterone quickly demonstrated its usefulness in the persistent estrus problem. A single injection of 0.5–1.0 mg interrupted spontaneous persistent estrus for two to four days, while subsequent daily treatment with even smaller amounts was accompanied by surprisingly regular cycles, usually with luteinization (Everett, 1940a,b). Similar treatment of rats exposed to continuous illumination demonstrated that progesterone would sustain normal cyclic ovarian function under those conditions, preventing the onset of persistent estrus for as long as the daily injections were continued (Everett, 1940a).

The logical progression from these findings was to determine whether the regular daily supply of progesterone was essential or whether progesterone might be particularly important during diestrus or proestrus once the steady state of persistent estrus had been interrupted. The latter

proved to be the case, for regular cycles could be sustained simply by injecting progesterone during each successive proestrus (Everett, 1943). From this
fact it was an easy step to demonstrating a positive effect in cyclic females
of both the DA strain and a normal strain derived from Osborne–Mendel
stock. In 5-day cyclic females, progesterone injection on the third day of
diestrus advanced ovulation 24 hours (Everett, 1944*a*, 1948).

Discovery of the comparable advancement of ovulation by estrogen
treatment (Everett, 1948) resulted from trials with combinations of estrogen
and progesterone treatments in persistent-estrous DA rats. Although injection of estradiol benzoate during persistent estrus had failed to induce ovulation, it seemed possible that, if the persistent estrus was first interrupted
by a progesterone injection, treatment with estrogen during the ensuing
diestrus might be effective. However, that also failed. But estradiol benzoate
given to 5-day cyclic Osborne–Mendel rats on diestrus day 2 resulted in
ovulation 24 hours early.

Comparisons of corpora lutea from formerly persistent-estrous DA
rats that had been rendered cyclic by progesterone therapy, on the one
hand, with corpora lutea from cyclic rats of the normal strain, on the other
hand, presented distinct histologic and histochemical differences (Everett,
1944*b*). In the former case the cell volume was distinctly smaller and the
amount of Schultz-positive lipid (cholesterol) was far less than that in the
normal animals. These differences suggested a moderate degree of
luteotropic prolactin stimulation in the Osborne–Mendel rats and its
absence in the others. The obvious next step was to treat persistent-estrous
rats with small amounts of prolactin after a set of corpora lutea had been
induced by progesterone. By using a fluctuating daily dosage, inadequate to
maintain a pseudopregnancy, it was possible to reproduce the histologic and
histochemical features of the normal corpus luteum (Everett, 1944*b*, 1945).
In fact, it was possible to sustain ovulatory cycles in sequence by continuing
the treatment, provided that one set of corpora lutea had first been induced
by progesterone. In their absence the prolactin treatment was ineffective
and persistent estrus returned. This clearly indicated that the maintenance
of cycles was due to a moderate secretory activity of the corpora lutea and
not to gonadotropin contamination of the prolactin (ICSH activity was not
detectable in hypophysectomized subjects).

Comparatively large amounts of daily prolactin, on the other hand,
produced pseudopregnancy, characterized by enlarged corpora lutea
containing little visible lipid. Investigation of mechanisms involved in the
accumulation of lipid stores in corpora lutea led to the administration of
estradiol benzoate in normally pseudopregnant and pregnant rats and, thus,
to the finding that such treatment would induce ovulation (Everett, 1947).
Administration of estradiol benzoate on day 4 (the fourth day of leukocytic

vaginal smears) resulted in ovulation during the second night and the deposition of large amounts of Schultz-positive lipid in the corpora lutea, provided that the pituitary glands were intact. Similar effects were produced by LH when injected on day 5 at the time of hypophysectomy, but not in rats hypophysectomized the previous day. The ability of corpora lutea to store cholesterol in response to LH was shown to require the luteotropic action of prolactin and to be counteracted by a prolactin excess.

At this point it was appropriate to re-examine the refractoriness of DA rats to estrogen for LH release. Functional interrelationship between estrogen and progesterone had been indicated by the fact that for inducing ovulation in the persistent-estrous animal progesterone was most effective in late diestrus or proestrus (Everett, 1943). Several persistent-estrous rats were made "pseudopregnant" by daily injection of 1.5 mg progesterone (Everett, 1948). The administration of 50 μg estradiol benzoate on the fifth day usually induced either ovulation or luteinization with trapped ova. Thus it had become abundantly clear that in this species the induction of gonadotropin release and ovulation results from an increment of estrogen and that progesterone facilitates this estrogen effect.

It was also apparent that the progesterone effect is exerted on the day of its administration, whereas the effect of estrogen is delayed some 24 hours, suggesting a lengthy intermediary chain of events. It was also recognized that a relatively long-acting form of estrogen must be used. Estradiol-17β had proven ineffective (25 μg in oil) unless in a form allowing slow release (as a crystal or in a beeswax pellet).

Whatever the time of steroid injection, if ovulation was induced, the new corpora lutea were consistently in a common stage of development at a given time later that day and were very similar to the new corpora lutea of spontaneously ovulating animals. Hence the responsible gonadotropic stimulation must have occurred at comparable hours in all cases. Boling and associates (1941a) had related the progress of follicle maturation and the time of ovulation to the onset of behavioral estrus. Although they did not link the ovarian events with time of day, it had been shown by others (Hemmingsen and Krarup, 1937) that the onset of heat behavior is associated with the daily activity rhythm. Thus the Boling data indirectly coupled ovulation with clock hours. In a group of 28 normal 4-day cyclic rats autopsied during the early morning of the day following proestrus, I found ovulation between 0100 h and 0230 h, direct evidence indeed for that relationship (Everett, 1948).

Meanwhile Sawyer, Markee, and associates (1947, 1949) had demonstrated that in rabbits the coital stimulus for ovulation could be blocked by rapid intravenous injection of Dibenamine or atropine sulfate within a few minutes after coitus. If administration of either drug was delayed 5 min, ovulation was not prevented. Sawyer and I had been closely associated during studies of serum cholinesterase in rats as influenced by hormonal status. There was mutual interest in each other's work on ovulation in the rabbit and rat. We speculated about the possibility of blocking ovulation in rats by means of the drugs that would block the ovulation reflex in rabbits. Our first experiments in rats with Dibenamine were carried out in late November 1947 in pregnant animals injected with estradiol benzoate on day 4 (Sawyer, Everett, and Markee, 1949). Dibenamine administration on either that day or the next morning usually prevented the ovulation expected during the second night. The first trials in cyclic rats soon followed; Dibenamine injection during the morning or early afternoon of proestrus often prevented ovulation, while injection late in the afternoon usually failed to interfere (Everett, Sawyer, and Markee, 1949). Thus it was evident that some event subject to interruption by this drug takes place during the afternoon of proestrus about 12 hours before ovulation. Subsequently, by use of atropine sulfate in massive subcutaneous dosage, it was possible to define the proestrus "critical period" more precisely. When given before 1400 h, atropine uniformly blocked ovulation and failed to interfere when given at 1600 h. It was also more uniformly effective than Dibenamine in the pregnancy experiments. We did not attempt to delimit a critical period in the estrogen-induced ovulation in pregnant rats, possibly because we were puzzled to find that one rat of five had two luteinized follicles in spite of the fact that atropine had been injected at 0800 h. In retrospect, that evidence of a very early beginning of the induced LH surge may now be ascribed to the ongoing progesterone secretion, since in 4-day cyclic rats progesterone injection very early on the day of proestrus (0530 h) has occasionally caused partial ovulation despite atropine injection at 0800 h (Redmond, 1968).

Inasmuch as the spontaneous ovulation of rats can be blocked by the same drugs that can block the reflex ovulation of rabbits, it appeared that we were dealing in both species with hypothalamic mechanisms and with the neurovascular linkage of the hypothalamus to the adenohypophysis. Green and Harris (1947) had recently proposed that the various secretions of the pars distalis are regulated by chemotransmitters passing to the gland via the hypophyseal portal vessels. The blocking experiments with Dibenamine, an adrenergic blocking agent, had been interpreted as evidence that the chemotransmitter for LH might be a catecholamine. Since the atropine-sensitive link in the coital reflex in rabbits is more rapidly completed than the Dibenamine-sensitive link, it was considered that atropine acts more centrally than the adrenergic blocker (Sawyer, Markee, and Townsend, 1949).

Early in 1949 Hans Lowenbach of the Department of Psychiatry at Duke presented a seminar on the effects of hypoxia on hypothalamic

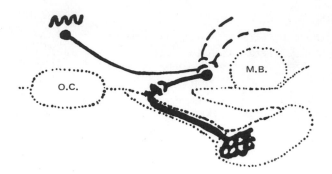

FIGURE 1. A schematic diagram presented at a seminar in 1949 to illustrate the concept of a diurnally rhythmic physiologic clock in the rostral hypothalamus governing the ovulatory discharge of gonadotropin. *O.C.* = optic chiasma; *M.B.* = mammillary body.

temperature in cats. The fact that pentobarbital had been used as anesthetic led to consideration of the drug's influence on the hypothalamus. That discussion is directly responsible for our use of pentobarbital as an agent for blocking ovulation in rats. My journal records, as of March 1949, the simple question: "Can ovulation of [4-day cyclic] rats be blocked by Nembutal at 3 thru 5 PM ?" The affirmative answer to the question led within a few weeks to the finding that not only is the ovulatory discharge of gonadotropin normally confined to the afternoon of proestrus, but the "LH-release apparatus" in rats has an inherent 24-hour periodicity (Everett and Sawyer, 1950).

Hillarp (1949) reported the induction of persistent estrus in rats by large, bilateral anterior hypothalamic lesions, thus confirming Dey's earlier finding in guinea pigs (1940). Hillarp also noted that the effect could be produced by much smaller lesions close to the arcuate nuclei. This crystallized our view that spontaneous ovulation involves a signal from the brain analogous to the reflexly induced signal in the rabbit. In view of the fact that by pentobarbital sedation during the proestrus critical period and then on successive days at similar hours one could produce a follicular cycle (a sort of persistent estrus), it seemed that the diurnally cyclic mechanism might reside in the rostral hypothalamus. With that thought in mind I made the rough lantern slide sketch shown in Figure 1 for presentation in a local seminar. The broken lines converging on the representative tuberal (arcuate) neuron were intended to represent whatever hormonal and afferent neural input might be essential to sustaining the day-to-day gonadotropic activity of the follicular phase of the cycle (activity later termed "tonic" by Barraclough and Gorski, 1961).

The 24-hour rhythmicity involved in rat ovulation had first been recognized in our analysis of the advanced ovulation induced by progesterone administration to 5-day cyclic rats on diestrus day 3 (Everett and Sawyer, 1949). That effect could be blocked by atropine injection at 1400 h, although progesterone had been given six hours earlier. We discussed three alternative hypotheses, as follows: (1) "Neurohumoral stimulation of the hypophysis occurs at a regular time each day and . . . response of the gland depends entirely on local modification of its threshold of activation by the sex steroids." (2) "A principal site of action of the sex steroids is in the tuberal region and (or) the median eminence, where they serve to lower thresholds to a variety of afferent impulses. . . . [Given] adequate steroid levels at these sites, stimuli from the 24-hour 'clock' administer the coup de grace." (3) "The center in the rostral hypothalamus is characterized by an (intrinsic?) diurnal rhythm of sensitivity, but its own threshold of excitation is determined by local action of sex steroids." These hypotheses remain current. They are not mutually exclusive.

In view of present-day moves to extend neuroendocrine studies to species other than rabbits and rats, it is appropriate to recall certain precautions stated by Everett and Sawyer (1950), as follows: "A diurnal rhythm of excitability of the LH-release apparatus may exist in only certain species, while in others the neural mechanism may be continuously near threshold for perhaps several days during each cycle. If periodic excitability is actually the rule, it may in some species be demonstrable under only the most rigid control of (physical and social) environmental conditions. Conceivably there are species in which [the specific ovulating stimulus to the hypophysis] may extend for a much longer time than in rats." We also emphasized that the ovulation-blocking capability of a barbiturate is not closely related to its depressant effect on motor activity, pointing out that ovulation can be blocked by phenobarbital at dosage levels producing barely detectable ataxia.

During a visit to our laboratories by Geoffrey Harris in 1950 many of the above ideas were discussed. He mentioned that Bard had recently told him of an experiment in which the hypothalamus of a bitch had been surgically isolated from the rest of the brain. The animal had subsequently come into heat. We speculated about whether she may also have ovulated. Recent developments in rats (Halász, 1969) and monkeys (Knobil, 1974) make it likely that she did.

Another discussion with Harris during that visit concerned an experiment by Westman and Jacobsohn (1938) which had greatly puzzled me. *After* cutting the pituitary stalk in rats and inserting a metal foil barrier, they had stimulated the cervix and apparently induced pseudopregnancy thereby. The solution of the puzzle became apparent when I later read

Desclin's (1950) paper describing the induction of pseudopregnancy by estrogen administration to hypophysectomized rats bearing hypophyseal grafts on the kidney. Neither Desclin nor Westman and Jacobsohn had tested for pseudopregnancy after simply isolating the hypophysis from the brain by transplantation or stalk sectioning. The outcome of such experiments was essentially certain. I soon found that the transplanted gland can recover promptly and, while losing most of its trophic activities, can maintain corpus luteum function for weeks and even months (Everett, 1954, 1956). There was thus an implied increase in prolactin output and, in turn, an implied inhibitory influence of the hypothalamus on that one secretion of the pars distalis.

It was logical at that point to ask whether normal secretory functions would return to such a transplant if it was regrafted under the brain. Harris and Jacobsohn (1952) had found that hypophyseal homotransplants, placed under the tuber cinereum at the time of hypophysectomy in female rats, rapidly acquired vascular connection from the median eminence. Normal estrous cycles soon resumed. The retransplantation experiment was to differ from this in that the animal's own pituitary gland was first to be transferred to the kidney capsule where it would become established for several weeks as a prolactin secreting tissue. Then it would be returned close to the median eminence. The experiment was skillfully accomplished by Miroslava Nikitovitch-Winer, who came to my laboratory as a graduate student in 1955. Reasonably normal estrous cycles returned not long after the second operation and many of the animals became pregnant (Nikitovitch-Winer and Everett, 1958, 1959). Thyrotropic and corticotropic activities, essentially lost by grafts remaining on the kidney, were also restored in the retransplanted glands. The functional repair was accompanied by renewed cytologic differentiation.

Another aspect of the interrelationship of the control mechanisms for gonadotropin and prolactin secretion was seen in the *delayed pseudopregnancy* phenomenon, regularly encountered after infertile mating in pentobarbital-blocked rats (Everett, 1952, 1967). Although the stimulus (coitus) took place during the infertile cycle, its effect was expressed only when a new cyclic ovulation had taken place several days later—pseudopregnancy beginning then lasted for the usual 12 to 14 days.

The mating trials that led to delayed pseudopregnancy were actually intended to determine whether reflex ovulation could be demonstrated in pentobarbital-blocked rats. That had been suggested by the report of Dempsey and Searles (1943) that corpora lutea were formed after copulation in rats that became persistent-estrous under continuous illumination. My intent was to block spontaneous ovulation with pentobarbital on the proestrus afternoon, to place the female with a known fertile male overnight, and to give the usual blocking dose of pentobarbital (or phenobarbital) on the second afternoon. The rationale was that if the female copulated during the intervening night and if copulation induced an ovulatory discharge of gonadotropin, this could be detected on the third morning by the presence of corpora lutea whose approximate age could be evaluated histologically. As it turned out, the majority of the females copulated and some of them ovulated in response (Everett, 1952, 1967). However, the frequency of success was disappointing and it seemed that if the question of provoked ovulation was to be further pursued, the better experimental subject would be the rat with light-induced persistent estrus. In the summers of 1955 and 1956 a medical student, J. P. Bunn, attempted to repeat the experiments described by Dempsey and Searles, with the intent of determining whether the reflex ovulation could be induced either by an observed copulation or possibly by artificial stimulation of the cervix. After weeks of failure we decided to try stimulating the brain through an indwelling electrode. This gave immediate success, as reported the following year (Bunn and Everett, 1957). In most cases the electrode tip rested in the amygdala, while in one rat it was in the septum. It did not occur to us that the pentobarbital-blocked, cyclic rat might be a suitable experimental subject.

Critchlow (1957, 1958), perhaps at the urging of C. H. Sawyer, his mentor, was more venturesome and demonstrated that pentobarbital anesthesia was actually no hindrance. Stimulation through a pair of electrodes deep in the hypothalamus immediately over the median eminence was regularly followed by ovulation in spite of the pentobarbital. This was a breakthrough and since that time the pentobarbital-blocked proestrous rat has become an important tool in neuroendocrine research.

In 1958, R. L. Riley and I undertook to repeat Critchlow's experiment, planning to see whether ovulation could be induced during diestrus or pseudopregnancy. After mediocre success in the proestrous animals when electrodes were in the tuberal region, we explored areas farther forward, finding far more predictable results with electrodes in the medial preoptic area. Preoptic stimulation was also effective in late diestrus in the 5-day cycle (Everett, Riley, and Christian, 1959), inducing advanced ovulation, although a more intense stimulus was then required. It was also possible to induce ovulation during pseudopregnancy, especially toward its close but sometimes as early as day 5 (unpublished). Two years later, with the aid of some 500 rats and with the valuable collaboration of J. R. Harp, J. W. Holsinger, and H. M. Radford, the following information had been revealed (see Everett, 1961, 1964; Everett and Radford, 1961): (1) Effectiveness of stimulation with a wide variety of pulse patterns was related to size of an electrolytic lesion produced thereby. (2) The apparent stimulative action of the lesion was probably not due to interruption of an inhibitory pathway, since only a unilateral lesion was needed. Furthermore, comparable preoptic damage by mechanical or radio-frequency lesions failed to induce ovulation. (3) An iron deposit from the stainless steel electrode was always present in the effective lesion. (4) Microinjection of $FeCl_3$ reproduced the effect of the electrochemical lesion. (5) Continuous direct current electrolysis was as effective as monophasic pulses. (6) The larger amount of electric current needed on diestrus day 3 compared with that on proestrus was represented by a proportionately larger electrochemical lesion. (7) Electrochemical stimulation of the septum could also induce ovulation, provided that a comparatively large electrochemical lesion was introduced. (8) Mapping studies suggested a highly dispersed neuronal system originating in the septal complex, continuing as a diffuse system through the medial preoptic area and anterior hypothalamus, and finally converging sharply to the medial basal tuber. (9) For inducing ovulation only a part of this system need be activated.

About 10 years were to pass before the electrochemical stimulation technique came into use in other laboratories. Even yet we do not know how its stimulative action comes about. Meanwhile, I demonstrated that ovulation can be induced by nonlesioning biphasic pulse trains delivered through platinum electrodes, provided that stimulation continues for 45–60 minutes (Everett, 1965). Both methods should continue to prove useful in further study of the central neural controls for ovulation.

It has been instructive to review the old records during the writing of this essay. There is much unfinished business, a good deal of which has awaited development of techniques that have only recently become available. The challenge of the persistent estrus phenomenon has not been forgotten. In fact, we have recently been comparing persistent-estrous and cyclic rats with respect to the relative amounts of LH discharged following either treatment with LRF or electrical stimulation of the hypothalamus. The primary defect seems to be in the brain and not the pituitary gland. Such a conclusion fits with early evidence that persistent-estrous rats rarely show estrous behavior (Everett, 1939; Boling, *et al.* 1941*b*).

ACKNOWLEDGMENTS

It is a pleasure to name the following persons who gave valuable technical assistance at different times from 1939 to 1965: Charles Erixon, Mahlon Hedrick, William Wilson, Sibyl Yost, Mary Bercowitz, H. B. Thurston, Betty Dalehite, Hill Grimmett, Steven Lang, John Snow, John Gehweiler, Mary Gibson, James Townsend, Elbert Mundy, George Ploza,

Paul Eckman, Ronald Everett, John Sadler, William Fore, Daniel Tucker, Terence George, David Spitler, Janice Everett, Matthew Patton, Michael Temko, Donald Craft, James Booher, Clara Flanagan, Roger Poor, Edward Robe, Sandra Osinchak, Peter Duke, Beverley Champion, Frank Cowherd, James Fuqua, Fred Daugherty, and Grover Henderson.

Research in my laboratory from 1949 to 1959 was variously supported by the Research Council of Duke University and the Committee for Research in Problems of Sex, NAS-NRC. Subsequent support was by grants from the National Science Foundation.

REFERENCES

Barraclough, C. A., and R. A. Gorski (1961). Evidence that the hypothalamus is responsible for androgen-induced sterility in the female rat. *Endocrinology* **68:** 68.

Boling, J. L., R. J. Blandau, A. L. Soderwall, and W. C. Young (1941*a*). Growth of the Graafian follicle and the time of ovulation in the albino rat. *Anat. Rec.* **79:** 313.

Boling, J. L., R. J. Blandau, B. Rundlett, and W. C. Young (1941*b*). Factors underlying the failure of cyclic mating behavior in the albino rat. *Anat. Rec.* **80:** 155.

Browman, L. G. (1937). Light in its relation to activity and estrus rhythms in the albino rat. *J. Exp. Zool.* **75:** 375.

Bunn, J. P., and J. W. Everett (1957). Ovulation of persistent-estrous rats after electrical stimulation of the brain. *Proc. Soc. Exp. Biol. Med.* (N.Y.) **96:** 369.

Critchlow, B. V. (1957). Ovulation induced by hypothalamic stimulation in the rat. *Anat. Rec.* **127:** 283.

Critchlow, V. (1958). Ovulation induced by hypothalamic stimulation in the anesthetized rat. *Am. J. Physiol.* **195:** 171.

Dempsey, E. W., and H. F. Searles (1943). Environmental modification of certain endocrine phenomena. *Endocrinology* **32:** 119.

Desclin, L. (1950). À propos du mécanisme d'action des oestrogènes sur le lobe antérieur de l'hypophyse chez le Rat. *Ann. Endocrinol.* (*Paris*) **11:** 656.

Dey, F. L. (1940). Ovarian and uterine changes in guinea pigs with hypothalamic lesions. *Anat. Rec.* **76** (2) (Suppl.): 86.

Everett, J. W. (1939). Spontaneous persistent estrus in a strain of albino rats. *Endocrinology* **25:** 123.

Everett, J. W. (1940*a*). Persistent estrus, correlated with a failure of spontaneous ovulation, appearing in early life in a certain strain of rats. *Anat. Rec.* **76** (2) (Suppl.): 87.

Everett, J. W. (1940*b*). The restoration of ovulatory cycles and corpus luteum formation in persistent-estrous rats by progesterone. *Endocrinology* **27:** 681.

Everett, J. W. (1943). Further studies on the relationship of progesterone to ovulation and luteinization in the persistent-estrous rat. *Endocrinology* **32:** 285.

Everett, J. W. (1944*a*). Evidence in the normal albino rat that progesterone facilitates ovulation and corpus-luteum formation. *Endocrinology* **34:** 136.

Everett, J. W. (1944*b*). Evidence suggesting a role of the lactogenic hormone in the estrous cycle of the albino rat. *Endocrinology* **35:** 507.

Everett, J. W. (1945). The microscopically demonstrable lipids of cyclic corpora lutea in the rat. *Am. J. Anat.* **77:** 293.

Everett, J. W. (1947). Hormonal factors responsible for deposition of cholesterol in the corpus luteum of the rat. *Endocrinology* **41**: 364.

Everett, J. W. (1948). Progesterone and estrogen in the experimental control of ovulation time and other features of the estrous cycle in the rat. *Endocrinology* **43**: 389.

Everett, J. W. (1952). Presumptive hypothalamic control of spontaneous ovulation. *Ciba Found. Colloq. Endocrinol.* **4**: 167.

Everett, J. W. (1954). Luteotrophic function of autografts of the rat hypophysis. *Endocrinology* **54**: 685.

Everett, J. W. (1956). Functional corpora lutea maintained for months by autografts of rat hypophyses. *Endocrinology* **58**: 786.

Everett, J. W. (1961). The preoptic region of the brain and its relation to ovulation. Pages 101–112 in C. A. Villee, ed. *Control of Ovulation.* Pergamon Press, New York.

Everett, J. W. (1964). Preoptic stimulative lesions and ovulation in the rat: 'Thresholds' and LH-release time in late diestrus and proestrus. Pages 346–366 in E. Bajusz and G. Jasmin, eds. *Major Problems in Neuroendocrinology.* S. Karger, Basel/New York.

Everett, J. W. (1965). Ovulation in rats from preoptic stimulation through platinum electrodes. Importance of duration and spread of stimulus. *Endocrinology* **76**: 1195.

Everett, J. W. (1967). Provoked ovulation or long-delayed pseudopregnancy from coital stimuli in barbiturate-blocked rats. *Endocrinology* **80**: 145.

Everett, J. W. (1970). Photoregulation of the ovarian cycle in the rat. Pages 387–403 in J. Benoit and I. Assenmacher, eds. *La Photorégulation de la Reproduction chez les Oiseaux et les Mammifères.* CNRS, Paris.

Everett, J. W., and H. M. Radford (1961). Irritative deposits from stainless steel electrodes in the preoptic rat brain causing release of pituitary gonadotropin. *Proc. Soc. Exp. Biol. Med.* (*New York*) **108**: 604.

Everett, J. W., R. L. Riley, and C. D. Christian (1959). Ovulation after stimulating the rat hypothalamus late in diestrus. *Proceedings of the Endocrine Society,* 41st Annual Meeting.

Everett, J. W., and C. H. Sawyer (1949). A neural timing factor in the mechanism by which progesterone advances ovulation in the cyclic rat. *Endocrinology* **45**: 581.

Everett, J. W., and C. H. Sawyer (1950). A 24-hour periodicity in the "LH-release apparatus" of female rats, disclosed by barbiturate sedation. *Endocrinology* **47**: 198.

Everett, J. W., C. H. Sawyer, and J. E. Markee (1949). A neurogenic timing factor in control of the ovulatory discharge of luteinizing hormone in the cyclic rat. *Endocrinology* **44**: 234.

Green, J. D., and G. W. Harris (1947). The neurovascular link between the neurohypophysis and adenohypophysis. *J. Endocrinol.* **5**: 136.

Halász, B. (1969). The endocrine effects of isolation of the hypothalamus from the rest of the brain. Pages 307–342 in W. F. Ganong and L. Martini, eds. *Frontiers in Neuroendocrinology,* Oxford Univ. Press, New York.

Harris, G. W., and D. Jacobsohn (1952). Functional grafts of the anterior pituitary gland. Proc. R. Soc. London Ser. B, **139**: 263.

Hemmingsen, A. M., and N. B. Krarup (1937). Rhythmic diurnal variations in the oestrous phenomena of the rat and their susceptibility to light and dark. *K. Dan. Vidensk. Selsk., Biol. Medd.* **13** (7): 1.

Hillarp, N.-Å. (1949). Studies on the localization of hypothalamic centres controlling the gonadotrophic function of the hypophysis. *Acta Endocrinol.* **2**: 11.

Knobil, E. (1974). On the control of gonadotropin secretion in the rhesus monkey. *Recent Prog. Horm. Res.* **30**: 1.

Nikitovitch-Winer, M., and J. W. Everett (1958). Functional restitution of pituitary grafts retransplanted from kidney to median eminence. *Endocrinology* **63**: 916.

Nikitovitch-Winer, M., and J. W. Everett (1959). Histocytologic changes in grafts of rat pituitary on the kidney and upon re-transplantation under the diencephalon. *Endocrinology* **65**: 357.

Phillips, W. A. (1937). The inhibition of oestrous cycles in the albino rat by progesterone. *Am. J. Physiol.* **119**: 623.

Redmond, W. C. (1968). Ovulatory response to brain stimulation or exogenous luteinizing hormone in progesterone-treated rats. *Endocrinology* **83**: 1013.

Sawyer, C. H., J. W. Everett, and J. E. Markee (1949). A neural factor in the mechanism by which estrogen induces the release of luteinizing hormone in the rat. *Endocrinology* **44**: 218.

Sawyer, C. H., J. E. Markee, and W. H. Hollinshead (1947). The inhibition of ovulation in the rabbit by the adrenergic blocking agent Dibenamine. *Endocrinology* **41**: 395.

Sawyer, C. H., J. E. Markee, and B. F. Townsend (1949). Cholinergic and adrenergic components in the neurohumoral control of the release of LH in the rabbit. *Endocrinology* **44**: 18.

Terasawa, E., and C. H. Sawyer (1969). Electrical and electrochemical stimulation of the hypothalamo-hypophysial system with stainless steel electrodes. *Endocrinology* **84**: 918.

Westman, A., and D. Jacobsohn (1938). Endokrinologische Untersuchungen an Ratten mit durchtrennten Hypophysenstiel. VI. Production und Abgabe der Gonadotropen Hormone. *Acta Pathol. Microbiol. Scand.* **15**: 445.

8

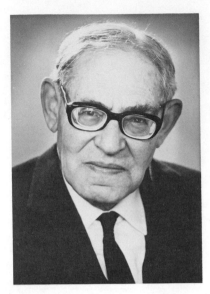

Hans Heller

Hans Heller was born in September 1905, at Brunn, Czechoslovakia, which was Austrian until 1918. He graduated Dr. rer. nat. in Prague in 1927 and from 1928 to 1934 held an appointment in the Department of Pharmacology, University of Vienna, which was punctuated by a spell in England.

After leaving Austria in 1934 he qualified in medicine at Cambridge in 1938 and was awarded a Beit Memorial Fellowship in the following year. In 1942 he became Lecturer-in-Charge of the Department of Pharmacology of the University of Bristol and later Professor and Head from 1949 until his retirement in 1971. He passed away in December, 1974.

Hans Heller edited the *Journal of Endocrinology* from 1963 to 1974 and had been chairman of the Society for Endocrinology since 1971. He was president of the European Society for Comparative Endocrinology from 1965 to 1969 and was a member of the Central Committee of the International Society of Endocrinology and of the Advisory Committee for *General and Comparative Endocrinology*.

Along with his research work, Hans Heller edited *The Neurohypophysis* (Butterworths, 1957); *Oxytocin*, with R. Caldeyro-Barcia (Pergamon Press, 1961); *Neurosecretion*, with R. B. Clark (Academic Press, 1962); *Comparative Endocrinology*, with U.S. von Euler (Academic Press, 1963); *Pharmacology of the Endocrine System: The Neurohypophysis*, with B. T. Pickering (Section 41 of International Encyclopaedia of Pharmacology and Therapeutics; Pergamon Press, 1970); and *Subcellular Organization and Function in Endocrine Tissues*, with K. Lederis (Mem. Soc. Endocr. 19, Cambridge University Press, 1971).

Ned Opes Ned Vires Sed Artis Aceptra Permanent*

HANS HELLER

At the beginning of 1928, Professor E. P. Pick, head of the Institute of Pharmacology of the University of Vienna, was looking for a research assistant with a degree in organic chemistry. I had obtained such a degree the previous year by studies which included a year of research in the field of organic arsenic compounds. This had led me to the work of Paul Ehrlich, whose hypotheses on the selective binding of dyes and dyelike arsenic compounds made a deep impression on me. Pharmacology seemed therefore to be the right subject for me: I applied for the post and obtained it. At that time Pick was interested in the findings of several workers that extracts of duodenal mucosa produce a hypoglycemic effect and that they do so even when given by mouth. The latter statement was of special interest to him because a friend of his, Msgr. Ignaz Seipel, formerly a professor of theology in the University of Vienna and thus a colleague of his, and later Federal Chancellor of the Republic of Austria, was a diabetic and had complained to him about the discomfort caused by the injection, several times daily, of soluble insulin, the only preparation then available. I was able to confirm that extract of the upper third of the small intestine lowered the blood sugar of rabbits when given parenterally and that the dried extract when given in very much larger doses was also orally active. Moreover, because it proved impossible by standard methods to extract insulin from the intestinal mucous membrane, I came to the somewhat daring conclusion that my intestinal principle acted by releasing insulin (see Heller, 1931). This hypothesis could not be verified, since, of course, at that time methods for measuring insulin in the blood were not available. When—more than 30 years later—this became possible, the release of insulin from the pancreas by inte-

---

* Neither wealth nor power but the rules of learning remain. (Inscription on Tycho de Brahe's tombstone in the Teyn Church at Prague.)

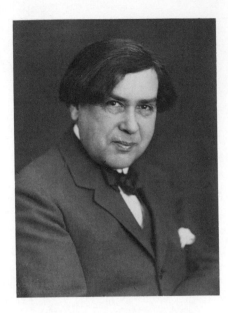

FIGURE 1. Alfred Fröhlich, in the early 1930s.

stinal extracts both *in vivo* and *in vitro* was demonstrated by many investigators. However, whether this activity is exerted by one or a combination of the known intestinal hormones (secretin, pancreozymin, enteroglucagon) or yet by another factor has even now not been established, according to the most recent review of the subject (Pfeiffer, Raptis, and Fussgänger, 1973).

While occupied with this laborious work—the mucosa from miles of cattle gut from the slaughter house had to be scraped off—I kept my ears open when other members of the department discussed their work around the tea table in the afternoon. The company was stimulating and varied and was still very much under the influence of Pick's predecessor, Hans Horst Meyer, who had retired in 1924. Meyer had come from Germany to Vienna and had retained his pronounced East Prussian accent. He had an incisive and sparkling mind. Although a smallish man, he had a magnificent, sharp-beaked head reminding me of the old Norman knight, de Aquila, whom Kipling in *Puck of Pook's Hill* describes as "pouncing in his talk like an eagle, but always binding fast." Indeed, he had some of the fierceness of a bird of prey. When, some years later, he was told by E. P. Pick that I intended to marry, he is reputed to have said: "Throw him out: A married research assistant does not work properly." Historically speaking, Meyer's greatest merit was probably the fact that in his famous textbook, *Die experimentelle Pharmakologie als Grundlage der Arzneibehandlung* (Experimental Pharmacology as Basis of Drug Therapy), published in 1910, he was one of the first to divorce pharmacology decisively from materia medica by grouping drugs according to their site of action rather than according to their chemistry.

Other permanent members of the departmental staff were Alfred Fröhlich, the associate professor, and two younger men, Hans Molitor and Richard Rössler. Also present were usually some visiting workers from abroad and some clinicians who, because of poor facilities in their respective hospitals and clinics, did their experimental work in the department of pharmacology. Fröhlich (Figure 1) had become famous when, as a young man, he described the syndrome of adiposogenital dystrophy which still bears his name. The patient, a boy of 14, had been suffering from attacks of vomiting and headaches for $2\frac{1}{2}$ years and during that time had been rapidly gaining weight. When seen by Fröhlich in September 1901 he was blind in the left eye and vision in the right eye was also diminishing. Fröhlich diagnosed a tumor in the neighbourhood of the brain stem and suggested that it had originated in the pituitary. He recommended surgical intervention. An operation was performed at which a cystic tumor of the pituitary was found and drained. An excellent photograph of the patient before the operation is included in Fröhlich's original publication (1901). According to a note (p. 272) in John F. Fulton's *Biography of Harvey Cushing,* the patient was still alive in 1939.

At the time I worked in Vienna, Fröhlich—who presented an unusual picture since he wore his hair long, which then was only done by the more eccentric type of artist—had a modest office in the basement of the institute. Like many associate professors in the Austrian universities, he had little in the way of research facilities. In fact, his graduate research assistant, Dr. Feher, was paid by a well-to-do clinician, Professor E. Zack, with whom Fröhlich collaborated. As the brilliantly clever son of a rich Jewish family, Fröhlich had traveled widely before the First World War and had spent some months in Liverpool in Sherrington's laboratory where he met Harvey Cushing, who became his lifelong friend. He had joined H. H. Meyer in 1906 and became a *Dozent* in 1910. He had maintained his interest in the pituitary for some years—having been one of the first to confirm Dale's discovery of the oxytocic effect of neurohypophysial extracts—but by the time I knew him he was mainly interested in cardiovascular problems. He left Vienna in 1939 and went to the United States where he worked in the May Institute for Medical Research in Cincinnati until his death in 1952. However, other members of the department were deeply interested in the neurohypophysis. Beginning in 1925 Pick himself and his senior lecturer, Hans Molitor, published a series of papers in which they advanced the hypothesis that body water is regulated by a center situated in the mid-brain which they called "water center." They postulated that this center was under the inhibitory influence of the cerebral cortex and assumed further that removal of this restraining influence either by surgical means or by certain hypnotics led to overactivity of the center which in that state could no longer be inhibited by posterior pituitary extracts. They upheld their hypothesis of a central effect of the antidiuretic hormone in spite of the observation by Starling and Verney in 1925 that posterior pituitary extracts decrease urine flow in a heart-lung-kindney preparation and a report of Janssen (1928) that such extracts retained their inhibitory action in animals whose brain had been removed down to the level of the corpora quadrigemina. In fact, they disregarded the possibility of a renal action of a neurohypophyseal hormone, although they themselves had shown earlier that dogs with chronic kidney lesions produced by corrosive poisons no longer responded to posterior pituitary extracts.

Another part of the water center hypothesis was the assumption that a decrease in the water content of the plasma led to its stimulation, which then caused the tissues to liberate water into the blood. Some diuretics like caffein and organic mercurials were thought to mobilize water in the same manner and this hypothesis was apparently supported by the results of one of the part-time clinical workers in the department, Fritz Brunn, who, stimulated by Pick, had found in 1921 that posterior pituitary extract caused water retention in frogs. In 1929 it was suggested to me to investigate further this "Brunn effect" (as it is frequently called to this day). This work led to two papers (Heller, 1930a, 1930b). In the first I came to the conclusion that, contrary to the prevailing opinion in the laboratory, the Brunn effect was not caused by a "change in the physicochemical state of tissue colloids" and that it was associated with an inhibitory action of the posterior pituitary extract on the frog kidney. The second paper recorded the then very puzzling finding that both oxytocin and vasopressin exerted a pronounced Brunn effect in frogs. (The explanation came many years later when it was shown—as discussed further on—that the main neurohypophyseal hormone in frogs is vasotocin, a polypeptide whose chemical constitution is intermediate between that of the two mammalian hormones.) The results reported in these two papers were statistically evaluated, i.e., I calculated the significance of differences by a method similar to Student's t test, which was at that time very unusual. When I—rather proudly—showed the manuscripts to E. P. Pick, he said "My dear boy, why did you go to all this mathematical trouble. If your results are clear, you do not need it, and if you do not see at a glance what they show, statistics will not help."

The laboratory was often visited by workers from other universities. The most regular visitor was probably Otto Loewi who, on his way home to

Graz, often passed through Vienna. I remember in particular one occasion when he had attended a meeting of the German Pharmacological Society. He was invited to tea and Meyer, Pick, and Loewi discussed the meeting and started to demolish the scientific reputation of a good many of their senior colleagues. The moment Loewi had left, Pick—usually the kindest of men—turned to Meyer and said, "I don't know why Loewi should be so critical. After all, he is not so marvelous himself." This happened, of course, before Loewi had received the Nobel prize.

Loewi was the first of the founders of the theory of the humoral transmission of nervous impulses I met. His brilliant personality and singleness of purpose did not fail to have an influence on me. However, I was already too dug in in my work to accept his advice to drop the work I was then doing and to try to identify his *Vagusstoff*. He remained a friend, nevertheless, and years later when he was exiled from Austria, I had the sad privilege to welcome him to my house in Oxford and to meet him again when he was living in New York. Having in 1949 accepted a visiting professorship at New York University College of Medicine in Homer Smith's laboratory, I visited the pharmacology department of that institution soon after my arrival and found Loewi, then in his 77th year, sitting in front of an isolated frog heart preparation busy—as he says in his autobiographic sketch (1960)—tidying "leftovers from earlier problems." He ceased experimental work in 1955 but he retained his liveliness well beyond his 80th year. When I met him last in 1958 he discoursed so animatedly on German poetry—he wrote poems himself—that it was difficult to get a word in edgeways.

There were usually also several visitors from abroad working in the department and two of them, F. H. Smirk (later knighted for his services to medicine in New Zealand) and C. Stanton Hicks (later knighted for his services in establishing the Australian Army Catering Corps and subsequently the British and U.S. Army Catering Corps), had an important influence on my life. I had never been quite happy in Vienna about the general attitude to medical research. It seemed to me that, in spite of much good work, the overall approach was too speculative. I was therefore deeply impressed by the sober and critical way in which Smirk and Stanton Hicks treated scientific problems and decided to ask them to help me to go to Cambridge where I wanted to study for a medical degree. After I was accepted by Emmanuel College as a medical student for the session 1930/31 my tutor, T. S. Hele (a biochemist and later master of the college), arranged for me that I could work after hours in the Department of Pharmacology. Pharmacology in Cambridge was then taught by W. E. Dixon, the first to show that vagal stimulation liberates an *inhibitory substance*. In the report on his findings which he published in 1907 in an out-of-the-way journal (*Medical Magazine* **16**: 454) Dixon stated that the substance like muscarine was completely antagonized by atropine. He interpreted his findings as meaning that some inhibitory substance is stored up in that portion of the heart to which we refer as a *nerve ending*. J. A. Gunn (1932) in his obituary for Dixon says that he had asked Dixon why he had not pursued this work further and was told that Dixon was deterred by the universal skepticism with which his views were received. This may well have been one factor, but having known Dixon, I wonder whether another was the pressure of a multitude of brilliant ideas which made it difficult for Dixon to concentrate for too long on a particular subject. In 1924 Dixon, together with F. H. A. Marshall, was the first to postulate a connection between neurohypophyseal and ovarian function. Being still interested in this problem he suggested to Peter Holtz (who was spending the first part of a Rockefeller Foundation scholarship in Cambridge and some years later became widely known as the discoverer of dopa decarboxylase) and me to find out whether estrogens sensitize the mammalian uterus to the action of oxytocin. (Curiously enough, the interaction between estrogen and oxytocin is still far from clear so that even now—45 years later—I am still working on this problem.)

Although negative, the results of this study interested H. H. Dale (later Sir Henry), the discoverer of the oxytocic action of posterior pituitary extracts, sufficiently to invite me to discuss our findings. Thus I had the opportunity to meet yet another of the pioneers of the humoral transmission concept. A few months before that I had also met T. R. Elliott, who in 1904 had suggested that sympathetic nerves might act by liberating adrenaline at the myoneural junction. Dixon, Loewi, Elliott, and Dale are clearly men who laid much of the foundation of neuroendocrinology since it soon became likely that the principles of humoral transmission of nervous impulses were as valid for the central nervous system as they are for stimuli to the autonomic nerves. Moreover, there is now good evidence that the peripheral neurotransmitters (catecholamines, acetyl choline) are also concerned with the transmission of cerebral impulses.

After relatively few years of outstanding physiological research which gained him election to the Royal Society, Elliott had been diverted by his service during the First World War to clinical medicine. Having been appointed to a full-time professorship of medicine at University College Hospital Medical School, he did not continue experimental work but never failed to encourage and to support young people to do so. His wide knowledge, clarity of mind, and critical ability were of great help when one intended to submit a paper. My work with F. H. Smirk (1932) in Elliott's department led to a further analysis of the mechanism of action of vasopressin, showing in particular that the inhibition of water diuresis produced by this hormone is not caused by interference with water absorption from the gut. Having been happily occupied in both Cambridge and London, I left England at the beginning of August to spend a holiday in the Dolomites. However, shortly after my arrival, I received the news that Walter Dixon had suddenly died at the age of 61. What now? Without his help continuing work at Cambridge would be very difficult. Fortunately, having heard about Dixon's death, E. P. Pick was kind enough to offer me an assistant lecturership in his department. I returned to Austria, both sad and happy, realizing that the old temptress Vienna still had a hold on me, and plunged once more into research work, continuing at the same time—in a rather desultory fashion—my medical studies. Two papers published at that time might be mentioned. One, in collaboration with a Japanese colleague, G. Kusunoki (1933) showed that Pitressin injected intracisternally into dogs had a pronounced pressor action while other vasoactive substances like adrenaline, acetylcholine, histamine, and adenosine, in spite of their smaller molecular weight, had no effect on the blood pressure when injected into the cerebrospinal fluid; we adduced reasons for believing that vasopressin had a direct central effect. These findings led to an exchange of letters with Harvey Cushing (then a man of 64), who had made similar experiments in man, but they remain a puzzle. Another paper (with F. F. Urban, 1935) reported the results of a very laborious investigation into the fate of ADH *in vitro* and *in vivo*. It was the first systematic study of this subject and yielded a number of new findings, e.g., (1) the very fast clearance of the hormone from the circulation contrasted with slow inactivation in defibrinated blood and serum *in vitro*, (2) the excretion of antidiuretic activity in the urine after the *in vivo* injection of postpituitary extracts, and (3) the preferential inactivation of the ADH by liver and kidney *in vitro*.

While this work was in progress the political situation in Austria became darker and darker. There was an outbreak of fighting in the spring of 1934 between the extreme right-wing Heimwehr and the Socialist workers, during which the former shelled municipal blocks of flats not very far from where we (I had married in 1933) were living. There was no fighting near the university but all public transport was halted; the tramcars abandoned in the streets presented a curious picture on my long way from an outer suburb. However, this did not mean that the university precinct remained quiet. Although the tension between the workers and the government-supported fascist militia died down, the strong Nazi element among the students became more riotous every day. On one occasion we watched—helplessly because the doors of the institute were locked—how the Nazis forced some of their fellow students to jump out of a first floor window into the courtyard of the adjacent anatomy department, which led to many injuries amongst the victims. On another occasion the trouble was more personal. Pick, who was personally quite fearless, accepted against the advice of his friends who knew that his Jewish origin would make this a "provocation," the deanship of the Medical Faculty. It was the practice for one of the younger lecturers to see him in the morning in his office in the main building of the university to receive messages for the department. On one such occasion when it was my turn, I was set upon by over a dozen Nazi students who knocked me down with knuckle-dusters. Although I was bleeding copiously from a scalp wound, neither the senior staff inside the building nor the police outside dared to come to my help.

Foreseeing a takeover of Austria by the Nazis, I had already been thinking of leaving Vienna again and this episode helped me to make up my mind. Accordingly, I asked Emmanuel College whether I would be permitted to return to Cambridge to continue my medical studies. When this was granted we left for England in the autumn of 1934. A hard year of studying followed, mine being the common experience that it is much more difficult to pass examinations as a "mature" student than as a youngster. Having worked there before, it was natural to choose University College Hospital for my clinical work, especially as T. R. Elliott put a room at my disposal where I could do research. However, I soon found out that a medical student in his clinical years has little time for anything but his routine work. Moreover, the political situation on the Continent made it more than likely that the subsidy we received from my wife's and my own parents would cease at any moment. This was an ample incentive to qualify as quickly as possible in order to obtain paid employment. Having obtained my Cambridge M.B. in 1938, I immediately started to look for a post but this was not an easy matter. Medical schools at this time were small—most pharmacology departments had no more than two or three established posts, research posts were scanty, and quite a number of these had been generously awarded to older and more experienced scientists who, like myself, had to leave their posts on the Continent for racial or political reasons. This being so, I was advised by Elliott to apply for a Beit Memorial Fellowship for Medical Research (£400 per annum at that time) which I was lucky enough to obtain, starting with the session 1939/40. However, even before I was due to take it up the war was upon us. I had volunteered for the Emergency Medical Service earlier in the year and had been posted to the Peace Memorial Hospital at Watford as blood transfusion officer and this is where I went when the war started. There was little to hold me back in London: My family had been evacuated to South Devon as guests of Dame Harriet Chick and experimental work at UCH was no longer possible because Charles Harrington, who as head of the Department of Clinical Pathology was in charge of the animal house, had all animals killed in case they escaped during an air raid.

In Watford I duly organized the Blood Transfusion Service but after a few weeks of the "phoney war" found no further useful occupation. I applied for release from the EMS which was not granted, but a request for unpaid leave was. Much relieved, I moved to the Department of Pharmacology at Oxford where J. H. Burn had offered me facilities. This lively laboratory which was dominated by autopharmacology (i.e., inquiries concerned with the pharmacology of neurotransmitters and hormones) proved to be very stimulating. However, I did not stay in the field of neurohypophyseal research but branched out into clinical work and was able to show (with the kind help of Chassar Moir, the professor of obstetrics) that, although newborn infants could concentrate their urine to a considerable extent, their kidneys were less sensitive to posterior pituitary extracts than those of adults (Heller, 1944). I concluded (as it turned out later, correctly) that this was mainly due to the immaturity of the renal tubules.

Another series of investigations led me into the field of comparative endocrinology. I had noted that the presence of antidiuretic activity in the pars nervosa of cold-blooded vertebrates had not been demonstrated and that quantitative determinations of the hormone content had only been recorded for cat and human glands. Referred to body weight, considerably less antidiuretic activity was found in the pituitary of all nonmammalian classes of vertebrates but the significance of this finding became clear only when, in a second paper (Heller, 1941), the activities of nonmammalian pituitary extracts were compared by several assay methods. I came to the conclusion that the neurohypophysis of frogs (and probably also that of birds and fishes) elaborated a principle which, though chemically related to the mammalian hormones, was not identical with either of them. This conclusion was rather daring, since at that time class or species differences in the amino acid composition of neurohypophyseal hormones had not been suspected. For this reason, perhaps, the postulated existence of the water balance principle (as I had tentatively called the amphibian hormone because it was more active in the Brunn test than vasopressin) was regarded with skepticism for many years. I remember, for instance, that even 17 years later in 1959 I received a telephone call from Leonard Bayliss (who was rewriting his father's famous textbook) asking whether I still believed in the "water balance principle." Fortunately, I was able to reply not only that there was no reason to doubt the existence of this principle but also that, in collaboration with B. T. Pickering (Heller and Pickering, 1960, 1961), I had established its amino acid composition, which was that of 8-arginine oxytocin(= vasotocin, see later). The 1941 paper not only showed for the first time the existence of a neurohypophyseal hormone other than oxytocin and vasopressin (and thus a phyletic polymorphism of this group of principles) but also established the usefulness of the *multiple assay technique* which, as later (1955) formalized by J. H. Gaddum, led eventually to our discovery of further new neurohypophyseal biologically active peptides.

This may be the place to discuss briefly why so many pharmacologists have been attracted to neurohypophyseal research. The main reason seems to me that measurements of the effects of the posterior pituitary hormones required experimental procedures that were more easily available to experimental pharmacologists than to any other group of workers. Moreover, during the first half of the century, led by such men as Trevelyan, Gaddum, Burn, and Schild, pharmacologists were better used to bioassay techniques and their statistical evaluation.

In the middle of the war I moved to Bristol, where I had been appointed to the headship of the newly founded Department of Pharmacology with the princely salary of £550. At its inception, the department consisted of a largish classroom, a small room for the lecturer-in-charge and a storeroom. There was practically no equipment since the professor of physiology, from whose department pharmacology had been split off, had—as was his right—removed everything but a kymograph, a balance, and some glassware. When, on being appointed, I was asked whether I wished to make any remarks and I said, very diffidently, that more accommodation was needed, I was told by the vice-chancellor, Dr. Loveday: "Don't worry. We have the money and we shall start building a new medical school immediately after the war." It took over 20 years to implement this promise. During that period I tried—with some success, I believe—to build up the department and, more importantly, to recruit workers who were also interested in neurohypophyseal problems. Many of these (e.g., S. E. Dicker, M. Ginsburg, R. J. Fitzpatrick, K. Lederis, S. M. A. Zaidi) made notable contributions to this field and were destined to occupy chairs in other universities. Personally, I continued work on the hormonal regulation of the water metabolism of newborn infants and animals. The results of these studies were summarized in lectures given in the Department of Pediatrics of Harvard University (Heller, 1951) and later to the German Pediatric Society (Heller, 1958). Some advance was also made in the study of the fate of neurohypophyseal hormones. In collaboration with M. Ginsburg (1953) the very short half-life of vasopressin in the circulation of the rat could be demonstrated with precision and it could also be shown *in vivo* that the liver and kidneys are the main organs removing the hormone from the blood. This study served as a model for many subsequent investigations of the metabolic fate of peptide hormones. In it, it was also shown that hemorrhage releases large amounts of vasopressin, a procedure which later proved a useful tool in the hands of many other authors.

In 1955, the Colston Research Society, which obtains its support from the citizens of Bristol, asked me to direct one of its annual symposia. I chose *The Neurohypophysis* as the subject, and it would seem that this symposium, held in the University of Bristol from April 9th to April 12th, 1956, was the first international meeting devoted exclusively to this subject. Sir Henry Dale gave the introductory lecture and this was followed by papers by some of the most prominent workers in the field of neurohypophysial research, including B. Andersson, W. Bargmann, H. B. van Dyke, S. J. Folley, M. Pickford, W. H. Sawyer and others. In the neuroendocrinological context the most important contributions were those of Wolfgang Bargmann, who showed that neurosecretory material could be demonstrated "in the entire distribution of the supraopticohypophysial tract, from the nuclear regions to where the fibers fan out in the posterior pituitary," and of Bertil Hanström, who made a brilliant comparison between vertebrate and invertebrate neurosecretory systems.

In 1957, stimulated by the important advances in the chemistry of the neurohypophyseal hormones of mammals, I resolved to continue work on the occurrence of these hormones in nonmammalian vertebrates. However, as almost invariably in comparative endocrinology, the first problem was the collection of sufficient material to start with. We could either collect a sufficient number of glands from any one species and apply methods which had proved their worth in the isolation of the mammalian hormones or we could try to elaborate techniques which allow separation of these peptides in micro quantities. We opted for the latter procedure even though, surprisingly enough, there was then no simple chromatographic technique available for this kind of work. However, I traveled to Exeter to discuss the matter with Prof. H. N. Rydon who, in 1952 with P. W. G. Smith (*Nature* **169:** 922), had shown that mixtures of micrograms of peptides could be separated and visualized by a simple chromatographic procedure. The sensitivity of this technique had since been increased by a modification introduced by the German chemists Reindel and Hoppe (*Ber. deutsch. chem Ges.* **87:** 1103, 1954). When applied to a mixture of mammalian hormones K. Lederis and I could show (*Nature* **182:** 1231, 1958) that as little as 10 mu of each hormone could be separated, eluted, and assayed. During the course of the next year Dr. B. T. Pickering and I applied this technique to extracts of fish, frog, and chicken neurohypophyses and found that all the extracts contained two components, both with a pronounced oxytocic action. Moreover, tested by the multiple assay technique, one of these hormones had also a marked pressor, antidiuretic, and frog water balance activity. We could therefore state with confidence that it was a hormone which did not occur in mammals (Pickering and Heller, 1959). On communicating these results to H. B. van Dyke and W. H. Sawyer we learned that they had obtained very similar results. Moreover, they had compared the new hormone with an analogue of the mammalian neurohypophyseal hormone called vasotocin (put at their disposal by Katsoyannis and du Vigneaud who had synthesized it in 1958) and had found that its pharmacological characteristics were indistinguishable from those of the synthetic peptide. Van Dyke and Sawyer agreed to a simultaneous publication of the Bristol and New York results to which du Vigneaud added a note pointing out that this was a "remarkable example of the synthesis of a polypeptide hormone before its identification as a natural product."

The occurrence of vasotocin in nonmammalian neurohypophyseal extracts was soon confirmed by amino acid analysis of the new hormone (Heller and Pickering, 1960) but for some years it was believed that the other biologically active peptide in such extracts was oxytocin. However, in 1960 two French workers, J. Maetz and F. Morel, showed Dr. Pickering and myself some bioassay results which suggested to us that teleost fishes elaborated not only vasotocin but yet another neurohypophyseal hormone different from the mammalian principles. On further investigation by B. K. Follett and myself, this assumption proved to be justified. The new peptide, which we named ichthyotocin, was a year later identified by R. Acher as 4-serine, 8-isoleucine oxytocin. Dr. Follett and I found further that the neurohypophyseal extracts of amphibians contained a hormone which was identical with neither ichthyotocin nor oxytocin. From its pharmacological properties we suggested (as it later turned out, correctly) that it was 8-isoleucine oxytocin. Moreover, we could show that neurohypophyseal extract of lungfish contained the same "amphibian" principle, a matter of some interest since these fish are related to the ancestors of all four-footed animals.

These and other related findings made my colleagues and me eager to study the distribution of the neurohypophyseal hormones throughout the vertebrate phyla. This seemed important because none of the other groups of polypeptide or protein hormone had—nor have to this day—been studied as comprehensively. However, as anybody knows who has worked in the field of comparative endocrinology, it is by no means easy to collect sufficient material from animals which are neither domesticated nor used for food even if, as in our case, only a few glands were needed to characterize the hormone by chromatographic and pharmacological methods. Friends all over the world were of immense help even if they did not always go quite as far as Bernardo Houssay, who arranged a special expedition to the Argentino-Brazilian frontier to catch South American lungfish for us.

Moreover, in quite a number of instances, I traveled to far places to collect pituitaries myself: to Uganda to obtain glands from a variety of wild pigs and other large mammals (and dissecting out an elephant's pituitary in the field using pangas and spears as dissecting tools was quite difficult); to Sicily, where we obtained glands from the primitive six-gilled shark *Hexanchus,* a six-foot slate-grey monster with large green eyes which lives in the depths of the Mediterranean and which we dissected on the black volcanic beaches between Catania and Messina; to the Cape Haze Marine Laboratory (then under the direction of Eugenie Clark), situated on a key off of Sarasota, Florida, on the Gulf of Mexico where sharks are so abundant that we caught over 50 in a few weeks!

As a result of these and similar ventures the pattern of distribution of the neurohypophyseal hormones from the most primitive vertebrates to man is now fairly clear, although it must be stressed that this knowledge has been gained not only by the work in Bristol but also by the important contributions of W. H. Sawyer (New York) and R. Acher (Paris) and their co-workers.

When working with pituitary glands from a number of related species we (Ferguson and Heller, 1965) came across a phenomenon that may deserve to be specially mentioned. We were analyzing neural lobes from South American peccaries, a group of piglike animals, and found that they contained lysine vasopressin. However, Professor Sawyer, who was doing similar work on peccary pituitaries from Arizona, wrote to us that he could only find arginine vasopressin. It occurred to us that both hormones might be present and on analyzing our glands and Sawyer's extracts (which he very generously put at our disposal) further, we found that this was indeed the case. This and subsequent work by Dr. Ferguson (1969) indicated that the two analogues might be present in the same gland—presumably that of heterozygotes—whereas homozygotes contained only one of the hormones.

Recently, in the opening address delivered at the Seventh Conference of European Comparative Endocrinologists (Heller, 1974) in Budapest, I discussed the phyletic variations in the amino acid compositions of the neurohypophyseal hormones from the point of view of molecular biology and biochemical genetics and—drawing also on the much scantier evidence available of variations in the primary structure of other groups of polypeptide hormones and prohormones—attempted to formulate some generalizations as to the evolutionary background of such molecular events. It seems possible that these generalizations will also apply to the group of releasing factors or hormones whose peptide nature has only been so recently recognized.

The European Society for Comparative Endocrinology was a by-product of the work discussed in the preceding pages. Realizing that there was no European forum at which short progress reports in the field of comparative endocrinology could be made, E. J. W. Barrington and I instituted conferences on the subject in 1962 and a European Society was founded in 1965. It has now 634 members from 40 countries.

When the general outlines of the phyletic distribution of the various neurohypophyseal hormones and chemical structure of these polypeptides had been more or less established by 1970, it became clear that most vertebrates elaborated more than one of these active principles. The physiological significance of the mammalian hormones can be approximately defined, in so far as vasopressin seems mainly concerned with the regulation of water excretion and oxytocin with reproductive functions. Arginine vasotocin—which has now been found in all vertebrate classes, although in mammals it appears to occur only before birth—seems, like vasopressin in mammals, to act as the antidiuretic hormone in nonmammalian vertebrates. There is, however, strong suggestive evidence for the fascinating phenomenon of an evolutionary shift from one type of renal receptor to another: In bony fishes the antidiuretic action of vasotocin seems to be purely vascular (Henderson and Wales, 1974), its renal action in amphibians and reptiles is a mixture of vascular and tubular epithelial effects, while vasotocin in birds (Skadhauge, 1964) and vasopressin in mammals in physiological doses affects only the water permeability of the renal tubules. This evolutionary recruitment of new receptors by a neurohypophyseal hormone is, of course, not unique. Another example is the effect of oxytocin on the mammary myoepithelium.

The physiological significance of the nonapeptides which are synthesized by the neurohypophysial tissue of nonmammalian vertebrates in addition to vasotocin is still obscure. My colleagues and I have now for several years searched for biological functions in which these hormones would be more effective than vasotocin (in the same way as vasopressin in mammals is a very much more potent antidiuretic agent than oxytocin) but so far without success.

While these comparative studies were under way more general aspects of neurohypophyseal research were not neglected. Up to 1951 the neural lobe of the pituitary remained somewhat of a puzzle, since by the standards of that time its cytology did not resemble that of an endocrine gland. In that year, however, W. Bargmann and E. Scharrer published a paper in which they formulated the concept that the neural lobe is only the site of hormone storage and release, and only a part of a neurosecretory system which originates in nuclei of the hypothalamus. This concept was soon supported by experimental evidence as well as by an upsurge of electron microscopical findings, and gained universal acceptance. However, numerous problems remained to be solved. One of these was the mechanism by which the hypothalamoneurohypophyseal system is able to release vasopressin and oxytocin in different quantities or, under some circumstances, only one hormone alone. The simplest assumption appeared to me (Heller, 1961) that separate neurons were responsible for the synthesis, storage, and release of each hormone or, as I put it, that there existed "vasopressinergic" and "oxytocinergic" fibres. In order to attempt to demonstrate their existence Dr. K. Lederis and I (1962) decided to isolate neurosecretory granules by ultracentrifugation of sucrose homogenates of mammalian posterior lobes and to control the purity of the appropriate fraction both by electron microscopy and by bioassay, which had not been done before. The granule fraction was then subjected to density gradient centrifugation. The results together with those of other workers—though not conclusive—are consistent with the view that vasopressin and oxytocin are produced in separate neurons.

This type of problem seems to me a good illustration of questions which arise not only in connection with the morphology and function of the hypothalamoneurohypophyseal complex but also with regard to any other system of peptidergic neurons as, for example, those which elaborate the releasing factors or hormones affecting adenohypophyseal secretion—some of which may be chemically related to the neurohypophyseal principles. It might be said that in this sense the many and laborious investigations concerned with the morphology and function of the neurohypophyses (to which the work on the biochemical genetics of neurohypophysial hormones and that on the neurophysins should be added) are not only of intrinsic interest, but can also be regarded as model studies, the results of which may be applicable to a wide variety of neurosecretory mechanisms both in vertebrates and in invertebrates and therefore to a wide area of neuroendocrinology.

REFERENCES

Dixon, W. E., and F. H. A. Marshall (1924). The influence of the ovary on pituitary secretion; a probable factor in parturition. *J. Physiol.* **49:** 276.

Elliott, T. R. (1904). On the action of adrenalin. J. Physiol. **31:** 20P.

Ferguson, D. R. (1969). The genetic distribution of vasopressins in the peccary (*Tayassu angulatus*) and warthog (*Phaecochoerus aethiopicus*). *Gen. Comp. Endocrinol.* **12:** 609.

Ferguson, D. R., and H. Heller (1965). Distribution of neurohypophysial hormones in vertebrates. *J. Physiol.* **180:** 846.

Fröhlich, A. (1901). Ein Fall von Tumor der Hypophysis cerebri ohne Akromegalie. *Wien. Klin. Rundschau* **15:** 883, 906.

Gaddum, J. H. (1965). In *Polypeptides which Stimulate Plain Muscle.* Livingstone, Edinburgh and London.

Ginsburg, M., and H. Heller (1953). The clearance of injected vasopressin from the circulation and its fate in the body. *J. Endocrinol.* **9:** 283.

Gunn, J. A. (1932). Obituary for Walter Ernest Dixon. *J. Pharmacol. Exp. Ther.* **44:** 3.

Heller, H. (1930a). Über die Einwirkung von Hypophysenhinterlappenextrakten auf den Wasserhaushalt des Frosches. *Arch. Exp. Pathol. Pharmakol.* **157:** 298.

Heller, H. (1930b). Über die Wirkung der getrennten Hypophysenhinterlappenhormone auf die Wasseraufnahme beim Frosch. *Arch. Exp. Pathol. Pharmakol.* **157:** 323.

Heller, H. (1931). Über das blutzuckersenkende Hormon der Darmschleimhaut (Duodenin). *Wien. Klin. Wochenschr.* **44:** 476.

Heller, H. (1941). Differentiation of an (amphibian) water balance principle from the antidiuretic principle of the posterior pituitary gland. *J. Physiol.* **100:** 125.

Heller, H. (1944). The renal function of newborn infants. *J. Physiol.* **102:** 429.

Heller, H. (1951). The water metabolism of newborn infants and animals. *Arch. Dis. Child.* **26:** 195.

Heller, H. (1958). Die Hypophysenhinterlappen- und Nebennierenrindenhormone wahrend der ersten Lebenszeit im Zusammenhang mit der Regulation des Wasserhaushaltes. *Monatsschr. Kinderheilk.* **106:** 81.

Heller, H. (1961). Occurrence, storage and metabolism of oxytocin. Page 3 in R. Caldeyro-Barcia and H. Heller, eds. *Oxytocin.* Pergamon Press, Oxford.

Heller, H. (1974). Molecular aspects in comparative endocrinology. *Gen. Comp. Endocrinol.* **22:** 315.

Heller, H., and G. Kusunoki (1933). Die zentrale Blutdruckwirkung des neurohypophysären Kreislaufhormons (Vasopressin). *Arch. Exp. Pathol. Pharmakol.* **173:** 301.

Heller, H., and K. Lederis (1962). Characteristics of isolated neurosecretory vesicles from mammalian neural lobes. In H. Heller and R. B. Clark, eds. *Neurosecretion. Mem. Soc. Endocrinol.* **12:** 35.

Heller, H., and B. T. Pickering (1960). Identification of a new neurohypophysial hormone. *J. Physiol.* **152:** 56P.

Heller, H., and B. T. Pickering (1961). Neurohypophysial hormones of nonmammalian vertebrates. *J. Physiol.* **155:** 98.

Heller, H., and F. H. Smirk (1932). Studies concerning the alimentary absorption of water and tissue hydration in relation to diuresis. Part III. The influence of posterior pituitary hormone on the absorption and distribution of water. *J. Physiol.* **76:** 283.

Heller, H., and F. F. Urban (1935). The fate of the antidiuretic principle of postpituitary extracts *in vivo* and *in vitro. J. Physiol.* **85:** 502.

Henderson, I. W., and N. A. M. Wales (1974). Renal diuresis and anti-diuresis after injection of arginine vasotocin in the freshwater eel (*Anguilla anguilla L.*). *J. Endocrinol.* **61:** 487.

Janssen, S. (1928). Über zentrale Wasserregulation und Hypophysenantidiurese. *Arch. Exp. Pathol. Pharmakol.* **135:** 1.

Loewi, O. (1960). An autobiographical sketch. *Perspect. Biol. Med.* **4:** 3.

Pfeiffer, E., S. Raptis, and R. Fussgänger (1973). Gastrointestinal hormones and islet function. Page 259 *in Handbook of Experimental Pharmacology,* vol. 34. Springer, Berlin/Heidelberg/New York.

Pickering, B. T., and H. Heller (1959). Chromatographic and biological characteristics of fish and frog neurohypophysial extracts. *Nature* **184:** 1463.

Skadhauge, E. (1964). Effects of unilateral infusion of arginine vasotocin into the portal circulation of the avian kidney. *Acta Endocrinol. (Kbh.)* **47:** 321.

9

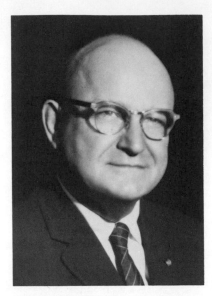

Joseph C(larence) Hinsey

Joseph C. Hinsey was born in Ottumwa, Iowa, on April 29, 1901. He attended public schools in Ottumwa and was enrolled in Iowa Wesleyan College from 1918 to 1920. He then transferred to Northwestern and obtained the B.S. with highest distinction in 1922 and an M.S. from this institution in 1923. He received his Ph.D. in Anatomy from Washington University in St. Louis in 1927. His first teaching post was as Assistant in Zoology at Northwestern and in 1923–24 he was an Instructor in Biology at Western Reserve University. On his move to Washington University he became an Assistant in the Department of Neuroanatomy and Histology and became an Assistant Professor there following the receipt of the Ph.D. degree in 1927. He was Assistant Professor and Associate Professor of Neuroanatomy at Northwestern from 1928 to 1930 and then moved to Stanford University as Professor of Anatomy. In 1936 he was appointed Professor and Chairman of Physiology at Cornell University Medical College. He became Professor and Chairman of Anatomy there in 1939, a post which he held until 1953. He also served as Dean of the School of Medicine from 1942 to 1953 and then became Director of the New York Hospital—Cornell Medical Center in 1953, a post which he held until retirement in 1966.

Dr. Hinsey has received many honors. He was president of the Association of American Medical Colleges in 1950 and chairman of its executive council from 1946 to 1954. He received the Abraham Flexner Award for distinguished service to medical education in 1958 and has received merit citations from Northwestern University, Washington University, and the University of North Carolina School of Medicine.

His interest in neuroendocrinology was an outgrowth of his other interests in the neurological sciences.

Recollections About the Neurological Sciences with Emphasis on Neuroendocrinology

JOSEPH C. HINSEY

As I review my investigative career, I find that it has dealt with the anatomy (gross, microscopic, comparative), physiology, embryology, pathology, chemistry, and pharmacology of the nervous sytem as well as neuroendocrinology, which was an outgrowth of other interests in the neurological sciences. Some review of the institutions where I have been and the responsibilities there is indicated.

I was born in Ottumwa, Iowa, on April 29, 1901, the son of a mother who had been a school teacher and of a father who was an executive in a chain of wholesale groceries. My grandfather, Joseph C. Hinsey, M.D., had been a pioneer physician in that community starting in 1854. After graduating from high school in Ottumwa, I was fairly well committed to preparing for a career in clinical medicine in that community. After the first two years of college at Iowa Wesleyan, I transferred to Northwestern University in Evanston, where I planned to enter medical school after one year. However, William Albert Locy, the professor of zoology, persuaded me to stay in Evanston for my senior year and to become a student assistant in his department. After graduation, I stayed on for another year and an M.S. degree, with a thesis dealing with amoeboid movement. The year of 1923–24 was spent as an instructor in biology at Adelbert College of Western Reserve

---

JOSEPH C. HINSEY ● Emeritus Professor of Anatomy, Cornell University Medical College, New York, New York.

University in Cleveland. In 1924, I became an assistant in the Department of Neuroanatomy and Histology, which had been established for Stephen Walter Ranson as chairman in the Washington University Medical School in St. Louis. I enrolled in the graduate school for a Ph.D. degree with Ranson as chairman of my committee and with Joseph Erlanger and Herbert S. Gasser representing my minors in physiology and pharmacology. In addition to the investigation for my thesis, which will be described later, I took and completed all courses taken by medical students in the basic sciences. This required, in addition to the courses taken there, courses in gross anatomy at Northwestern and Wisconsin, bacteriology at Wisconsin, and pathology at Michigan. In teaching I was in charge of one of three sections of 25 students in histology and neuroanatomy. I was awarded the Ph.D. degree in June of 1927 and was then made an assistant professor there. In June of 1926, I married Sarah (Sally) Callen, whom I met in my first year of college. She and our daughter, Elaine, and son, Joseph, have been understanding and supportive down through the years. In February of 1928 I went with Dr. Ranson to the Northwestern Medical School on the McKinlock Campus in Chicago to help him establish a new Institute of Neurology, where the staff engaged in full-time research and graduate teaching. I was made an associate professor of neuroanatomy in 1929. In September of 1930 I went to Stanford with the rank of professor of anatomy in a department headed by Arthur William Meyer and where Charles H. Danforth and Frank M. MacFarland were senior professors and Joseph Markee and Homer Violette were assistant professors. William W. Greulich was a graduate student in the department. I was responsible for the teaching of neuroanatomy and gave an elective course on the visceral nervous system. I participated in the teaching of other courses in the department. While at Stanford, where the first year and the first quarter of the second year of the medical course were then given on the campus in Palo Alto, I became much involved in university affairs. I was a member of the Lower Division Committee, the Scholarship Committee, the Faculty Athletic Committee, and later became the faculty representative in athletics to the Pacific Coast Conference. I was the faculty advisor for my college fraternity and served as one of three faculty members on the Interfraternity Board. During the year 1935–36 I was the president of the Stanford Research Club. I was advisor to the students in the lower division who were preparing for biology and medicine, and had a conference with each student before registration in each quarter. This was influential in my interest over the years in the problems related to the preparation for the study of medicine. In addition to all of this, an active research program was carried on in which a group of very able students were involved who later made significant contributions to medicine. In September of 1935 we moved into a new home, which we had planned and built on a plot on the Stanford Campus that had been leased by the university. Dr. Gasser had invited me to spend my first sabbatical year (1936–37) with him at the Rockefeller Institute and we had worked out a budget for my program. In December of 1935 I was invited to give a lecture at Cornell in New York City. When the offer of the chairmanship of the Department of Physiology there, which had been held by Graham Lusk and Herbert Gasser, came in January of 1936, I was reluctant to leave Stanford, where we were so happily situated. Looking back, it is difficult to see what caused me to change my mind but in March I decided to accept. In going to Cornell, I was determined to stay away from institutional administration. When Charles R. Stockard passed away in the spring of 1939, I was persuaded to become head of anatomy, and for one year I was in charge of both physiology and anatomy. Just as the work in the Department of Anatomy was going well for me, a few days after Pearl Harbor, I was thrust into the deanship at Cornell. Until July of 1953, I was chairman of anatomy and dean of the Medical College. Then I was made director of the New York Hospital—Cornell Medical Center, a position I held until my retirement in July of 1966. For three more years I was asked to serve as a consultant. From 1956 to 1967 I held the title of professor of neuroanatomy and continued participation in the teaching in this field during that time.

My investigations in the neurological sciences have been involved with two main areas, postural contraction (*muscle tonus*) of skeletal muscle and the visceral nervous system. My concern has been with the anatomical structures and how they function. It was my good fortune to have been a student of the men who developed the cathode ray oscillograph and to be able to collaborate in one of the first investigations where it was used in the analysis of function. Likewise it was a line of investigation in which I participated that led to the reintroduction of the Horsley-Clarke stereotaxic instrument into neurological investigations. These two investigative procedures have been most significant in the advancement of our knowledge of the nervous system. At the time I started with Dr. Ranson, there was great interest among neurologists and neurosurgeons in surgical procedures on the visceral nervous system that had been recommended for relief of exaggerated postural contraction of skeletal muscle and for a number of vascular disorders. Ranson's doctoral thesis had dealt with the components in peripheral nerves contributed from the dorsal root ganglia, and he was curious as to the meaning of the pericellular endings about dorsal root ganglion cells that had been described by Cajal and others. For a number of years, he did experiments to test the possibility that these pericellular endings were synapses of fibers of intraspinal origin traversing the dorsal roots. I spent the first year of graduate work trying to stain and delineate the meaning of these endings. I used various stains on the cells from many types of dorsal root ganglion cells, including those from fetuses. When I reported to Dr. Ranson that I could not establish that they were normal structures, he informed me that another student had spent a year on the same problem and had come to the same conclusion. Ranson did not give up until R. W. Barris (1934) established that they were not normal structures but were ones that appeared due to trauma. I then embarked on a study of the innervation of skeletal muscle and the blood vessels therein in cats in which I had isolated by degeneration procedures the dorsal root component, the ventral root somatic motor one, and the thoracolumbar sympathetic one. I found no hypolemmal thoracolumbar sympathetic fibers supplying striated muscle fibers, contrary to many observers at that time. By chance, I was able to demonstrate for the first time that the end plates on the intrafusal muscle fibers of muscle spindles were supplied by small fibers of ventral root origin. Later Eccles and Sherrington demonstrated that these were fibers of about 6 microns in diameter which left the spinal cord in the ventral roots. When I presented my findings at the spring meetings of the American Association of Anatomists in Nashville in 1927, there was critical discussion of them, but the extensive investigations of Drs. Marion Hines and Sarah Tower published later were in essential agreement.

These observations on skeletal muscle and the blood vessels (Hinsey 1927, 1928, 1934b) caused me to speculate as to what could be responsible for the pseudomotor contractions that had been described by Vulpian and Sherrington when skeletal muscle becomes sensitized by section of the somatic motor nerve fibers some 7 to 10 days previously. The dilatation of blood vessels in the extremities produced by stimulation of the dorsal roots, the reflex flare studied by Sir Thomas Lewis (later by Harold G. Wolff), and the herpetic eruptions studied so extensively by Henry Head all posed problems regarding a possible explanation. Otto Loewi had described the production of a chemical transmitter when the vagus nerve was stimulated, and along about this time, Walter Cannon produced evidence for the elaboration of sympathin when postganglionic sympathetic fibers were stimulated. Dr. Ranson insisted that I tone down some of my far-out speculations regarding humoral transmission in the first draft of my paper on blood vessels (Hinsey, 1928). I discussed with him the use of the cathode ray oscillograph in collaboration with Dr. Gasser to determine the nerve fibers involved in dorsal root dilatation and the Sherrington phenomenon. He advised me not to bother Dr. Gasser, who was busily involved in other investigations. When I discussed this with Dr. Gasser and outlined a suggested procedure, his response was to ask when I could bring the animals over and begin. At that time, Erlanger, Gasser, and Bishop had been concerned with perfecting the technique and studying the waves made by the potentials in the A-spike. The slower C-spike had not yet been found. In our first paper (Hinsey and Gasser, 1928), we concluded that the Sherrington phenomenon was mediated by small fibers, which was correct, but later evidence showed that these small fibers were not of dorsal root origin (Hinsey and Cutting, 1933).

After I left St. Louis in the early spring of 1928 to accompany Dr. Ranson back to Northwestern, Dr. Gasser and I continued our collaboration. I operated on the animals there and shipped them to St. Louis. Dr. Gasser blocked out his schedule and we did experiments day after day without interruption. In August of 1930, just before I left for Stanford, we finished experiments in which we were able to show that fibers whose conduction rate was about 2 meters per second and whose potentials were found in the C-spike of the action potential were responsible for both the Sherrington phenomenon and dorsal root dilatation (Hinsey and Gasser, 1930). We incorrectly concluded that they both arose in the dorsal root ganglia. I never was satisfied with this conclusion and after some 60 experiments done at Stanford with selective degeneration procedures, we were able to show that the Sherrington phenomenon was produced by conduction in postganglionic sympathetic fibers (Hinsey and Cutting, 1933). This differed from dorsal root dilatation, which depended on conduction in small fibers of dorsal root ganglion origin. When I sent our paper to Dr. Gasser for editorial review, he wrote that it was difficult for him to believe but that our evidence was conclusive. After I had gone to Cornell, one day Dr. Gasser called and told me that he had just had a visit with Sir Henry Dale, who had told him that Dr. Burn had confirmed our conclusion in observations made on the dog.

I have gone on at some length to present these observations because they help to explain the suggestion Dr. Markee and I made for humoral transmission from the hypothalamus and the posterior pituitary to the anterior lobe. In the memorial note to the late Dr. Joseph E. Markee in 1971, Drs. Sawyer, Everett, and Hollinshead state, "In the early years at Stanford, a very fruitful collaboration was begun with Dr. Joseph Hinsey on neurological mechanisms involved in ovulation and pregnancy in reflexly ovulating rabbits and cats. In the course of their studies, Drs. Markee and Hinsey suggested in 1933 that nervous control of the anterior pituitary might be transmitted by a humoral mechanism some years before the anatomy and blood flow in the pituitary portal system had been correctly described. Their brief note in the *Proceedings of the Society of Experimental Biology and Medicine* is often quoted as a landmark in the budding field of neuroendocrinology." I was able to convince Dr. Markee that there was no direct nerve fiber connection between the hypothalamus and posterior lobe going to the anterior lobe. Although the pituitary portal system had not been correctly described, the arrangement of the vasculature was such as to provide possible channels for transmission. It was natural for me to think of humoral transmission in light of my work on the Sherrington phenomenon and dorsal root dilatation.

In the late twenties, Dr. Ranson and I did many experiments on the reflex patterns in the extremities of cats. In one paper (Ranson and Hinsey, 1930) we diagrammed for the first time an arrangement of premotor neurones in chains in which reverberating conduction could explain the prolonged afterdischarge we found present in deafferented extremities. Observations made later by Lorente de No in Golgi preparations demonstrated the anatomical basis for such an explanation. Until the fall of 1927, decerebrate preparations in our laboratory were always made according to the anemic technique of Davis and Pollock. We were perplexed to observe in decerebrate animals of this type that crossed extensor reflexes in deafferented muscle exhibited prolonged afterdischarges instead of the abrupt relaxations described by members of the Sherrington School. During the summer of 1927, I was invited by a group at the University of Wisconsin (Drs. Walter Sullivan, Otto Mortenson, and Joseph Gale) to observe some experiments on unilaterally sympathectomized goats to repeat the often-quoted experiments of Hunter and Royle. These goats were decerebrated according to the transection method of Sherrington. The Australian observers believed that skeletal muscle fibers received two hypolemmal innervations, one from somatic motor fibers and one from postganglionic sympathetic fibers. Their experiments led them to believe that the exaggerated postural contraction in decerebrate goats was reduced when postganglionic sympathetic pathways were interrupted. They recommended sympathectomies in cases where there was exaggerated postural contraction in man. They had some enthusiastic supporters among American neurosurgeons. After trials and much serious debate, it was abandoned but it did serve to focus attention to other approaches to the surgery of the visceral nervous system.

Dr. Hunter was responsible for sending the late Dr. Herbert J. Wilkinson to work with me at Northwestern and he was able to confirm my observations that there was no hypolemmal innervation to skeletal muscle from fibers originating in postganglionic sympathetic neurons. When I returned that fall, I convinced Dr. Ranson that we should repeat our experiments on the crossed extensor reflexes in deafferented muscle and use the transection method. This was done at a level in the rostral portion of the midbrain at a higher level than that produced by the anemic method. We found that when this was done, we confirmed the earlier observations showing the abrupt relaxation at the termination of the stimulus. We found that we could confirm our earlier experiments showing prolonged afterdischarge by making a more caudal section in the same animal (Ranson and Hinsey, 1929). This caused us to explore the rostral portion of the midbrain to try to explain what we had observed. When the section was made so as to include a wedge of the hypo- and subthalamus rostral to the midbrain, we were surprised to find that these animals could stand and walk. After many months of work, we published on the role of the hypothalamus and midbrain in locomotion (Ranson, Hinsey, and McNattin, 1930). At the same time, we stimulated the rostral surface of the midbrain in the area of the red nucleus and the surrounding reticular formation and recorded the postural responses elicited. It is of interest that it was in the study of this area and its rostral connections that Dr. Magoun made his significant contributions. In our experiments, we located the points of stimulation by inserting cat hairs and later studied the microscopic sections (Hinsey *et al.,* 1930). Such a method left much to be desired and the decision was made to have a Horsley-Clarke stereotaxic instrument built by an expert instrument maker at the University of Chicago. We had seen the instrument in use in the hands of Dr. Edward Fincher from Atlanta who was working as a fellow with Dr. Ernest Sachs in St. Louis. Dr. Sachs had brought the instrument back when he returned from work with Horsley, in which he had used it with experiments on the thalamus. I have been told that this instrument was given to Dr. Magoun at a later time. Our instrument was to become available about the time I left for Stanford. Dr. Ranson had not wanted me to leave; he offered to meet the Stanford offer. He stated that I was leaving a great opportunity to work with the new instrument in solving questions which I had helped to raise. Dr. W. R. Ingram came to the institute that fall and was followed subsequently by Drs. Magoun, Fisher, Hare, Hetherington, Barris, Berry, and others. After careful preliminary studies, Ingram and others mapped the midbrain and the thalamus, and among the first studies made were repetitions of our earlier ones dealing with control of postural contractions. It was of interest that our earlier observations were fairly accurate. The reintroduction of the Horsley-Clarke instrument and the methods for accurate localization of the point of stimulation, the placement of discrete lesions, and the localization of lead-off electrodes opened up great new opportunities in the neurological sciences and for answering the problems of neuroendocrinology. The bound volumes of the publications from the Institute of Neurology at Northwestern give testimony to this. My complete set of these volumes is now in the Papanicolaou Library of the Department of Anatomy at Cornell. The history of the development of this method was told in an Alpha Omega Alpha lecture at the University of Minnesota (Hinsey, 1961).

At Cornell, we were fortunate to be joined by Drs. Kendrick Hare and Charles Berry, and we utilized the Horsley-Clarke instrument in experiments there. I had been concerned about the proper control of the stimuli in experiments of this kind. Many of the earlier experiments had been done with a Harvard inductorium. It was my good fortune to be joined by William A. Geohegan during the last half of his first year in medical school at Cornell. He was a graduate of electrical engineering at Cornell who qualified later for his medical degree. He proved to be one of the finest colleagues with whom I have ever worked. He built a stimulator in which it was possible to study the three characteristics of the stimulus, strength, configuration, and frequency through a wide range, keeping two constant and varying the third. We found that the ordinary 60-cycle 110-volt line with proper resistance gave us stimuli which were very effective. With the background of a rather extensive series of studies, we built a stimulator to be used in neurological work in the military services (Geohegan and Hinsey, 1948). Mr. Raymond Phipps built about 250 of these in our physiology shop at Cornell for use in the military services all over the world. We reported on observations made on somatic responses obtained by stimulating the hypothalamus and surrounding regions with our controlled stimulation techniques (Hinsey, 1940). Our studies on the effectiveness of methods of stimulation were very helpful in observations Geohegan, Wolf, Aidar, Hare, and I (1942) made on the preganglionic pathways to the upper extremity and to the eye of cats and monkeys. Geohegan and I were fortunate to be joined by the neurosurgeon, Dr. Bronson S. Ray, in doing similar work on man in some 20 cases where surgical procedures made possible the stimulation of appropriate ventral roots in man (Ray, Hinsey, and Geohegan, 1943). Geohegan and Aidar (1942) described a reorganization of the terminations of preganglionic nerve terminations in sympathetic chain ganglia. This phenomenon has been rediscovered recently some 30 years later. During World War II, our group was involved in studies on nerve regeneration where we combined anatomical observations with ones made with the cathode ray oscillograph analysis. Dr. Geohegan and I worked with Mr. Hugh DeHaven and Dr. Eugene DuBois on Crash Injury Studies in Military Aviation. One of the products of this program was an inertia lock for shoulder harness control. This was manufactured by the American Seating Company in Grand Rapids, Michigan. Modifications of this lock are still in use. Later this work dedicated to reducing injuries in military aviation was extended into automotive safety at Cornell Medical College, and we shared the Sperry Award for our contributions to automotive safety with the Cornell Aeronautical Laboratory at Buffalo.

The Department of Anatomy at Stanford was housed in a building designed to be a museum. A laboratory adequately but modestly equipped for experimental neurology was provided. The animal quarters were excellent with attached outdoor pens. This made possible long-term chronic experiments. The first year and the first quarter of the second year of the medical course were presented on the campus in Palo Alto in scattered buildings. The remainder of the medical course was centered mainly in quarters near the Stanford Hospital in San Francisco. The Lane Library there was a great asset. Most of the cost of our investigations was provided from departmental funds with very modest support from a Rockefeller Foundation grant for fluid research made to Stanford University and Dr. Markee had a grant from the Sex Division of the National Research Council.

We continued observations on the reflexes involved in standing and walking in opossums, rabbits, cats, and monkeys. Dr. C. C. Cutting studied these reflexes in a series of 100 newborn babies in the Department of Pediatrics at Stanford. We did many experiments to determine whether there were efferent fibers of intraspinal origin which traversed the dorsal roots (Hinsey, 1933). In studies of long duration, we examined the role of dorsal root and postganglionic sympathetic fibers in trophic innervation, using the rate of growth of hair as the indicator. Changes in the hip joint were described in this series. A great deal of interest was directed to the anatomy and physiology of the visceral nervous system (Hinsey, 1934a, 1939).

At that time, my colleague, Dr. Joseph Markee, was observing changes in endometrial transplants into the anterior chambers of eyes in rabbits and monkeys. Our discussions led us into experiments designed to learn the role of the nervous system in ovulation in rabbits, cats, and monkeys (Hinsey and Markee, 1932, 1933, 1935; Markee and Hinsey, 1933, 1935a,b, 1936; Markee, Wells, and Hinsey, 1936). The nature of our observations was such that we were able to describe what takes place at the rupture point in ovulation. A ring of dilated blood vessels surrounds the rupture point and the wall of the ovary is so weakened that a portion of the ovarian wall is extruded ahead of the ovum. When I presented these observations before a section of the anatomists at their meeting at Duke in the spring of 1936, I was taken over the coals by Dr. Edgar Allen, who believed that it was a blowout phenomenon produced by pressure within the ovary. I was most fortunate that Dr. Carl Hartman, Dr. George Bartelmez, and Dr. Everett Evans strongly supported the interpretation which we had placed on our observations. As has been mentioned, we were most fortunate to have made the early interpretation of the role of humoral transmission in the activation of the anterior pituitary lobe (Hinsey and Markee, 1933).

In the summer of 1932, while Dr. Markee was in the Middle West on vacation, I observed a case of superfetation in a unilaterally sympathectomized cat which was undergoing observations over a long period. Thirteen days after two kittens were born, two more of normal size were delivered. I did an autopsy which was observed by Drs. Meyer and Danforth and carefully preserved the tissues with particular attention to similar treatment of the two uterine horns. When Dr. Markee returned and we had studied the tissues, we decided to do a series of experiments to determine the factors in uterine growth. Using a planimeter, we devised a method by which we could determine the volume of each of the layers in the uterine horns (Hinsey and Markee, 1933, 1935; Markee and Hinsey, 1936). We learned that there is a local factor of distension which plays an important role.

I treasure those years of collaboration with Dr. Markee and I regret that he has not lived so that he could describe what took place in our association. We had a lot of fun as we let serendipity guide us along. At Cornell, our attention was turned to other fields. Dr. Hare and I studied some rabbits in which the pituitary stalk was cut and ovulation did not occur as it did in four animals where the section was incomplete. Reference was made to these observations in a review which I wrote in 1937 (Hinsey, 1937) but a final publication was never prepared. The last year I was at Stanford, I renewed a friendship with Dr. Robert A. Phillips, whom I had first known as a medical student in St. Louis. He accompanied me to Cornell, where we carried on a series of observations on diaphragmatic sensation. These produced proof for the mechanism of referred pain from that area (Hinsey and Phillips, 1940). While at Cornell, Dr. Phillips began some of the work which later led him to his significant contributions to our knowledge of cholera which he made as a naval medical officer.

In 1939, after I succeeded Dr. Stockard as chairman of anatomy, I was able to expedite and find support for Dr. Papanicolaou's resumption of his studies on the cytologic method in cancer detection. It should be remembered that his work with Stockard on the use of vaginal smears in studies of the estrous cycle proved to be very valuable to Drs. Allen and Doisy in their pioneer work on ovarian endocrinology. I have oftentimes wondered what would have been the course of our work if Dr. Markee and I had remained together for a number of more years, after we separated in 1936.

In 1945, I was elected to the executive council of the Association of American Medical Colleges and became its chairman in 1946 for a term that lasted until 1954. During this time, we carried on a vigorous campaign to improve the quality and increase the quantity of medical education in the United States. A series of teaching institutes held annually with participation of all member institutions was devoted to improving the work of each department in our schools and to increasing the participation of faculty members in the work of the AAMC. Our efforts to get federal financial aid for our programs resulted in the legislation of 1956 for research facilities and much later in 1963 and 1965 for teaching facilities. I served a term on a research committee of the Institute for Neurological Diseases and Stroke and was also a member of the first committee on review for teaching facilities. The National Fund for Medical Education was started in 1947. A survey on medical education was conducted by Drs. John Deitrick and Robert Berson and one on the preparation for the study of medicine by Drs. Aura Severinghaus, Harry Carman, and William Cadbury. We raised the money to build a central headquarters building for the AAMC on ground donated by Northwestern University in Evanston. This later was moved to Washington. I served on the Truman Commission on the Health Needs of the Nation under the chairmanship of Dr. Paul Magnuson. There have been a number of commissions to study health needs in subsequent years. I think it is important to recognize that medical educators have endeavored to anticipate many of the problems that are with us today and have accomplished much that is reflected in the forward march of work in the neurological sciences.

As I have reviewed my experiences in Academia, I remember with great gratitude the opportunities made possible by the institutions with which I have been connected. I have had the good fortune to have had many gifted teachers and have gained so much in my associations and companionship with colleagues in many institutions in addition to the ones in which I have served. The various national scientific and educational associations have provided a forum for discussion and enlightenment. I owe much to the students and the junior colleagues with whom I have worked. I still continue to "reap the unseen harvests" made possible by their careers in many branches of the health sciences and medical care.

I am convinced that a basic scientist on a medical faculty should have a concern for his relation to clinical medicine, particularly in the teaching. Much of the investigation with which I have been involved was inspired by questions raised by patient care. I commend the reading of Dr. Denny Brown's closing remarks made at the Conference on Education in the Neurological Sciences (Denny Brown, 1967) where he describes the neurophysician. Contrary to many of the recommendations made at the present time, it would be a mistake to place the basic sciences in the liberal arts departments. In addition to my own experiences with neurophysicians and neurosurgeons, I can cite the careers of my colleagues, Drs. Papanicolaou and du Vigneaud, to support my argument for a close physical and intellectual relationship with the clinical sciences for the good of teaching, research, and patient care. There are so many other examples to support this point of view.

I have observed the development of the various clinical specialties and have had a particular interest in the neurological sciences. Dr. Aura Severinghaus has recently described (Severinghaus, 1971) in excellent fashion the forward march of the neurological sciences and the part played by the Institute for Neurological Diseases and Stroke. I was privileged to serve as a member of the commission which planned the Conference on Education in the Neurological Sciences held at White Sulphur Springs, West Virginia, in November of 1966 under the chairmanship of Dr. James O'Leary. In my final summary (Hinsey, 1967), after reviewing some philosophical considerations, I referred to a statement made originally by Drs. Aura Severinghaus, Joe Brown, and myself on academic responsibility. I paraphrased it as follows, "First, all of us in the academic field must assume the responsibility for advancing the frontiers of knowledge. Second, we need to know how to put the new things we learn into context with what we already know, the established body of knowledge. Thirdly, we need to teach this to students who will become the future practitioners and academicians. Fourthly, if there is any application to patient care, we must see to it that it is applied as soon as possible." Today, there is much pressure from political and public sources to greatly increase the number of students in the health sciences. As far as the teaching of medical students is concerned, I have tried to be dedicated to the development of the individual student. I have a similar dedication to the principle of caring for one patient at a time. There is no substitute for quality and excellence in either instance.

REFERENCES

Barris, R. W. (1934). Frequency of atypical neurons in spinal ganglia under normal conditions and after lesions of roots, nerves or ganglia. *J. Comp. Neurol.* **58:** 325.

Denny Brown, D. E. (1967). Closing remarks before Conference on Education in the Neurological Sciences. *Arch. Neurol.* **17:** 586.

Geohegan, W. A., and O. J. Aidar (1942). Functional reorganization following preganglionectomy. *Proc. Soc. Exp. Biol. Med.* **50:** 365.

Geohegan, W. A., and J. C. Hinsey (1948). A stimulator for neurosurgery. *Arch. Neurol. Psychiatry* **60:** 536.

Geohegan, W. A., G. A. Wolf, Jr., O. J. Aidar, K. Hare, and J. C. Hinsey (1942). The spinal origin of preganglionic fibers to the limbs of the cat and monkey. *Am. J. Physiol.* **135:** 324.

Hinsey, J. C. (1927). Some observations on the innervation of skeletal muscle. *J. Comp. Neurol.* **44:** 87.

Hinsey, J. C. (1928). Observations on the innervation of blood vessels in skeletal muscle. *J. Comp. Neurol.* **47:** 23.

Hinsey, J. C. (1933). The functional components of the dorsal roots of spinal nerves. *Q. Rev. Biol.* **8:** 457.

Hinsey, J. C. (1934a). The anatomical relations of the sympathetic system to visceral sensation. *Proc. Assoc. Res. Nerv. Ment. Dis.* **15:** 105.

Hinsey, J. C. (1934b). The innervation of skeletal muscle. *Physiol. Rev.* **14:** 514.

Hinsey, J. C. (1937). The relation of the nervous system to ovulation and other phenomena of the female reproductive tract. *Cold Spring Harbor Symp. Quant. Biol.* **5**: 269.

Hinsey, J. C. (1939). Autonomic nervous system. *Annu. Rev. Physiol.* **1**: 407.

Hinsey, J. C. (1940). The hypothalamus and somatic responses. *Res. Publ. Assoc. Res. Nerv. Ment. Dis.* **20**: 657.

Hinsey, J. C. (1961). Ingredients in medical research. The story of a method. The Pharos of Alpha Omega Alpha, January 1961, p. 13.

Hinsey, J. C. (1967). Final summary before Conference on Education in the Neurological Sciences. *Arch. Neurol.* **17**: 583.

Hinsey, J. C., and C. C. Cutting (1933). The Sherrington phenomenon. IV. A study of some of the possible antagonists. V. Nervous pathways. *Am. J. Physiol.* **105**: 525.

Hinsey, J. C., and H. S. Gasser (1928). The Sherrington phenomenon. I. The nerve fibers involved in the sensitization of the muscle. II. The nerve fibers which produce the contracture. III. Antagonism by adrenaline. *Am. J. Physiol.* **87**: 368.

Hinsey, J. C., and H. S. Gasser (1930). The component of the dorsal roots mediating vasodilatation and the Sherrington phenomenon. *Am. J. Physiol.* **92**: 679.

Hinsey, J. C., and J. E. Markee (1932). A search for neurological mechanisms in ovulation. *Proc. Soc. Exp. Biol. Med.* **30**: 136.

Hinsey, J. C., and J. E. Markee (1933). Pregnancy following bilateral section of the cervical sympathetic trunk in the rabbit. *Proc. Soc. Exp. Biol. Med.* **31**: 270.

Hinsey, J. C., and J. E. Markee (1935). I. Does thoracolumbar sympathectomy affect the growth of the pregnant cat uterus? *Anat. Rec.* **61** (Suppl): 253.

Hinsey, J. C., and R. A. Phillips (1940). Observations on diaphragmatic sensation. *J. of Neurophysiol.* **3**: 175.

Hinsey, J. C., S. W. Ranson, and H. H. Dixon (1930). Responses elicited by stimulation of the mesencephalic tegmentum. *Arch. Neurol. and Psychiat.,* **24**: 966–977.

Markee, J. E., and J. C. Hinsey (1933). Internal migration of ova in the cat. *Proc. Soc. Exp. Biol. Med.* **31**: 267.

Markee, J. E., and J. C. Hinsey (1935*a*). A case of probable superfetation in the cat. *Anat. Rec.* **61** (Suppl): 241.

Markee, J. E., and J. C. Hinsey (1935*b*). II. A local factor in the growth of the pregnant cat uterus. *Anat. Rec.* **61** (Suppl): 311.

Markee, J. E., and J. C. Hinsey (1936). Observations on ovulation in the rabbit. *Anat. Rec.* **64**: 309.

Markee, J. E., W. M. Wells, and J. C. Hinsey (1936). III. A local factor in the growth of the rabbit uterus. *Anat. Rec.* **64** (Suppl): 221.

Ranson, S. W., and J. C. Hinsey (1929). The crossed extensor reflex in deafferented muscle after transection of the brain-stem at different levels. *J. Comp. Neurol.* **48**: 393.

Ranson, S. W., and J. C. Hinsey (1930). Reflexes in the hind-limbs of cats after transection of the spinal cord at various levels. *Am. J. Physiol.* **94**: 471.

Ranson, S. W., J. C. Hinsey, and R. F. McNattin (1930). The role of the hypothalamus and mesencephalon in locomotion. *Arch. Neurol. and Psychiatry* **23**: 1.

Ray, B. S., J. C. Hinsey, and W. A. Geohegan (1943). Observations on the distribution of the sympathetic nerves to the pupil and upper extremity as determined by stimulation of the anterior roots in man. *Ann. Surg.* **118**: 647.

Severinghaus, A. E. (1971). Neurology. A medical discipline takes stock. DHEW Publication No. (NIH) 72–175.

10

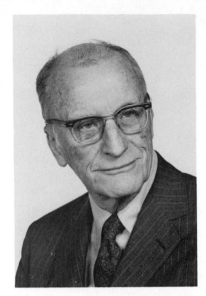

Hudson Hoagland

Dr. Hudson Hoagland, a physiologist, is cofounder and president emeritus of the Worcester Foundation for Experimental Biology. He holds his bachelor's degree from Columbia, his master's from MIT and his Ph.D. from Harvard. He has honorary Doctor of Science degrees from six other colleges and universities—Colby College, Wesleyan University, Clark University, Bates College, Boston University, and Worcester Polytechnic Institute. Dr. Hoagland has taught at Harvard, Cambridge University, and Clark University and, in 1944, he and his colleague, the late Dr. Gregory Pincus, started the independent Worcester Foundation for Experimental Biology and became its codirectors. This nonprofit organization, employing over 250 people, is engaged in research in the biomedical sciences and has an active postdoctoral teaching program. Dr. Hoagland has published or edited a number of books and many scientific papers. He has served as president of the American Academy of Arts and Sciences and of the Society of Biological Psychiatry, and has been a trustee or director of a number of scientific institutions. He was recipient of a Modern Medicine Award for Distinguished Achievement and was named "Humanist of the Year" in 1965 by the American Humanist Association. In 1969 Dr. Hoagland was given the Worcester Engineering Society's Award for Scientific Achievement. The Society of Biological Psychiatry gave him its Gold Medal Award in June of 1973.

Reflections

HUDSON HOAGLAND

I was a miserable prep school student, much more interested in sports and a good time than in study. In 1916, at the age of 16, I claimed I was 18, the minimal admission age, and went to the Plattsburg summer training camp for army officers, since World War I, for us, was just over the horizon. In the following year I enlisted in the army, missing the entire last year of high school, so in a sense I was a school dropout. Having enlisted in a new National Guard artillery battery and having been to Plattsburg, I was made a line sergeant, since most of the enlisted men and some of the officers had had little or no military experience.

I look upon my year in the army (1917–18) as the most valuable educational year of my life. I, of course, had had no trigonometry, which was a senior high school course, but a subject one needed to aim artillery effectively and, as a section sergeant in charge of three horse-drawn '75s and their caissons, I had to learn it the hard way—by myself. This brought home with a jolt the practical importance of mathematics on which people's lives, including my own, would depend.

Young as I was, I had become engaged at 17 to Anna Plummer, and three years later we were married and remained so for the next 53 years until her death in May 1973. When the war was over, there was a question of my going back to high school, a thought I couldn't abide as an ex-sergeant and engaged to be married—and, of course, I couldn't possibly have passed college entrance board examinations. Fortunately for me, Columbia University had for the first time put in scholastic aptitude tests for returning veterans and I passed the tests and was admitted as a freshman. In college I worked hard and received my bachelor's degree in 1921, with a major in mathematics, in three years instead of the usual four.

It had been taken for granted that I would become an engineer and

HUDSON HOAGLAND ● Worcester Foundation for Experimental Biology, 222 Maple Avenue, Shrewsbury, Massachussets.

enter my family's manufacturing business making rolling mill machinery, so I attended MIT and received a master's degree in chemical engineering in 1924. During my last year at MIT I was assigned a practical problem at the Lackawanna Steel Company in Buffalo, which was one of several stations for our graduate practice work. However, I found myself little interested in my assigned problem and did some desultory reading in the Buffalo Public Library. There I came across an article by the late Professor L. T. Troland of the Harvard psychology department on the nature of the nerve impulse. I knew nothing of biology or of the nervous system and was astonished and delighted to learn that one could record photographically by string galvanometer or capillary electrometer electrical nerve messages and thus learn exciting new things about the way the machinery of the body works. So deeply was I moved by this discovery that after the MIT commencement in June, I enrolled as a graduate student in psychology at Harvard under Troland and took a summer course in physiology at the Harvard Medical School. Fortunately both my wife and I were comparatively well off financially. Indeed, our four children were born while I was a graduate student either at MIT or at Harvard during the 1920s.

Troland was killed in a moutain-climbing accident a year or two after I had arrived at Harvard and the psychology department kindly permitted me to work on my thesis in the laboratory of the late Professor W. J. Crozier, who had established a new Department of General Physiology as part of the then Division of Biology. His training in physical chemistry and his great knowledge of zoology and animal behavior made him a fascinating teacher and, although I took my doctorate in psychology, my thesis was in physiology under his direction. This was followed by a year as a National Research Council Fellow and two years as an instructor in physiology and tutor in biology at Harvard in Crozier's department.

In 1930–31, on a Harvard traveling fellowship, my wife and I went for a year to Cambridge University to enable me to work in the laboratory of E. D. Adrian, who was then Royal Society Professor of Physiology and who later became Lord Adrian of Cambridge, now chancellor of the university, a Nobel Laureate, past master of Trinity College, and the recipient of many other honors. It was a great privilege to be with him for a year shortly after his pioneering work in recording electrical activity in single nerve fibers. Our lasting friendship with the Adrians and my work in his laboratory were very happy experiences.

Before leaving for England I had accepted, in 1930, a position as professor and head of the Department of Biology at Clark University in Worcester and, on returning in 1931 I established a laboratory of neurophysiology there. I had received this offer since the Department of Psychology at Clark at that time was heavily weighted in favor of experimental and physiological psychology and it desired all its Ph.D. students to do a minor in physiology. I had given a seminar at Clark, had a degree in psychology, and had published a half-dozen papers in neurophysiology that were well received and interested senior members of the psychology department. The Clark Department of Biology had lost its chairman who was a general physiologist. Thus, for a variety of reasons, the job was offered to me despite my age of thirty years.

In the early thirties funds for science were extremely hard to come by. The university was financially poor and its budget for biology meager. I was fortunate to receive modest grants from several sources, particularly the Rockefeller Foundation, to aid my work in neurophysiology and I was also fortunate in attracting a few able graduate students, and especially Dr. Ladd Prosser, who was with me as an assistant professor from 1934 to 1939. Prosser is today a very distinguished physiologist.

At Harvard, Gregory Pincus and I had received our Ph.D. degrees in 1927 and had become warm friends. He had remained as an assistant professor in Crozier's department after I left, but after two 3-year terms his appointment was not renewed despite his brilliant work. I was eager to have him join me at Clark and together we raised sufficient funds from various outside sources to make it possible for him to come as a visiting professor. By 1936 he had published his book, *The Eggs of Mammals,* and also a number of papers which reported for the first time successful parthenogenesis in a mammal, i.e., rabbits that had mothers but no fathers. This received much attention from both the scientific and lay press, but it was met by less than enthusiasm by some conservative members of the university. I found Pincus's interest and knowledge of steroid hormones exciting. He had already developed improved methods of determining urinary steroids and applied these to endocrine problems.

STUDIES OF PHYSIOLOGICAL RHYTHMS

My work at Clark had been in studies of electrical responses in sensory nerve fibers from the skin to appropriate stimuli. It also involved an analysis of electrical responses from the sensory lateral line nerve of fishes and of taste responses in their facial nerves. During the early thirties I studied the electroencephalogram (EEG) and particularly the relation of the frequencies of alpha rhythms to brain metabolism. An opportunity presented itself to study in man the effects of insulin in changing brain oxygen and sugar utilization on the EEG. The late Ewen Cameron, research psychiatrist at the Worcester State Hospital in the mid-thirties, following

Sakel's reports from abroad, was the first in America to use insulin shock therapy on schizophrenic patients and I collaborated with him in studies of their brain metabolism and EEG frequencies. My interest in this study stemmed from earlier work on determinants of physiological rhythms.

At Harvard with Crozier, and later at Clark, we had made many studies of temperature effects on various frequencies of events in poikilothermous animals. The Arrhenius equation described these frequencies as well as oxygen consumption, and carbon dioxide production of many tissues and yielded multimodal values of activation energies which we ascribed to specific enzyme controlled slow steps in sequential controlling chemical steps of respiration and of heartbeat frequencies, rhythms of appendage movements, cilia beats, and respiratory movements in many diverse "cold-blooded" animals. Nearly all of some 300 activation energies of such processes fell in some 10 well-defined modes, suggesting a limited number of enzyme systems acting as chemical pacemakers for a variety of physiological processes.

In collaboration with physicians at the Worcester State Hospital in the early 1930s I studied effects of temperature elevated by diathermy on the EEG alpha frequencies of general paretic patients and found the Arrhenius equation described these frequencies as a function of temperature and yielded three different activation energies depending upon the severity of the disease. The three values I found corresponded to three of the most prominent peaks of distribution we had earlier found with primitive organisms.

Subsequently, by use of the temperature analysis, I was able to show that the human time sense also follows the Arrhenius equation and gives an activation energy corresponding to one of the minor modes of distribution but different from those of alpha rhythms. I was therefore especially pleased to observe effects of insulin in depriving the brain of sugar and observe the correlated decrease of alpha frequencies and recovery on giving intravenous sugar, confirming the EEG changes with brain respiration.

J. R. Bergen, in my laboratory at the Worcester Foundation, developed a procedure for measuring blood flow through the head of rats and calculated that some 70% of the measured flow was flow through the brain. A comparison was made by Bergen and me in 1953 of blood flow through the heads of normal and adrenalectomized salt-maintained rats and we found that adrenalectomy considerably decreased the blood flow. The decreased blood flow could be restored to normal in two hours with adrenal cortical extract, Δ^5-pregnenolone, or cortisone, but not with desoxycorticosterone. Arterial-venous oxygen measurements showed that although the adrenalectomized rat utilizes more oxygen per blood cycle through the head, the circulatory slowing results in a marked reduction of oxygen consumption by the tissues. Restoration of oxygen consumption is also aided by adrenal cortical extract and Δ^5-pregnenolone, but not by desoxycorticosterone. The reduction in brain oxygen consumption following adrenalectomy is accompanied by reduction of the electrocorticogram frequency, which is restored by the same steroids that restore blood flow and oxygen consumption.

Studies of blood flow through the brain itself made by tapping the vein draining the transverse sinus at its point of emergence from the skull also showed marked reduction of brain blood flow in adrenalectomized rats as compared to normal rats. These blood flow studies combined with measurements of the oxygen content of arterial and venous blood, the latter taken directly from the transverse sinus, showed a reduction of brain oxygen consumption in adrenalectomized rats of 18%. Cortisone fully restored to normal the brain blood flow and oxygen consumption as well as the EEG frequency.

Space does not permit a review of studies by my colleagues and me of electrolyte studies in brain and muscle of normal and adrenalectomized rats before and after stressful swim tests and before and after hormone replacement therapy in the adrenalectomized rats.

HUMAN STRESS STUDIES

In 1940 World War II was rapidly descending upon us and we were impressed, from work of Hans Selye and Ann Forbes, with the importance of the adrenal cortex in meeting stress. I was invited to spend a summer at the Naval Air Training Station in Pensacola to work in collaboration with a group of physiologists and psychologists to see if we could find better methods of selecting pilots. Some 30% of the cadets were flunking out of their training courses and no one knew why. Hallowell Davis and the late Alexander Forbes, then both of Harvard, and I took with us our EEG recording equipment to see if any EEG properties might be found to be related to flying ability. No such correlations were forthcoming, however, but I was impressed with the fact that flight instructors were able to work for relatively few hours a day because of the tensions and stresses involved in teaching cadets to fly.

On returning to Worcester, Pincus and I were intrigued with the possible role of the adrenal cortex in meeting military and workaday stresses, and at Clark in 1941 we set up experiments to study urinary and blood variables that at that time were the standard measurements of the adrenocortical response to stress in man. We developed a battery of stressful tests, including a pursuit meter imitating formation flying of an airplane.

Operating and scoring well for long periods on this machine were stressful and fatiguing. Our first subjects were paid volunteers at the college but later, in 1941, we were able to obtain the services of a squadron commander at Gunter Field in Alabama to investigate adrenal function in his flight instructors. I shall not belabor details of our various tests. Suffice it to say that we did obtain some interesting correlations between various stress measurements, fatigue, and adrenocortical function. We also studied the properties of Δ^5-pregnenolone as a possible antifatigue agent. This substance was used because preliminary work (subsequently confirmed) had indicated that it might be a precursor of cortisone, which at that time was quite unavailable for clinical use and hydrocortisone was still in the offing. Pregnenolone, even in very large doses, had no untoward side effects. Of course studies of effects of this substance were double-blind, placebo-controlled. We studied (1941–42) not only aviators but also several groups of industrial workers doing piece-rate work and compared their performance on placebos and on pregnenolone. We also investigated adrenocortical responses in Pratt and Whitney test pilots flying new planes under dangerous conditions. We extended our investigation to submarine personnel through the cooperation of Charles Shilling, then commander and medical director at the New London submarine base. These wartime results indicated that workaday stresses do enhance adrenocortical output and that those men best able to resist fatigue in general called least on their adrenals when stressed. We found, in general, pregnenolone better able than placebos to improve performance in most of the tests in which it was used.

It occurred to me that it would be worth investigating adrenocortical stress responses in schizophrenic patients since it was thought that the stresses of living were contributory to the development of the psychosis. Evidence published elsewhere indicated a genetic component in the disorder which might be reflected in biochemical indices of abnormal enzyme function. We had, nearby, the Worcester State Hospital which, for a generation, had been a center for research in schizophrenia by many able scientists. Pincus, Fred Elmadjian, and I accordingly used our stress studies on several hundred volunteer male schizophrenic patients matched with male controls of comparable age, and we found statistical differences in various urinary and blood cell indices of steroid metabolism following ACTH administration and under conditions of experimental stress. The finding of diurnal rhythms of adrenocortical function was a product of this work and we used it as a corrective to standardize steroid measures obtained at various times of the day. It was known that in severe adrenal insufficiency, and also in excessive overproduction of corticoids by tumors, that psychological and behavioral disturbances may occur and some of these resemble aspects of schizophrenia. The differences we found in several adrenocortical indices between groups of schizophrenic patients and groups of controls were statistically significant but there was considerable overlap in our measures and no satisfactory diagnostic index emerged from these extensive investigations. There were hints from our work that the administration of certain types of steroids might be therapeutically beneficial but therapeutic studies yielded negative results. Later direct measurements of corticoids in adrenal vein blood showed little difference between patient and normal groups and the differences we found were primarily in urinary steroids, indicating some abnormalities in the metabolism of the adrenocorticoids after their release from the gland. These differences we thought might result from genetic differences in the two populations. We were unable to find that the modified adrenal metabolites in schizophrenics were causally related to the disorder. For controls we used not only "normal" persons but also other groups of hospitalized mental patients.

Our studies of adrenocortical function in schizophrenia lasted from 1944 to 1954. Over the last two decades the foundation's work on schizophrenia has continued but along very different lines. My colleagues and I have been interested in the role of biogenic amines, especially one or more that appear to be bound to certain blood globulin molecules. This work is continuing and has promise, but no new therapy is as yet in sight.

In connection with our studies of adrenocortical function in stress and in schizophrenia, there were some valuable by-products. Pincus, Louise Romanoff, and other collaborators at the Worcester Foundation studied urinary steroids in some 600 normal men and women ranging in age from the second to the ninth decade and their findings were useful in establishing standard norms to compare with endocrinopathies. Some corticosteroids showed little change in secretion rates with age compared to the output of some sex hormone steroids.

In 1941–42 I had a sabbatical year of work with the late Walter B. Cannon, which I regarded as a great privilege. Also, during the mid- and late forties, I studied, with several colleagues, the control of potassium and sodium in brain and muscle in adrenalectomized and intact rats and in adrenalectomized rats given various forms of steroid replacement. Electrical activity of peripheral nerve and of the EEG were also correlated with adrenocortical function or its lack in this series of experiments.

THE WORCESTER FOUNDATION FOR EXPERIMENTAL BIOLOGY

Pincus and I were able to attract research grants and young scientists to work with us. However, space was, as always, a problem and we found it necessary at Clark to convert a barn into a laboratory. This barn belonged to property near the campus I rented from Clark as our family living accommodations. The situation was far from satisfactory, however, and Pincus and I discussed the possibility of breaking entirely free from the university and establishing a research institute of our own supported entirely by grants and gifts. I was the only one of our research group in physiology who was paid by Clark and my position carried tenure, but the challenge of starting a new enterprise was great and led me to obtain a Guggenheim fellowship and resign from Clark. Thus in 1944 the Worcester Foundation for Experimental Biology came into being with Pincus and me as its codirectors, and so we functioned until his death in 1967. We were, and are, a not-for-profit educational and research institution and our board of trustees was composed of friends who were business and professional men and women, including a number of distinguished scientists.

We had attracted to Clark on grants some dozen people, including several with the doctorate, for work in endocrinology and neurophysiology, and it was this initial group that formed the nucleus of our new institution. We had no endowment, no earnings, no student or patient fees and knew that we must exist entirely on grants and gifts. Fortunately we were just entering the "Golden Age of Science" in which, at increasing rates, grants from federal sources were becoming available to universities, hospitals, and research institutions. Pincus and I were also in our early forties and had both published extensively and were known to our colleagues.

I had been given a small grant from the G. D. Searle Company of Chicago to investigate anticonvulsant drugs in animals. When this work was finished I requested that the grant be transferred to Gregory Pincus to be used to carry on basic endocrine studies, and in this way the Searle Company came to know of his talents. With this company's developing interest in endocrinology, he was given an appointment as consultant and spent two or three days every four or five weeks in Chicago discussing endocrine problems with representatives of the company. This relationship with Searle proved to be of increasing value over the years since they gave Pincus generous grants to pursue basic research on steroids under conditions similar to those that would be given by a private philanthropic foundation. It was understood that they would have prior knowledge of his findings, but work done under their grants would be published in the usual media.

Shortly after the advent of the Worcester Foundation, I received contracts from the Office of Naval Research which financed my studies of stress in relation to the adrenal cortex, electrolyte metabolism, and EEG activity mentioned earlier.

As time went on, our annual working income increased with support from the National Institutes of Health, Atomic Energy Commission, grants and contracts for nonclassified work with the armed forces and later with the National Science Foundation. We also had support from a number of private foundations and generous annual gifts from individuals. Our initial income from grants to support our group of a dozen people was approximately $75,000 per year. Our trustees in 1945 gave or raised $50,000 to purchase an attractive residence in Shrewsbury, a suburb of Worcester, which we converted into laboratories. Compared to the barn at Clark, we felt we had ample space, but as our work advanced, the space problem grew apace, and it became clear that more buildings were necessary. We had originally been confined to 12 acres and 2 buildings. At its peak activity in 1970, the budget exceeded $5 million and we employed over 300 people. Today the Worcester Foundation has a research budget of $4 million, with a tract of some 130 acres of desirable residential land in Shrewsbury and, in addition to the original house and garage, we have erected 10 new buildings and acquired several more when we purchased our enlarged estate. Our personnel numbers around 250, with about 100 holding the doctorate. These include fellows who come to us for training purposes as well as our permanent staff.

Dr. Pincus and Dr. M. C. Chang were both outstanding in the field of reproduction physiology and attracted a number of able young scientists. During the late forties and early fifties we had become increasingly aware of the unprecedented upsurge in population growth rates in the underdeveloped countries, and Pincus and Chang started work on what they hoped might be a practical oral steroid contraceptive. This research seemed at first impossible to finance for political reasons. Neither federal agencies nor big foundations would touch it nor was industry at all interested, and the research, we knew, would be very expensive.

I had known the late Mrs. Stanley McCormick for some years since we were both interested in schizophrenia and one day she came to my office and I learned of her deep concern about the "population explosion." She had heard of Pincus's work in reproduction studies and hoped that he might wish to seek an oral contraceptive. To make a long story short, Mrs. McCormick was the primary source of funds that led to the discovery by Pincus and Chang of "the Pill." She contributed some two million dollars over a 12-year period for this work. Pincus and Chang found a group of 19-norsteroids that block ovulation in rats and rabbits without untoward side effects. Pincus then asked Dr. John Rock of the Harvard Medical School to cooperate in administering the most promising of these substances to a small group of volunteer women and testing them for ovulation while on the pills. The success of these modest clinical tests led Pincus, in collaboration with Dr. Celso-Ramon Garcia and the Planned Parenthood organization of Puerto Rico to study some 15,000 women volunteers in Puerto Rico and

Haiti in tests of the effectiveness of the pill along with any possible deleterious side effects. The history of the happy outcome of these studies is too
well known to require repetition here.

Ralph Dorfman was with us from 1951 to 1964 as our director of laboratories. He left to become director of the Institute of Hormone Biology of
the Syntex Corporation and is now president of Syntex. Pincus and
Dorfman built strong groups in basic steroid hormone research, some of it
with application to medical problems including cancer, cardiovascular
studies, and nervous and mental disorders earlier mentioned. Many of these
people are still with us, but others have left. Some distinguished members of
the latter group in the steroid field are Erwin Schwenk, here from 1952 to
1961, past director of research of the Schering Corporation, now retired;
Howard Ringold (1960–67), research director of Syntex; James and Sylvia
Tait (1958–70), discoverers of aldosterone; Oscar Hechter (1944–66); Ian
Bush (1964–67); Eli Romanoff (1946–70); and Fred Elmadjian (1947–63). A
considerable amount of our work involved clinical studies in collaboration
with investigators at several hospitals in Worcester, two in Boston, and one
in Chicago. We also had postdoctoral training programs for a number of
years in the fields of mammalian reproduction, psychobiology, and steroid
chemistry. Hundreds of young scientists from many countries were trained
at the Worcester Foundation in these programs, remaining in residence with
us from one to three years.

I had planned to retire in 1967 at the age of 67, but Pincus's unexpected death that year led me to continue as president for another year,
while Mason Fernald, who had been administrative director of the laboratories of the pharmaceutical company, Smith, Kline and French, came to us
in 1967 as administrative director. At the end of his first year I retired and
he became the chief executive officer. Fernald was not a professional
scientist and the times had become very difficult since government grants
were slowly drying up and the "Golden Age of Science" was slowing down
from the point of view of liberal government financing. Fernald agreed with
me and other trustees that what was needed was a scientist of distinction
who could develop a new program, while supporting and maintaining the
current successful ones. A search committee of scientists on our board of
trustees was chosen to find such a man. Fernald had an attractive offer from
elsewhere and wished to accept it. A number of people were considered for
the directorship but the first choice of the committee, with which I personally had nothing to do, was that of my son, Dr. Mahlon Hoagland, who
was professor and head of the biochemistry department at Dartmouth
Medical School. Several years earlier, as scholar in cancer research of the
American Cancer Society at the Massachusetts General Hospital and
associate professor at Harvard Medical School, he had been senior investi-

gator in the discovery of transfer RNA and the activating enzyme systems involved in its function. He was thus internationally known as a molecular biologist. Initially he turned down our offer. Several years before, Pincus had also tried to entice him to the foundation and he had declined since he was then immersed in his research at Harvard and didn't want to interrupt it. However, in 1970, to my surprise, he informed me that, if the job were still open, he would like to be reconsidered and the trustees were unanimous in renewing their invitation to him to come as our director. He brought with him from Dartmouth a very able associate director, Dr. Federico Welsch, and at the time of this writing he has attracted some 30 young scientists to join our staff to engage in basic studies of growth with emphasis on malignant growth.

As I look back over my own career in science, I think that the work that interested me most—which was the most fun—was my early work in neurophysiology. This could not be considered neuroendocrinology, which came later. The particular study I enjoyed most over the years was my investigation of possible biochemical mechanisms in the brain that determine our sense of time flow and duration. Space does not permit a discussion of these problems, but I found them very exciting.

As often happens, I derived much pleasure from my friends and colleagues in various organizations, particularly as a member of the board of directors of the American Association for the Advancement of Science and, as a member since 1934 and president from 1961 to 1964, of the American Academy of Arts and Sciences. During the last 10 or 15 years my publications have not dealt with new experimental material but with social and philosophical problems related to the development of science and technology. Services as a director or trustee of a number of institutions have also been rewarding in my later years, but as one gets older, it is startling to find how fast a subject (with which one was once familiar and a contributor to its advancement) progresses, and also how young people come in and carry the ball when it has fallen from the hands of the older generation. Most of my professional friends are either dead or retired and this is an inevitable experience if one lives long enough. A friend, given a party on his 75th birthday, was warmly congratulated. When he got up to speak, he said, "There's really nothing to congratulate me about—all I did was get old and anybody can do that if he has enough time."

11

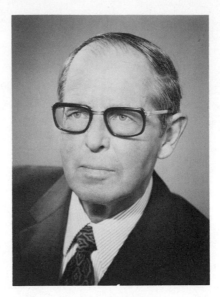

Walter J. M. Hohlweg

Walter J. M. Hohlweg was born on October 10, 1902, in Vienna, where he grew up and later studied chemistry at the Technical University. In 1926 he became an assistant at the Biological Research Institute of the Austrian Academy of Science in Vienna, where he started research work in endocrinology.

From 1928 on, he worked in the main laboratory of Schering AG in Berlin and in 1930 became head of the research group for hormones. He obtained the degree Dipl. Ing. Chem. from the Technical University in Berlin in 1931, and in 1937 from the Technical University in Vienna received the doctor's degree summa cum laude for the thesis, *The isolation of an estrogen from* Butea superba *and its biological effects*. In 1945 he was appointed head of the laboratories of the University-Hospital for Women at the Charité in Berlin, where he became Professor of Endocrinology in 1952. In the same year a new Institute for Experimental Endocrinology at the Humboldt University in Berlin was founded and he was nominated as Director. Ten years later he returned to Austria as head of the hormone laboratory at the Women's Hospital of the University of Graz and continued research work in endocrinology until 1973.

Professor Hohlweg has published 182 papers in medical, endocrinological, and chemical journals and wrote the article *The Hormones of the Gonads* (114 pages, 71 illustrations, and 1498 literary quotes) in the *Handbuch der Biologie und Pathologie des Weibes,* (Urban und Schwarzenberg, 1953).

The *Deutsche Nationalpreis* was presented to him in 1960, while in 1972 he became honorary member of the *Gesellschaft fur Endokrienologie und Stoffwechselkrankheiten* in the GDR and in 1974 honorary member of the *Deutsche Gesellschaft fur Endokrienologie* in the FRG.

The Regulatory Centers of Endocrine Glands in the Hypothalamus

WALTER HOHLWEG

In a speech to the Royal and Imperial Society of Physicians in Vienna in 1912 Bernhard Aschner closed with the following words:

> Not only hypophysectomy, but even a mere wound in the base of the thalamencephalon leads to atrophy of the gonads in male and female dogs. The extent to which the hypothalamus can be regarded as a regulatory center for endocrine glands must therefore be decided after further research has been carried out.

In the *Handbuch für Innere Sekretion,* 1929, however, Leon Asher proves beyond doubt:

> The endocrine glands are autonomous organs and as such are by definition independent to a great extent of the nervous system.

Three years later, however, W. Hohlweg and K. Junkmann (1932*a*) state:

> Internal secretion from the anterior pituitary and the gonads is controlled by a nervous system.

On which research results was this new theory based?

I had just finished my chemistry studies in Vienna in 1926 when a friend told me that Prof. E. Steinlach, director of the physiological department of the Biological Experimental Unit of the Academy of Sciences in Vienna, was looking for a chemical scientist in the field of sex hormone research. Since I was greatly interested in biology and medicine, besides

WALTER HOHLWEG • Professor Emeritus, Humboldt Universität, Berlin. Present address: Prevenhueberweg 25, 8042 Graz, Austria.

chemistry and mathematics, I applied for the position and was engaged as assistant.

My first task was the isolation of follicular hormone from bovine placenta. Apart from the chemical work, I carried out all the Allen-Doisy tests on extracts, made vaginal smears, and stained and studied them under the microscope. The chemistry laboratory was poorly equipped and financial means were limited. Many pieces of laboratory equipment such as mixers for chemicals I made myself, with the aid of a technical construction kit which I had been given years before as a Christmas present. My isolation work was successful, as was reported in the *Akademischen Anzeiger* of December 1927.

The research work in the biological unit was supported by Schering AG in Berlin, and the company made a contract with me which bound me to move to Berlin, should the experiments in their main laboratories make this necessary. This happened in 1928. Since I love the Alps and am an enthusiastic mountaineer I was reluctant to leave Vienna. Berlin seemed so far away from the peaks and snows of my homeland!

Prof. W. Schöller, the director of the main laboratory, encouraged endocrinological research wherever possible. In the Department for Hormone Research, of which I became head in 1930, I had well-equipped chemistry laboratories and a histological and a biological laboratory at my disposal, as well as room for several thousand rats plus rabbits and monkeys. My field of work was extensive. It was composed of isolating and testing estrogens, developing orally effective estrogen preparations, testing and producing a pure form of corpus luteum hormone, and isolating and testing FSH (follicle stimulating hormone), ICSH (interstitial cell stimulating hormone), or LH (luteinizing hormone), and HCG (human chorionic gonadotropin).

It was also possible to carry out purely fundamental research in the main laboratory. What interested me in this area was the following problem: Hypophysectomy leads to histologically demonstrable atrophy of the gonads, since their activity is dependent on the influence of hypophyseal gonadotropins. Zondek described the anterior pituitary as the motor of gonadal function. In older publications I had read that histological changes of the pituitary occur after castration. *Castration cells* appear in the anterior lobe, but what did these castration cells show about the function of the pituitary? Did they secrete gonadotropins in relation to the hormone secretion of the gonads and what was this relationship? I decided to find an experimental explanation for the interdependence of pituitary and gonads.

I discovered that after gonadectomy not only sexually mature but even infantile rats developed castration cells in the anterior pituitary. The pituitaries of normal and castrated rats were then tested for their gonadotropin content. Pituitary glands with castration cells had significantly higher gonadotropin values than normal pituitaries. Fourteen days after castration the pituitaries of infantile rats contained more gonadotropin than those of mature females!

The occurrence of castration cells and the increased gonadotropin content in the pituitary could be prevented or reversed by giving males and females estrogens or androgens. The amounts of hormones necessary depended on the age and sex of the animals. For example, 3-week-old female rats were given 0.015 μg estradiol or 15 μg testosterone daily in order to prevent the appearance of castration cells, whereas it was necessary to give sexually mature females 20 times this amount of hormone.

These experiments had brought to light a feedback mechanism, which can be briefly defined thus: The gonadotropic function of the pituitary is kept within physiological limits by an inhibiting reaction of the gonadal hormones.

I found it especially remarkable that both the pituitary and the gonads of infantile animals are as well able to function as those of mature animals. The hormonal and germinative function of infantile gonads comes into action when enough gonadotropins are present to trigger them, and the pituitary of infantile castrates produces more gonadotropins than that of the normal adult animal. Therefore *pubertas praecox* ought to occur if an infantile ovary is implanted into an infantile female 14 days after castration. The following experiment confirmed my theory (Figure 1).

Of 30 infantile female rats 15 were castrated and the remaining 15 were castrated 14 days later. The females castrated 14 days previously and the females which had just been castrated each received one freshly collected ovary implanted into the kidney. Thus 5-week-old castrated females had an ovary of corresponding age implanted in the kidney.

The implantation of an ovary immediately after castration did not cause any reaction, whereas all the females that received an ovary 14 days after castration reacted with signs of *pubertas praecox*. The vagina opened and estrus occurred, as was shown by vaginal smears. This was not, however, a true pubertas praecox, since the estrus did not recur. The estrogen secretion of the implanted ovary had reduced the gonadotropic function of the pituitary to a level normal for its age once more. Five weeks later, when the female rats reached the usual age of puberty, the implanted ovaries began to function in both groups and regular estrus cycles occurred.

My experiments had proved the following: The quantitative hormonal relationships which exist between the gonadotropic function of the pituitary and the gonads are such that certain amounts of gonadotropins lead to the

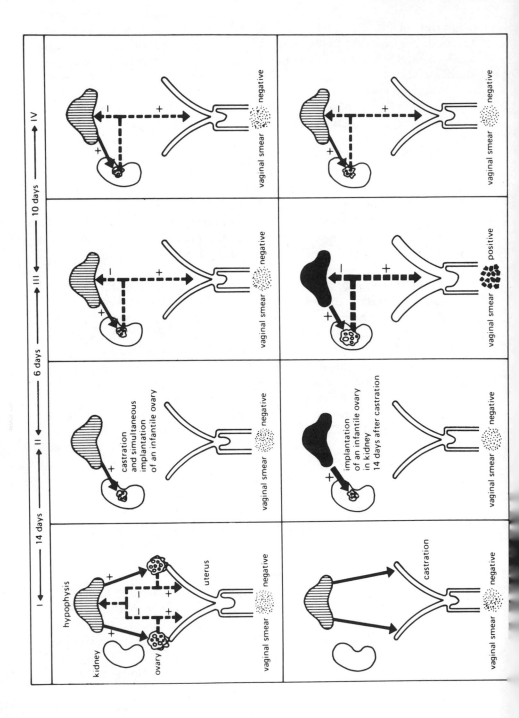

FIGURE 1. The most important phases of the experiment are shown, in which it was proved that the implantation of an infantile ovary in an infantile animal at the time of castration had no visible effect. When the implantation was carried out 14 days after castration, temporary sexual maturity was prematurely induced:

Phase I (upper): Normal equilibrium between the anterior pituitary and gonads of an infantile animal. *Phase I (lower):* Removal of the infantile ovary. *Phase II (upper):* Castration and the simultaneous implantation of an infantile ovary in the kidney of an infantile female rat. *Phase II (lower):* Implantation of an infantile ovary in the kidney of an infantile rat of the same age which had been castrated 14 days before. The implanted ovary comes under the influence of a gonadotropically highly active castration pituitary. *Phase III (upper):* The implanted ovary immediately takes over the function of the ovary which has been removed. The hormone condition does not change. *Phase III (lower):* Under the influence of the enhanced gonadotropin secretion by the pituitary gland of the castrated infant the ovary matures. Large follicles are formed and these produce estradiol, causing the development of the genital tract and inducing a state of estrus. This, in turn, has an inhibiting reaction on the function of the pituitary. *Phase IV (upper):* Unchanged infantile condition. *Phase IV (lower):* The inhibiting reaction of the follicular hormone has stopped the gonadotropic hypersecretion of the anterior pituitary. Estrus does not occur again until the normal age of puberty is attained.

production of certain amounts of sex hormones in the gonads, and that due
to the direct or *indirect* reaction by the sex hormones only a limited amount
of gonadotropins can be secreted.

The cybernetic feedback mechanism was thus indicated for the first
time as a regulatory principle of internal secretory glands. Why did I think
an indirect influence was possible? From the results of the ovary implantation experiments I assumed that a regulatory center existed apart from the
gonads and pituitary. The problem was to prove this.

I sought the assistance of K. Junkmann, the pharmacologist of the
main laboratory, who considered that it would be too difficult to denervate
the pituitary. We then came to mention the father of endocrinology,
Berthold, who in 1849 drew the following conclusion from the results of his
transplant experiments:

> The prevention of castration effects by a testis implanted in another place, where it has
> no connection with its original nerves, can only be due to a product of the testis which is
> secreted into the bloodstream.

We decided to investigate the reaction capacity of pituitary glands implanted in "another place." It was demonstrated that pituitary glands transplanted to the kidney showed no signs of alteration after castration. If the
pituitary glands of castrated animals were transplanted into the kidney of
castrated rats it was impossible to observe castration cells in the anterior
pituitary after 3 weeks.

We felt these results proved that a nervous center plays a part in the
relationship between pituitary and gonads. The hormone production of the
gonads, which is related to the production of gonadotropins by the pituitary,
affects a nervous sex center which regulates the gonadotropic function of the
pituitary on the basis of impulses received. When the level of sex hormones
in the bloodstream falls, this causes increased secretion of gonadotropins by
the pituitary by way of the sex center, which has the effect of causing
increased production of sex hormones by the gonads. Should the level of sex
hormones in the bloodstream exceed the normal range, the secretion of
gonadotropins is reduced in the same way and thus the hormone production
of the gonads is also reduced. The hormonal and germinative functional capacity of the gonads depends on the setting, that is the sensitivity, of the sex
center.

Due to histological findings made in a hyperplastic deformity of the
tuber cinereum which had caused precocious maturity, Driggs and Spatz
(1939) were of the opinion that the sex center must operate on the basis of
hormones.

Implantation experiments by Harris and Jacobsohn in 1952 confirmed
the existence of a neurohormone which travels to the anterior pituitary by

way of the portal vessels of the hypophyseal stalk, and in the following years a gonadotropin releasing factor (GRF) was successfully isolated from hypothalami, identified as a decapeptide and synthesized (McCann and Taleisnik, 1961; Igarashi and McCann, 1964; Schally, Arimura, and Baba, 1972).

As early as 1932 the feedback mechanism between the hormone production of the thyroid and the thyrotropic function of the pituitary was revealed in the experiments carried out by Junkmann and myself (Hohlweg and Junkmann, 1932*b*). Our supposition that this regulatory system is also influenced by a nervous center was later confirmed. In 1959 Shibusawa, Yamamoto, Nishi, Abe, and Tomie indicated the existence of a thyrotropin releasing factor (TRF). In the same way the hormone secretion of the adrenal cortex is controlled by a hypothalamic center with the aid of the corticotropin releasing factor (Guillemin and Rosenberg, 1955).

The discovery of the cybernetic control of endocrine glands gained clinical significance (see Figure 2). In the adrenogenital syndrome two regulatory systems are concerned. As the result of an enzyme disturbance in the adrenal cortex, extremely large amounts of androgens are formed in the process of glucocorticoid synthesis which inhibit the function of the ovaries via the sex center and lead to virilization. By the application of *physiological* amounts of glucocorticoids (cortisone, cortisol), the function of the adrenal cortex is suspended and the production of androgens inhibiting the sex center stops. The pituitary can now produce gonadotropin and the ovaries start to function.

In 1934 I discovered, during an attempt to produce an atrophy of the ovaries by estrogen treatment, the positive estrogen feedback mechanism. The ovaries of sexually mature rats which had been given 800 μg estrone s.c. daily for 4 weeks were not atrophied but revealed numerous large corpora lutea. The anterior pituitary of these females was greatly enlarged and had a characteristic histological picture. It was not possible, however, to establish the presence of FSH or LH (ICSH) in these "estrogen pituitaries."[*] I carried out further experiments based on these observations, which showed that a dose of estrogen triggers the secretion of LH from the anterior pituitary and leads to ovulation and the formation of corpora lutea. Even in juvenile female rats, corpora lutea can be found in the ovaries 7 days after a single injection of 4 μg estradiol (Hohlweg and Chamorro, 1937).

The *Hohlweg Effect* is sex specific for females, i.e., the injection of estrogen into males does not cause secretion of LH (ICSH), as was proved by experiments by Dörner and Döcke (1964).

---

[*] In 1962 I discovered for the first time that these estrogen pituitaries contain large amounts of luteotropic hormone (LTH) = prolactin.

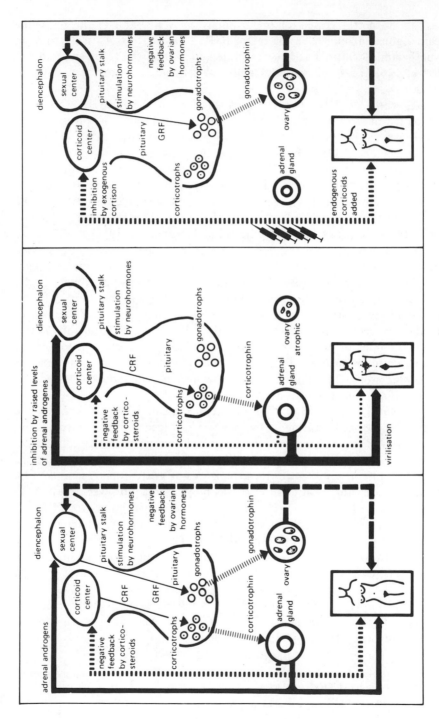

FIGURE 2. The neuroendocrine basis of the adrenogenital syndrome.

The sex center and pituitary react primarily as "female," independent of the chromosomal sex. The changeover to "male" is determined by the testosterone secreted from the fetal testis and is only completed some days after birth. If males are castrated immediately after birth and given implanted ovaries, these ovaries react by developing corpora lutea after estrogen injection at the right age. Females whose mothers were treated with testosterone during pregnancy, or which were given an injection of 1.25 mg testosterone propionate up to 5 days postnatally were sterile for life, since they did not ovulate or form corpora lutea (Barraclough, 1961). The females also demonstrate male psychosexual behavior patterns, just as males castrated on the day of birth prove to be genuine homosexuals.

In 1934 I published a further finding which is important for the therapeutic application of sex hormones. After long term administration of a sex hormone "the sex center becomes habituated to the higher level of sex hormone in the bloodstream. Due to the desensitization of the sex center an increased function of the gonads is made possible when hormone administration is ceased."

Twenty years later, American clinicians recorded a *rebound phenomenon.* In patients with oligospermia, testosterone treatment leads to azoospermia. After the discontinuation of treatment, however, spermiogenesis recommences and the number of sperms even exceeds the initial number.

The inhibition of ovulation by "the Pill" is also based on the negative estrogen feedback to the sex center (Figure 3) (Hohlweg, 1972). Pincus's supposition that progesterone or progestagens inhibit ovulation was incorrect. With *sequential therapy* estrogens alone are given, even after the calculated time of ovulation and only the last 5 pills contain a mixture of estrogen and progestagen.

My attempts, in cooperation with H.-H. Inhoffen, to develop an orally effective estrogen preparation led after many years to the synthesis of ethinyl estradiol in 1938. When given to women orally, this substance is 10 times as effective as an injection of estradiol benzoate. Ethinyl testosterone (syn.:pregneninolone), which was afterward synthesized, proved to be not androgenically but gestagenically effective when given *per os* (1938,1939)! The Pincus Pill contained ethinyl estradiol as its estrogen and ethinyl-nortestosterone as the progestagen. Even today every Pill on the market contains either ethinyl estradiol or its methyl ether.

In 1943 the andrologist H. Zahler informed me that H. Greene and M. Burrill had observed with testosterone an atrophy of the testes with microgram doses, and a hypertrophy with milligram doses after long term treatment of juvenile rats, compared with control animals. Since in my opinion the administration of testosterone could lead only to testis atrophy,

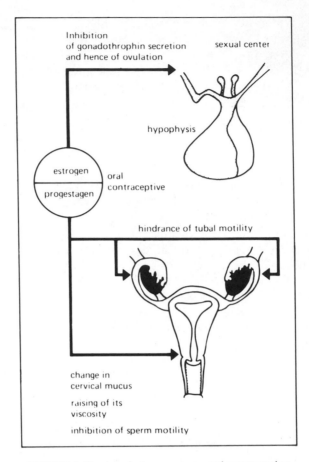

FIGURE 3. Physiological responses to oral contraceptives.

via the inhibition of the sex center, I checked this information—but found it correct. Histological inspection of the testes demonstrated that large and small doses of testosterone inhibited the interstitial cells and thus the production of testosterone. The tubules, and with them the germinative testis function, were, however, only inhibited by small doses of testosterone. Large doses had a stimulating effect!

These findings led to the assumption that testosterone and not FSH is responsible for the function of the tubules and spermiogenesis. This hypothesis was confirmed by unilateral intratesticular testosterone implantation. The implantation of 1 mg testosterone in the testis of an infantile rat led to atrophy of the interstitial cells but to stimulation of the tubules to the point of full spermiogenesis, whereas in the contralateral testis the interstitial cells and tubules atrophy.

The germinative function of the testes is not directly dependent on a hypophyseal gonadotropin. LH leads in the Leydig cells to the formation of testosterone, which acts as a local hormone with a direct stimulating effect on spermiogenesis. A report on the gametokynetic effect of testosterone was first published in 1946 because the manuscript and proofs were burned in Leipzig in 1944.

After the debacle of 1945 Schering had no vacancies for scientists. The equipment was badly damaged and what remained was confiscated down to the last book in the library. I became the head of the research laboratory in the Charité, Gynecological Hospital, as S. Aschheim's successor. In 1952 the Institute for Experimental Endocrinology of the Humboldt University was founded and I took over as its director until 1962. During these 10 years my students, my colleagues, such as E. Daume, G. Dörner, G. Knappe, and U. Laschet, and myself carried out and published extensive research work. The following are only a few examples.

A rebound phenomenon as the result of desensitization of the relevant hypothalamic regulatory center was observed in the thyroid gland after the discontinuation of long term administration of thyroxine and in the adrenal cortex after discontinuation of cortisone administration. An overproduction effect was discovered by which prepuberal administration of gonadotropins can increase the gonadal function and thereby raise the level of androgen or estrogens for long periods of time. Discontinuation of gonadotropin administration leads to increased gonadotropin secretion by the pituitary due to the desensitization of the sex center and thus to a genuine pubertas praecox.

My student and successor as director of the institute, G. Dörner, continued research work in the field of neuroendocrinology with great success. In his monograph *Sex Hormone Dependent Differentiation of the Brain and Sexuality* (Springer-Verlag, Wien/New York, 1972) he reported sensational results. This work also contains an extensive list of references.

I had returned to my own country, Austria, in 1962, where I took up residence in the capital of the Steiermark, Graz. Here I had an ideal position as endocrinologist in the newly built hormone laboratories of the university's Gynecological Hospital which I had helped to plan, and nearby were the cliffs of the Hochschwab range to climb.

REFERENCES

Aschner, B. (1912). Zur Physiologie des Zwischenhirns. *Wien. Klin. Wochenschr.* **27**: 1042.
Barraclough, C. A. (1961). Production of anovulatory, sterile rats by single injections of testosterone propionate. *Endocrinology* **68**: 62.

Dörner, G., and F. Döcke (1964). Geschlechtsspezifische Reaktion des Hypothalamus-Hypophysenvorderlappensystems der Ratte nach einmaliger Oestrogenapplikation. *Zentralbl. Gynäkol.* **86:** 1321.

Driggs, M., and H. Spatz. (1939). Pubertas praecox bei einer hyperplastischen Missbildung des Tuber cinereum. *Virchows Arch. Pathol. Anat. Physiol.* **305:** 567.

Guillemin, R., and B. Rosenberg (1955). Humoral hypothalamic control of anterior pituitary: A study with combined tissue cultures. *Endocrinology* **57:** 599.

Harris, G. W., and D. Jacobsohn (1952). Functional grafts of the anterior pituitary gland. *Proc. R. Soc. Ser. B* **139:** 263.

Hohlweg, W. (1934a). Veränderungen des Hypophysenvorderlappens und des Ovariums nach Behandlung mit grossen Dosen von Follikelhormon. *Klin. Wochenschr.* **13:** 92.

Hohlweg, W. (1934b). Propgynon und Sexualzyklus. *Med. Mitt. Schering-Kahlbaum* AG **6:** 9.

Hohlweg, W. (1972). Wirkungsmechanismus der hormonellen Kontrazeption. *Medical Tribune (Ausg. f. Deutschland)* **7:** 11.

Hohlweg, W., and A. Chamorro (1937). Über die luteinisierende Wirkung des Follikelhormons durch Beeinflussung der endogenen Hypophysenvorderlappensekretion. *Klin. Wochenschr.* **16:** 6.

Hohlweg, W., and M. Dohrn (1931). Beziehungen zwischen Hypophysenvorderlappen und Keimdrüsen. *Wien. Arch. Inn. Med.* **21:** 337.

Hohlweg, W., and H.-H. Inhoffen (1939b). Pregneninolon, ein neues per os wirksames Corpus Luteum-Hormonpräparat. *Klin. Wochenschr.* **18:** 77.

Hohlweg, W., and K. Junkmann (1932a). Die hormonal-nervöse Regulierung des Hypophysenvorderlappens und der Keimdrüsen. *Klin Wochenschr.* **11:** 321.

Hohlweg, W., and K. Junkmann (1932b). Über die Beziehungen zwischen Hypophysenvorderlappen und Schilddrüse. *Pflügers Arch. Gesamte Physiol.* **232:** 148.

Igarashi, M., and S. M. McCann (1964). A hypothalamic follicle stimulating hormone-releasing factor. *Endocrinology* **74:** 446.

Inhoffen, H.-H., and W. Hohlweg (1938). Neue per os wirksame weilliche Keimdrüsenhormon-Derivate: 17-Aethinyl-östradiol und Pregnen-in-on-ol-17. *Naturwissenschaften* **26:** 96.

McCann, S. M., and S. Taleisnik (1961). The effect of a hypothalamic extract on the plasma luteinizing hormone (LH) activity of the estrogenized, ovariectomized rat. *Endocrinology* **68:** 1071.

Schally, A. V., A. Arimura, and Y. Baba (1972). Isolation and properties of the FSH- and LH-releasing hormone. *Endocrinology* **129:** 246.

Shibusawa, K., T. Yamamoto, K. Nishi, C. Abe, and S. Tomie (1959a). Urinary excretion of TRF in various functional states of the thyroid. *Endocrinol. Japan.* **6:** 131.

Shibusawa, K., T. Yamamoto, K. Nishi, C. Abe, and S. Tomie (1959b). Studies on the tissue concentrations of TRF in the normal dog. *Endocrinol. Japan.* **6:** 137.

12

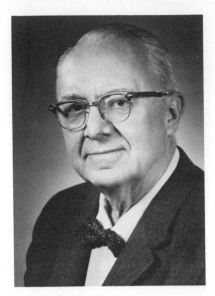

Walter R. Ingram

Walter R. Ingram was born on February 12, 1905, in Liverpool, England and later became a United States citizen after his family immigrated to the Dakotas. He was educated in the public schools in North and South Dakota and then enrolled in Grinnell College, where he obtained the B.A. degree in 1926. He then entered the graduate school at the University of Iowa in the Department of Zoology. He obtained the M.S. in 1927 and the Ph.D. in Zoology in 1929. He served as Instructor in Zoology at Syracuse from 1929 to 1930 and then moved to Northwestern where he served as Instructor and later as Assistant Professor in the Institute of Neurology from 1930 to 1936. He then returned to Iowa as an Assistant Professor of Anatomy and rose to the position of Professor and Chairman of Anatomy which he held from 1940 to 1966. Since that time he has been Professor and then Professor Emeritus and is currently Visiting Professor in the Department of Pathology at the University of Arizona.

Dr. Ingram has done pioneering work in neuroendocrinology, particularly on the neurohypophysis.

A Personal Neuroscientific Development with Remarks on Other Events and People

WALTER R. INGRAM

The course of one's constructive behavior or career bears no mystical landmarks. Rather, it follows the lines of least resistance or easily accepted opportunity, directed in part by prejudice, preference, energy, good and bad advice, a strong element of lucky circumstance. A reasonably high effort: indolence ratio is usually important. These remarks introduce a very personal statement on an early phase of neuroendocrinological history.

My own career has been directed by all the above. I was British born, imported in 1909 at age four to the Dakotas, where my father was a good minister with the usual handicaps, including impecuniosity. The Dakota phase lasted until college time, and the education afforded was excellent. In spite of restrictions in the family economy my brother and I both attended a good college, Grinnell. We worked for most of our support. The family theology did not take hold in my case but some philosophical lodestones persisted. I am not sure why, but it was assumed that I should become a physician—a status symbol, perhaps? I never attained this goal because of circumstances, partly financial, some lines of attractive least resistance, coincident opportunities, and, perhaps, good fortune.

College experience was a beneficial circumstance—with considerable epigenetic input—and I am very grateful for those years. Prof. H. W. Norris charmed me into biology, with appropriate supporting studies. He was unusual since in spite of the teaching grind of a small college professorship he mounted a drive for research in comparative neurology which earned him the respect of such scientists as C. Judson Herrick. Norris was also produc-

WALTER R. INGRAM • Professor Emeritus of Anatomy, University of Iowa and Visiting Professor, Department of Pathology, University of Arizona.

tively interested in the hypophysis. He was an astute and interesting character who, although he would have disdained the idea, was a prototypic Mr. Chips. He gave me the run of the laboratory, problems to follow, and odd but appropriate jobs for pay. He had much perspicacity, and was the first to point out the peculiarities of the blood supply of the cat brain. This observation led to later descriptions of the carotid rete, now known to be an intriguing heat exchanger. Norris was a fine teacher and so I early developed the concept that no teacher is viably good unless he is also a contributing scholar.

My hope for a medical education was clouded by financial circumstances. My qualifications for an adequate scholarship at Harvard were good except for a requirement, discovered too late, that the recipient's parents reside in Iowa. Professor Norris had occasionally mentioned that graduate study might be suitable for an impecunious preacher's son, and this was finally one of my lines-of-least-resistance. He helped me get a $700 assistantship at the University of Iowa—of course just a stopgap until another line should open into medical school. This line never did open, partly because it became fogged by the attractiveness of what I was doing. Some years later, when I was busy with delightful research experiences at Northwestern and had acquired a smattering of medical subjects, I asked Dr. Ranson, my chief, for an opportunity to complete work for the M.D. He refused, indicating that I would be disappointed in the progress and results of such a delayed split effort. He may have been influenced, unconsciously I'm sure, by the red-hot state of the Neurological Institute's program. In any case, he probably afforded me one of the best of many favors. He was not altogether hardhearted in such matters—later he supported Charlie Fisher's quest in that direction.

Circumstantially, I arrived at Iowa at a favorable moment. A reorganization of the zoology department was being set up by a new head, W. W. Swingle, an aggressive, facile-minded endocrinologist. There was no neurological work going on and there was no way of acquiring modern experimental approaches but to try endocrinology. Swingle was a dynamic, rather attractive, mercurial person who was driven by intellectual and status-seeking ambitions. He was fiery, sensitive, and difficult to love, but had many admirable qualities, including interest in the progress of industrious and original graduate students. His adrenal program was adequately staffed, so some of us went in for other angles—thyroid, sex and reproductive physiology, and the hypophysis, which was just then being dramatically presented in new guise by the work of P. E. Smith, H. M. Evans, and their collaborators.

After a hectic orientation Swingle, an old amphibian man, suggested that I try to modify the life patterns of some neotenic amphibians. My M.S.

thesis was apparently the first report of the induction of metamorphosis in hypophysectomized and thyroidectomized axolotls by implantation of inorganic iodine, which indicated (for what it was worth) that such beasts are able to concoct a suitable adulthood hormone without the services of these glands. This may or may not have some teleological significance. I also had a brief run-in with the adrenal cortex in chickens—a character-building experience.

Time was flying, so I returned to amphibia. Swingle had told me that he once saw an extraordinary mitotic skin response to anterior lobe homografts. I collected *Rana clamitans* tadpoles and implanted frog anterior lobes intraperitoneally. The skin thing was a bust, but I was wise enough to examine the thyroids and so was one of the first (Uhlenhuth of Maryland was the other) to describe thyrotrophic effects which were so spectacular as to surprise Dr. Swingle. These hopped-up glands presented the same histological picture as thyroids from cases of exophthalmic goiter. I made measurements of growth changes, compared the effects of glands from adult and larval donors, and prepared a Ph.D. thesis which was published some six months before I was granted the degree. This was an inspiring period, in part because I was very much on my own. Swingle was wrapped up in adrenal and other crises and was glad to have me fumble the ball over the goal line in my own way.

I received my Ph.D. in August 1929—again lucky, because Dr. Swingle returned to Princeton in June. I passed my exam in the spring, but needed to acquire more symbolic graduate credits in summer school. No one seemed to wish to try teaching me but the delay gave me some credits and a timely salary for teaching general zoology.

The three years at Iowa were good and my education was expanded and focused. My chief was good to me in his way. We became good friends and I admire him. He was then variously preoccupied, and working with savage intensity on an adrenal cortical extract. There were also some professors whom I respected, including the late Emil Witschi. I had minors in biochemistry (under H. A. Mattill) and in mammalian physiology. I was a research assistant to Swingle for two years, which meant time for my own devices. I did assist in the last stages of preparation of an active cortical extract, guided by Joe Pfiffner, from whom I learned much. When Swingle and Pfiffner left for Princeton I prepared and tested the extract on adrenalectomized cats. This went fine until some dogs which were in the charge of another student got loose and mangled most of the cats. I was informed later that when Swingle heard of this he spoke feelingly of that student for some 15 minutes, and without undue repetition.

Service on the summer school faculty in 1928 and 1929 afforded needed financial support. I should mention that I owe much for the educational companionship of fellow graduate students, especially Hans Haterius, Fritz Yonkman, and Warren Nelson. Hans later became professor of physiology at Wayne and at Boston. He took a personal interest in my work on hypothalamicohypophyseal mechanisms, which we often discussed with reference to the anterior lobe. In 1937 he became the first to produce LH release from the anterior lobe by localized hypothalamic stimulation.

Dr. Swingle had backed me for a job at Syracuse. I found I had credit enough to borrow the price of a Model A Ford and enough extra, with luck, to get my bride, Lydia, to New York State. My father said the marriage lines, gratis. Dr. Bowen, my father-in-law, handed me an envelope as I revved up the Model A. At the moment I was speculating grimly as to how we'd eat until paid, but the envelope contained $500—much money in 1929. It tided us over the low spots for several years and two babies. I mention this because the editors of this volume expressed interest in the financing of the writers' experimental efforts.

At Syracuse I made some good professional friends. There were also some new and pleasant graduate students, Horace W. Magoun, called Tid, and Jean Jackson, later Mrs. M. This acquaintanceship became a lasting affection. I continued anterior lobe-grafting in my green frogs and described its dramatic effects on the Golgi apparatus of thyroid cells.

During those nine months some fortuitous and fortunate coincidences occurred. In March, F. F. Yonkman, then a pharmacologist at Boston University, invited us to motor to the federation meeting at the University of Chicago. This was my first big meeting and I was thrilled, but after obeisance to the lords of endocrinology I found myself charmed by talks by E. D. Adrian, S. W. Ranson, and other neurologists, although I did not understand them well. I attended the live demonstrations, spending the most time at one conducted by Ranson, who, incidentally, in those days affected high, severely stiff collars, and at another conducted by a large, loud chap named Hinsey who did not. This dealt with postural problems in spinal and decerebrate animals. It was a fine experience for one who was unhampered by knowledge of the subject.

Later I received word from Dr. Swingle that he had recommended me for a position in Ranson's Neurological Institute at Northwestern. I saw his most kind letter and I am eternally grateful for it. Dr. Hinsey was leaving Northwestern for expanding horizons at Stanford and since Dr. Ranson had no hopes of filling his place with anyone as qualified, he sought an unspoiled youngster who might be hammered into something useful. My salary was to be only $100 more, which Syracuse matched, but I'd have gone to such a job with no raise. I was to have a chance to improve my background, also.

I reported to the Neurological Institute on Labor Day, 1930. At that time the Institute was about two years old. In 1924, Dr. Ranson had been lured from Northwestern to a professorship at Washington University, where J. C. Hinsey also of NW, was a graduate student. In the meantime Northwestern received some large gifts, and out of this prosperity the Institute of Neurology was founded. It is my impression that it was set up to utilize the known talents of Walter Ranson, to the glory of NW. Dr. Hinsey came with him. The Institute was composed of basic science and clinical contingents, with a core of departmental structure of a few full-time people. The other participants consisted of neurologically minded members of the anatomy and physiology departments and of the departments of neurology and psychiatry, and surgery. The core of the Institute had its own budget, which was adequate during the deflationary years, and as the richness of the research product increased, outside funds were attracted—as, in about 1933, from the Rockefeller Foundation. The training program, placed on a purely graduate footing in 1931, was then made more attractive. However, as the years advanced into the 1940s the economics of the period and shrinking university support required unacceptable dependence on outside support. Whether or not Ranson's death in 1942 was contributory, this situation forced the closing of the Institute in 1948.

Back to 1930 again, the full-time staff consisted of Dr. Ranson, Dr. Weil, and me, plus four temporary research fellows. Arthur Weil was a German-trained neuropathologist, an excellent chemist and all-around technologist who made a very good contribution.

That first year must have been a nitty-gritty affair for me. My evenings and weekends were spent studying gross anatomy. I absorbed neurohistological and experimental surgical techniques. I did a vast amount of reading and slide study on brain stem structure and Dr. Ranson suggested I do some counting of exotic cells appearing in dorsal root ganglia after certain surgical procedures. A small dose of this effectively immunized me, and I was guilty of stalling in this instance—which Ranson knew. A new, but planned development rescued me. This was to require a strong effort on my part in exploring the use of a Horsley-Clarke stereotaxic instrument, which now became available to us.

The background for this episode was provided by Ranson's and Hinsey's interest in the physiology of the interior of the brain as it related to body posture and locomotion. Old methods of stimulation and lesion production were not adequate for reasons which all neurophysiologists now appreciate. They were aware of R. H. Clarke's design for a stereotaxic approach which had been published first in *Brain* in 1908. This involved the localization of points within the brain according to rectilinear coordinates determined by a central fixed point determined by the intersection of coronal, sagittal, and horizontal planes. These planes were established by the fixation of the stereotaxic instrument to the skull, and were made usable by prepara-

tion of charts based on suitably marked serial sections. This instrument had
been used only a few times between 1908 and 1930 by Horsley and Clarke,
Kinnier Wilson, E. Sachs, A. T. Mussen, and F. J. F. Barrington. With it
one could approach any desired point for purposes of stimulation or lesion
production, with minimal damage elsewhere.

Circumstances, including a Great War, were not propitious for the
development of this innovative method, although several instruments were
built in London and one was sold by Clarke to Johns Hopkins along with
figures of chart brain sections prepared by E. E. Henderson. Another, according to Clarke, was taken to the Rockefeller Institute by Barrington,
who had used it in England in 1925. A similar instrument was used by F. H.
Lewy in Germany in the 1920s. Perhaps an immediate stimulus to Ranson
was a Clarke-built machine brought to St. Louis from England by Ernest
Sachs. I say perhaps, because I never heard Ranson speak of this machine
or acknowledge its existence, although he and Sachs were apparently
friends. Ranson never discussed with me his early thinking with regard to
Clarke's instrument. I am certain, however, that this was a hush-hush
operation. Dr. Ranson's shrewd and suspicious nature would not allow leaks
of information which might give an edge to competitors, real or imagined.

At any rate, he undertook to have such an instrument made, taking advantage of the services, available at the moment, of a man named Gaddas, a
skilled machinist and former assistant to Bovie, a biomedical engineer. Gaddas was able with great cleverness to replicate in brass the original instrument as depicted in *Brain*. This background story and that of learning to
use the machine effectively are as long as the task was formidable. They are
mentioned here because nearly all the questions asked me about this stage
of the Institute's history have been concerned with this adventure. Gaddas
finished his work in the late fall of 1930. I had studied the publications on
its use which were known to us and we proceeded with the preparation and
study of cat brains. When the instrument became available, it was used to
mark the key horizontal and vertical planes by inserting wires which left
holes in the finished sections. This involved adjusting the machine to the
head, which was not an easy problem, especially since this model was
constructed without allowing adequate working room, nor was it offset
properly to allow for moving the vertical needle carrier laterally. These and
other defects were shortly overcome by replanning, and an improved model
made largely of stainless steel was built to our specifications by Mr. Kittle
at the University of Chicago. Kittle subsequently made many of these machines for laboratories over the country. Some had interchangeable adapters
for use with rats—it was found that no modifications were needed for use
with macaques. This model was quite accurate and it was years before more
facile instruments of other design but using the same coordinates were

produced. Most later machines were actually head holders with improved working space for surgery and provisions for multiple electrode mounts, and had to be preset, which may have reduced accuracy. Varieties of angle approaches were also designed.

Concern with individual animal variations led me to measure many cat heads and to attempt to correlate these measurements with instrument settings. It was necessary to make individual adjustments only for very large or small specimens. It was possible to calculate shrinkage due to processing, data which could be used in charts for localizing points for lesions or stimulation. While the charts were in preparation we tried stimulatory exploration of the brain stem point by point in lightly anesthetized cats. We also started to learn lesion-making methods. Hence at a meeting of the American Association of Anatomists at Northwestern in the spring of 1931, we were able to present a live demonstration. This did not attract as much attention as I had expected, but those who came to see it were somewhat startled. In retrospect I am amazed that the work progressed so rapidly, considering other obligations. I am now wise enough to realize that young people do work fast and make decisions faster. I can see now why Dr. Ranson was content to let the youngsters shed the blood—and tears. He interfered very little with this learning process. He stood by and observed, making occasional suggestions or criticisms and held me to the line. He had no advantage of experience in this expanding situation but was able to stabilize our goals of high precision and honest observation. As a matter of fact, I never saw him personally use the instrument of which he was so proud, although he showed and explained it reverently to distinguished visitors. Perhaps he did not wish to interfere with the sharpening skills which his young men were developing. Perhaps, also, at age 50 Dr. Ranson's health was starting the course it would follow in the remaining 12 years of his life. I am certain he had intimations that stressful problems should in his case be dealt with at the desk rather than on the firing line. He made good and bad suggestions and, being at heart a gadgeteer, often came up with Goldbergian devices which occasionally worked. He was also prone to l'idée fixe and these fixations sometimes formed roadblocks which required strategic or diplomatic footwork to evade, as may come out farther on. He was, nevertheless, very nice indeed during this phase. I hope—and think—that he enjoyed the adventure just as I did. He did establish a smoothly running organization for maximum effective use of the facilities available, offered continuing encouragement, and made important decisions. Wisdom in these situations must be considered broadly.

The rapidity of progress is indicated by the publication in 1931 of four communications concerned with the developing methods and some results. Those were hard, intense, and sometimes bitter months—a clear dispassionate backward look is not easy. However, the inevitable frustrations and balks were transitory and the total abiding impression is one of reward and reinforcement. Certainly Dr. Ranson was rewarded to the point where some exuberance leaked from cracks in his normal shell.

There were some spots of happy adventure during this and later periods. There was the hairy matter of electrodes. We did not make glass-sheathed wires as described by Clarke, for good reasons. In pioneering, fairly straight lengths of insulated copper wire with bare tips were used. These worked but deposited quantities of copper, and they bent. We were not equipped to develop platinum needles. However, I saw resistance wire being used for other purposes and asked the Driver-Harris Company for enameled nichrome stainless steel wire, 22 and 28 gauge, which they gave us. We learned to stretch and smooth this material to straightness but stretching cracked the insulation disastrously. The Driver-Harris man, who should have an appropriate 400-degree memorial, gave me some tung oil varnish and we learned to dip and bake the electrodes and to grind suitable tips. Such electrodes made splendid electrolytic lesions and in due course were used to pick up potentials. For exploratory stimulation it quickly became apparent that unipolar electrodes were not precise enough—there was too much and too variable a spread of stimulating effects. So we fashioned side-to-side bipolar electrodes of straight insulated 22- and 28-gauge wires fashioned parallel, reinsulated smoothly overall, and with the tips ground precisely to the desired gap. These were quite accurate and the spread of shock effect could be restricted to less than one millimeter. Suitable straight tubing for concentric electrodes was not easy to get and the use of such equipment was deferred.

Making lesions was another adventure. The electrolytic method had been preselected and we were equipped in advance with a long adjustable resistance coil and an expensive Becton milliammeter. I forget the energy source, but the first use blew the fancy meter all to hell. Our consultants were rank amateurs. Northwestern was an elitely amateur school in those days except in football. This was a grinding crisis and I sought a solution we could afford—and understand. On south State Street, at that time full of radio repair and supply shops, I found what we needed—an inexpensive volume control which was adequately adjustable without fancy footwork, an equally cheap milliammeter, and a 40-volt B battery. I built a console consisting of a vertical panel perpendicular to a broad plank base and mounted the control, meter, battery, and a toggle switch conveniently. It worked for years, eventually being made more compact. It was a long time before fancy lesion makers became commercially available. This particular gizmo required adjusting to maintain the current as resistance due to polarization built up. When I went to Iowa, Clinton Knowlton helped to correct this with an instrument using house current and consisting of a rectifier tube, an adjustable resister, a voltage regulator tube, milliammeter, and suitable switches, set up in a tackle box.

We did not at this time use high-frequency coagulating current for producing lesions. We used anodal electrolysis chiefly because of relative gas accumulation and polarization—and because Clarke said so, which was important to Dr. Ranson. Actually, the cathode is also very usable, and I'm sure it was often inadvertently used. Certainly there were anodal iron depositions, and postoperative electrochemical reactions which have been discussed recently. The latter reaction has been useful to such wise investigators as Sawyer in studying the induced release of certain anterior lobe hormone releasing factors. It is of short relative duration, however, and the destructive effects are quickly distinguishable from the irritative. Bipolar electrodes were used for lesion making only when large lesions were required. Methods for this were refined by Frank Harrison, who was the first person with any savvy in electronics to come to the Institute.

Various encephalotomic instruments have been found useful recently for producing isolated islands of brain tissue. These are variations of similar designs which were in use as early as the last quarter of the 19th century. Since Dr. Ranson had had experience with incisional experiments we had no difficulty in controlling impulses to use such instruments, useful though they may be for appropriate needs.

We found that microscopic examination was required for conscientious work in localizing lesions and stimulation points. The later development of rapid serial frozen tissue methods helped greatly in this. Naked eye examination was not adequate and became less so as morphological knowledge became more detailed. Location of stimulated points could be done by electrolysis at productive spots, but in extensive explorations the progressive trauma could distort the results. Estimation of shrinkage by markers in tissue before processing made it possible to locate points by measurement along electrode tracks. Careful postexperiment lesion and point identification became important to us very quickly. The stereotaxic coordinates carried sufficient variation to make microscopic check necessary. We were not impressed when distinguished investigators visited the lab to learn our coordinate methods so they could attempt to locate brain points by chart, and thus conclude an experiment at one sitting. I fear the literature is scarred with too many reports of this sort of effort.

There were other small but important problems which required practical and also diplomatic solutions. These were especially pertinent to survival experiments. For instance, in anesthesia our resources were limited. Inhalation anesthesia was a nuisance with the stereotaxic machine in place, especially under aseptic conditions. About 1930 sodium pentobarbital became available and the Abbott capsules were being used for sedation on the obstetrical service. However, the chief's idea of a nonvolatile anesthetic was chloral hydrate, and even with his luck and in his hands it was lethal. It so happened that Dr. Ranson went to Europe in the summer of 1931 and when he returned we had a well-controlled system of intravenous barbiturate anesthesia going which he accepted in good spirit and to which he afterward pointed with a modicum of personal pride.

Also, we had infection problems in those already polluted years—Chicago cats had stores of virulent organisms. Fortunately these did not often infect our personnel. I once acquired a tremendous axillary lymphadenia which intrigued the surgeons and hence gave me a salutary and immunizing experience with intern's disease. In our first use of the Clarke instrument the placement of receptacled ear plugs to receive the ear bars was made easier by incising the tragal portion of the pinna. As a result and in spite of cleanliness and ingenious aftertreatment, we had atrocious infections and serious losses. Because we had had fine accuracy while using this method it was difficult to get clearance to abandon it. Another trip to Europe was worth its cost because it was possible during this interphase to establish a noncutting procedure without any discussion or ulcer diathesis. This was also most gratifyingly accepted and pridefully incorporated in the ritual.

Other refinements were inevitable, evolutionary, and rewarding, especially as good young people joined us, first Tid Magoun and Ralph Barris, then Kendrick Hare, Frank Harrison, and Charles Fisher. Many others were later selected by Ranson's usually accurate judgments. There were also summer guests and visitors from higher levels of the establishment. Ideas were rife and there was constant awareness of the pressure of critical scrutiny. It was a fine atmosphere for creative life and living. As the number of students and visitors increased, Dr. Ranson was able to secure additional space. We were comfortable but always crowded. The contingent intimacy was happy and the friendships which were formed have given increasing pleasure. As remarked before, the technical aspects of the Ranson era have been stressed here because of general interest in the history of these matters. The basic developments have served the emerging science of neuroendocrinology as well as neuroanatomy and general neurophysiology. The more slowly constructed clinical applications have been very impressive to interested pioneers. I clearly recall how horrified Dr. Ranson was when a prescient visitor suggested that this method might one day be used with human patients. This was a time in the lives of all of us which was highly charged—the intensity of effort and the emotional mosaic can only be hinted. The growing cloud of economic depression was no minor distraction.

During the period of technical refinement, experimentation went forward. Results of exploratory stimulation in the interior of the brain stem were reported, as were the effects of chronic lesions. The ventral diencephalon was explored to an extent sufficient to indicate that it was a rich field for experiments which could extend and modify the stimulation work reported by W. R. Hess. This exploration was mainly carried out by Magoun, Kabat, and others. In spite of the crudities of the Harvard coil stimulation the results have been very durable and furnished the takeoff point for Magoun's career. Frances Hannett and I prepared a stereotaxic atlas of the cat diencephalon which was later followed by one for the macaque (with Donald Atlas). Our original interests in posture and locomotion were not abandoned and in the course of exploratory lesion placements for such experiments, approaches for study of sleep and catalepsy were established and the prospects for precise exploration of hypothalamic phenomena became attractive. We quickly learned the importance of bilaterally symmetrical lesions for studies of hypothalamic deficits which were observable as changes in sleep patterns, in temperature regulation, appetite, anorexia, cachexia and obesity, aggressions and other emotion-related behaviors, and in changes in water exchange. For the latter we were prepared because the food and fluid intake of our chronic animals was routinely recorded. As I recall it, the occurrence of polyuria was first noted while studying survey lesions for analysis of catalepsy. We had been aware of the problems of diabetes insipidus and of rediscoveries of Ramon y Cajal's supraopticohypophyseal fiber tract. When we observed consistent changes in water exchange, the literature was carefully searched and the hypothalamist versus hypophysist controversy examined—a study which was greatly aided by the addition of Charles Fisher to our group. The experiments which followed formed a good basis for analysis and partial comprehension of hypothalamic-posterior hypophyseal relationships. The value of the results was appreciated not only by Fisher and me but also by Dr. Ranson, who was not especially well informed on endocrine systems. The findings were so significant that Fisher and I were afforded sufficient time and facilities to pursue the subject in depth, although other lines of attack on hypothalamic physiology were not neglected. Dr. Ranson was so aware of the importance of the concepts involved that when the Oxford University Press—depression wary—backed off from publication of a monograph on diabetes insipidus he was willing personally to support a planographed production of the Fisher, Ingram, and Ranson book.

It is a pleasure to acknowledge the importance of Charles Fisher's contributions. He was a very perceptive person, good at sifting and organizing material. His major contribution involved the quantitation of posterior lobe hormones under varying experimental conditions. He was an invaluable colleague and I regretted that it was fairly clear even then that his future was not to be defined or confined by the laboratory. Not all of our distinguished Chicago colleagues were so perceptive, and we were sometimes plagued with bad advice.

At any rate, the problem was followed assiduously, and although the stereotaxic approach was essential for elegant elucidation of the supraopticohypophyseal system, direct surgical methods were also developed which made it possible to analyze delicately the hypophyseal aspects of the problem. Experiments in incising the median eminence at various levels showed that this structure contained and released antidiuretic substance. The occurrence of diabetes insipidus depended upon sectioning the supraopticohypophyseal fibers as close to their source as possible, or required destruction of both supraoptic nuclei. About this time and quite independently, Broers, a student of Cornelis Winkler in Holland, expressed views similar to ours in his dissertation. I am glad we were able to note this in the monograph.

Our findings could have been much more nicely and completely explained if the circumstances had been different. We were aware of the Scharrers' work, on neurosecretion but none of us was ready to see its theoretical pertinence. While Dr. Ranson's critical attitudes were generally cool, there was some prejudice here which prevented the formulation of a concept applicable to our work. The idea that neurons produce secretions and that chemical message-substances could migrate within nerve fibers was apparently too much. However, Ranson did take Gaupp, an associate of Scharrer, into the laboratory later—a sign that perhaps dogma was rifting. Other untoward circumstances which arose were false alarms over supposed structural changes in pituicytes when blood hydration was altered. Production of antidiuretic hormone by supraoptic neurons, rather than by pituicytes, was shortly indicated when Kendrick Hare and others at Cornell showed that extracts of the supraoptic region contained antidiuretic substance when severed from the neurohypophysis. The use of renal clearance techniques in dogs with diabetes insipidus provided a sensitive assay method. Later, at Iowa, D. Phillips found ADH to be present in the hypothalamus during the normal interphase which may occur early in experimental DI.

The examination of renal and metabolic aspects of DI (with Charles Winter) perhaps received too much of my attention after I went to Iowa in 1936. We were, however, able to show that the production and excretion of ADH could be modified by hydration changes in cats.

Our group at Northwestern never really thought that hormones originating in the hypophysis were blood-borne to the hypothalamus. We were acquainted with Wislocki's work indicating the direction of flow in the hypophyseal portal system but our group was not yet sufficiently focused on the anterior lobe to appreciate its significance. The current thought was that the posterior lobe might offer triggering mechanisms for anterior lobe hormones, under hypothalamic influence. Hinsey wrote in 1937, "The relationships of the portal venules are such that they could well serve to transport a humoral substance elaborated by nervous stimulation of the pituitary stalk on to the anterior lobe." Haterius, in the same Cold Spring Harbor Symposium, postulated "a neurovascular" mechanism to transmit stimuli from the pars posterior to the pars anterior, the former being stimulated via nerve fibers from the hypothalamus. We were eventually happy to see the work of John Green and Geoffrey Harris in England lead to subsequent appropriate advances.

While we thought for a time that viable anterior lobe was necessary for full-blown DI, we could discern no good evidence for existence of a "diuretic hormone." We early approached some aspects of the relationships of the hypothalamus and the anterior lobe. David Cleveland and I, with the support of Loyal Davis, offered evidence indicating that the Houssay phenomenon might be produced by hypothalamic lesions as well as by hypophysectomy. The suggestion was not well received at the time. Much later, however, this situation was clearly established and a variable arrangement of the scattered neurons involved was noted. Barris and I demonstrated that hypothalamic lesions can induce increased sensitivity to insulin—and even a first order hypoglycemia. We associated this with an effect on the anterior lobe because of Houssay's experiments. Years later, Basil Spirtos and Nicholas Halmi showed that increased insulin sensitivity in rats with hypothalamic lesions is related to deficiency of growth hormone.

We also in the early days offered some indirect evidence of hypothalamoanterior lobe relationships by showing that hypothalamic lesions could be associated with dystrophic changes in the adrenal cortex and gonads. There was good evidence that such dystrophic changes were functions of the location of the lesions. The glandular subnormalities were most frequent with medioventral and rostral lesions, as I recall. Dorsocaudal lesions involving descending hypothalamic pathways produced no dystrophies. To quote from one 1937 statement, "Possibly the changes are due to some influence upon the anterior lobe, because nervous lesions such as spinal cord transections or denervation of the glands do not necessarily produce such alterations . . . these subnormalities have not approached the absolute atrophy produced by hypophysectomy, and furthermore there is indication of dissociation of the effects produced; for instance, there may frequently be subnormal gonads with normal adrenals, and in one case the reverse was observed." More histological and physiological studies were later made by other workers in the Institute and undoubtedly contributed to neuroendocrine progress.

There is no suitable place here to comment upon my work in other phases of neurology, including behavioral studies, and reverting to experimental neuromorphology. Some of my later students have from time to time made neuroendocrine contributions. Dwight Sattler was able to extend the findings of Chang that the supraopticohypophyseal system was subject to vagal reflex influence. Robert Joynt is distinguished for studies of osmotic control of ADH production and release, and of the action potentials of the supraopticohypophyseal fibers. He recently has been involved in studies of the median eminence. Donald Nibbelink helped clarify the neuroendocrine relationships of the paraventricular nucleus. I have long appreciated association with Nicholas Halmi, and in recent years have enjoyed working with José de Olmos on experimental morphological problems with neuroendocrine bearing.

I am afraid I have made an unduly long story out of some rather simple annals. Some parts of it may seem overstated because I have given special treatment to things about which the most questions have been asked. One of the main subjects of inquiry in recent times has been Ranson himself. Some personal glimpses of the chief have been permitted to surface throughout this account in ways which also indicate the nature of the laboratory atmosphere at the time. Some may seem flippant and cynical, but this is not intended. Walter Ranson was an extraordinary person whose inbred diffidence, seclusiveness, and sensitivity greatly affected his outward personality and perhaps even his health. Some Chicago scientists were unfavorably impressed by him as indicated by Mackay in his *History of Neurology in Chicago*. His synoptic statement was derived from persons who did not know Ranson well, and Mackay wisely praised Ranson's humanity as well as his stature as "an earnest scientist . . . an indefatigable seeker and revealer of the facts!" This author also in his peroration stated that the brightest lights of Chicago neurology were the basic neuroscientists, Herrick and Ranson.

I had extraordinary opportunities to know Dr. Ranson, not only in confronting together new experimental problems but also in personal confrontations. I had the advantage of knowing him before the affairs of the Institute became complex. He often rode home with me during the first years and of course we talked—about problems, people, the Institute, colleagues, Chicago, past experiences, books, art, philosophies personal and general. He had a sense of humor somewhat inhibited by his personal sensitivity and standards of suitability—although he was not really a snob. I occasionally flunked here. He was perceptive and a judge of the promise and ability of persons. He had a good family life, in part due to Mrs. Ranson's delightful personality, and his relations with his children were pleasant. His son understandably developed emotional troubles when prematurely exiled to Harvard medical school. I was impressed by the way Dr. Ranson handled this.

Ranson was concerned for and usually loyal to his young men. A frequent question to me is, "How about it? I hear Ranson was just a slave driver." In a sense he was, as any strong leader may be, but not in the crude sense. He desired the greatest work output which could be comfortably achieved, not only for the sake of Ranson and the Institute, but proportionately for the credit of the worker. I recall how he once told me regretfully that he had just been very mean to Magoun by refusing him time off for a family doing. "I tried to make him see that such events would be the more enjoyed when his undoubtedly brilliant future is assured." If I know Tid Magoun, I must feel that he himself on later occasions may have acted in similar fashion, although expressing himself differently.

Ranson's sensitivity and prejudices were his chief defects, along with a chronic disposition to believe the worst of people. His drive for preeminence caused a few persons to believe that the sine qua non contributions of his working associates were deliberately obscured. He could not tolerate association with persons he thought to hold derogatory views of Walter Ranson. There were such people and when he encountered one as paranoid as he, it caused sticky situations and long bitter aftermaths which left enduring scars even on the personalities of persons not involved. A sad situation involved W. R. Hess, with whom Ranson was apparently not acquainted but of whom he was so inordinately jealous that he wouldn't cite his work if he could avoid it. Not for ignorance of it, for sure, because I had to claw my way through Hess's opaque German and epitomize his writings for Ranson's perusal. About 15 years ago I had a delightful visit with Professor Hess in Zurich. He was a sweet and warm person. He was quite deaf and since I was becoming so, we were simpatico. He was almost tearful when he asked me why Dr. Ranson had not liked him.

In spite of these animadversions, my feelings for Walter Ranson are affectionate and marked by respect for a very fine scientist. When Ranson died another coincidence occurred. After the service there was an unexpected meeting—Hinsey, Magoun, and myself. None knew the others were there—Magoun was on vacation, Hinsey had been visiting his family in Ottumwa, and I happened to be in Chicago visiting my parents.

My situation in the Ranson show was happy. There were small injustices, but I never considered myself unfavorably touched by the environment. Even so, I never regretted leaving it and my personal relationships with Dr. Ranson after 1936 were very warm, as our correspondence attests.

However, I may have been affected by it, accounting for an urge for self-construction—and a distaste for appearing to be competitive. I do not need to reassure myself by nostalgic projections. Those were fine times. I rather think we had more fun in our crude ways than seems possible amidst today's unkempt sophistication.

REFERENCES

Barris, R. W., and W. R. Ingram (1936). The effect of experimental hypothalamic lesions upon blood sugar. *Am. J. Physiol.* **114:** 555.

Davis, L., D. Cleveland, and W. R. Ingram (1935). Carbohydrate metabolism. The effect of hypothalamic lesions and stimulation of the autonomic nervous system. *Arch. Neurol. Psychiatry.* **33:** 592.

Fisher, C., and W. R. Ingram (1936). The effect of interruption of the supraoptico-hypophyseal tracts on the antidiuretic, pressor and oxytocic activity of the posterior lobe of the hypophysis. *Endocrinology* **20:** 762.

Fisher, C., W. R. Ingram, W. K. Hare, and S. W. Ranson (1935). The degeneration of the supraoptico-hypophyseal system in diabetes insipidus. *Anat. Rec.* **63:** 29.

Fisher, C., W. R. Ingram, and S. W. Ranson (1935). Relation of hypothalamico-hypophyseal system to diabetes insipidus. *Arch. Neurol. Psychiatry* **34:** 124.

Fisher, C. A., W. R. Ingram, and S. W. Ranson (1938). *Diabetes insipidus and the Neuro-Humoral Control of Water Balance. A Contribution to the Structure and Function of the Hypothalamic-Hypophyseal System.* Edwards Brothers, Ann Arbor, Michigan.

Ingram, W. R. (1937). The relation of the hypophysis and associated hypothalamic mechanisms to water exchange. *Cold Spring Harbor Symp. Quant. Biol.* **5:** 381.

Ingram, W. R. (1939). The hypothalamus: A review of the experimental data. *Psychosom. Med.* **1:** 48.

Ingram, W. R. (1940). Nuclear organization and chief connections of the primate hypothalamus. *Res. Publ. Assoc. Res. Nerv. Ment. Dis.* **20:** 195.

Ingram, W. R. (1946). Hypothalamic lesions and insulin requirement in diabetic cats. *Anat. Rec.* **94:** 540. (Abstr.)

Ingram, W. R. (1947). Hypothalamic obesity in the cat. *Anat. Rec.* **97:** 345. (Abstr.)

Ingram, W. R., and R. W. Barris (1936). Evidence of altered carbohydrate metabolism in cats with hypothalamic lesions. *Am. J. Physiol.* **114:** 562.

Ingram, W. R., and C. Fisher (1936). The relation of the posterior pituitary to water exchange in the cat. *Anat. Rec.* **66:** 271.

Ingram, W. R., and C. Fisher (1937). The effects of thyroidectomy, castration, anterior lobe administration and pregnancy upon experimental diabetes insipidus in the cat. *Endocrinology* **21:** 273.

Ingram, W. R., C. Fisher, and S. W. Ranson (1936). Experimental diabetes insipidus in the monkey. *Arch. Intern. Med.* **47:** 1067.

Ingram, W. R., F. I. Hannett, and S. W. Ranson (1932). The topography of the nuclei of the diencephalon of the cat. *J. Comp. Neurol.* **55:** 333.

Ingram, W. R., L. Ladd, and J. T. Benbow (1939). The excretion of antidiuretic substance and its relation to the hypothalamico-hypophyseal system in cats. *Am. J. Physiol.* **127:** 544.

Nibbelink, D. W. (1961). Paraventricular nuclei, neurohypophysis and parturition. *Am. J. Physiol.* **200:** 1229.

Ranson, S. W., C. Fisher, and W. R. Ingram (1936). The hypothalamicohypophyseal mechanism in diabetes insipidus. *Proc. Assoc. Res. Nerv. Ment. Dis.* **17:** 410.

Ranson, S. W., and W. R. Ingram (1931*a*). Sections prepared for use in determining the location of any structures in the cat's brain in terms of Horsley and Clarke rectilinear coordinates. *Anat. Rec.* **48** (Suppl.): 61. (Abstr.)

Ranson, S. W., and W. R. Ingram (1931*b*). A method of accurately locating points in the interior of the brain. *Proc. Soc. Exp. Biol. Med.* **28:** 577.

13

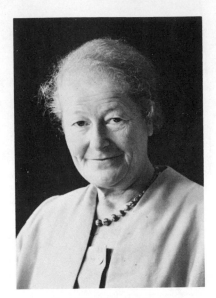

Dora Elizabeth Jacobsohn

Dora Elizabeth Jacobsohn was born in Berlin on March 1, 1908. She qualified in medicine at the Friedrich-Wilhelms University in 1933, but was not allowed to practice under the Nazi anti-Jewish regulations. After emigrating to Sweden in 1934 she worked with Axel Westman in Uppsala and in Lund. She was awarded the M.D. degree in Sweden in 1948 and a personal professorship in 1964.

My Way from Hypophysectomy to Hypophyseal Portal Vessels (1934–1954)

DORA JACOBSOHN

The story of my contribution to what nowadays is called *neuroendocrinology* begins with hypophysectomies in rabbits. This species is a *reflex ovulator*, and the study of the effects of the removal of the pituitary gland on ovulation and the formation and life-span of corpora lutea led straight into the problem of the neural control of the hypophysis.

The events that brought me in contact with endocrine research were, briefly, as follows: In January 1934 I had concluded my medical training in Berlin, when Germany was ruled by the Nazis. The authorities gave me a document (Figure 1) which confirmed that I had fulfilled the requirements for obtaining the medical licence. Because of the *Arier Paragraph* I was not to receive it, however, since I am a Jew. I emigrated to Sweden, where my mother had relatives, and I was supported by a private fund for intellectual refugees. As I hoped to become a practitioner in some other country, I went to Uppsala, a small university town near Stockholm, where I spent most of the time at the University Hospital, mostly at the Department for Obstetrics and Gynecology, which was headed by the late professor Axel Westman. Attached to the clinic was a small hormone laboratory for pregnancy tests and hormonal assays on mice, rats, and rabbits, which at that time was unusual and evidence of a progressive spirit.

As I was a foreigner, my activities were restricted to watching, listening, and reading. Westman was a vivid research worker, and I studied his papers, especially his most recent *Untersuchungen über die Abhängigkeit der Funktion des Corpus luteum von den Ovarialfollikeln und über die Bildungsstätte der Hormone im Ovarium"* (Westman, 1934). The paper,

DORA JACOBSOHN • Institute of Physiology, University of Lund, Lund, Sweden.

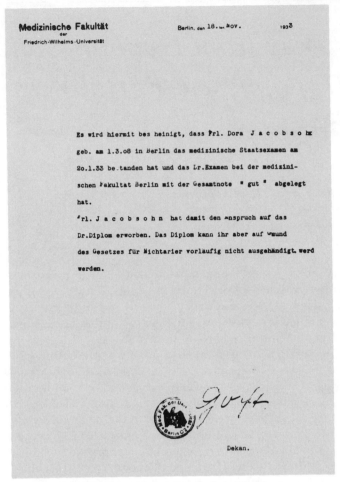

FIGURE 1 A. Notice of medical qualification.

which, incidentally, is quoted in extenso by G. W. Corner (1938), reports on experiments on rabbits. With a fine diathermy needle the ovarian cortex was destroyed, except for a single follicle. The fate of the remaining follicle and its hormonal function, as indicated by the reaction of the endometrium, were studied microscopically. The clearly presented problem and the well-designed and skillfully performed experiments of this work aroused my interest in research and animal experimentation. I also remember myself suggesting further work on hypophysectomized rabbits. At the time, Westman, who contrary to myself was an experienced researcher, thought it impossible to remove the pituitary gland in rabbits, but he agreed to try.

Nichtarier und akademische Prüfungen

Arische Abkunft eines Elternteils erforderlich

Der Amtliche Preußische Pressedienst teilt mit:

Zur Klärung von Zweifeln, die darüber entstanden sind, ob die zum weiteren Studium zugelassenen Studierenden nicht-arischer Abstammung ohne besondere Bedingungen auch zu den akademischen Prüfungen (Diplom-, Doktor-Prüfungen usw.) zugelassen werden dürfen, hat der Preußische Kultusminister Rust einen Erlaß herausgegeben, der ebenfalls auch über andere mit den Prüfungen nichtarischer Studierender zusammenhängenden Fragen Bestimmungen trifft. Nach diesen Bestimmungen wird zukünftig folgendermaßen verfahren werden:

Zu den Prüfungen sind diejenigen Reichsdeutschen nicht-arischer Abstammung unbeschränkt zugelassen, deren Väter im Weltkriege an der Front für das Deutsche Reich oder seine Verbündeten gekämpft haben, sowie Abkömmlinge aus Ehen, die vor Inkrafttreten des Reichsgesetzes gegen die Ueberfüllung deutscher Schulen und Hochschulen vom 25. April 1933 geschlossen sind, wenn ein Elternteil oder zwei Großeltern arischer Abkunft sind. Ferner sind zu den Prüfungen zugelassen diejenigen Studierenden nichtarischer Abstammung, die entweder zum Studium selbst zugelassen sind, oder denen das weitere Studium gestattet ist, und zwar auf Grund des Ausführungserlasses des Preußischen Kultusministers vom 16. Juni 1933 zur Ausführung des Gesetzes gegen die Ueberfüllung der deutschen Schulen und Hochschulen vom 23. April 1933.

Weiter trifft der Erlaß die Bestimmung, daß diejenigen Studierenden nichtarischer Abstammung, die bei Durchführung des erwähnten Ausführungserlasses vom 16. Juni 1933 bereits exmatrikuliert waren und die sonstigen Voraussetzungen zu einer Zulassung erfüllen, auf Antrag mit Genehmigung des Preußischen Kultusministers zu den Prüfungen zugelassen werden können. Allgemein ausgeschlossen von der Ablegung von Prüfungen sind alle diejenigen Studierenden arischer oder nichtarischer Abstammung, die aus der Liste der Studierenden gestrichen werden mußten.

FIGURE 1 B. Newspaper announcement that Jews would no longer be awarded licenses to practice medicine. (*Amtliche Preussische Pressdienst*)

With this began our joint work of about 10 years. That it was a joint work from the outset is due to Westman's generosity. He, certainly, had to carry the bulk of the responsibilities connected with at least the first half of the 22 papers published by us between 1936 and 1945.* Apart from this he made it possible that I, a foreigner of German birth but without a passport, got permission from the authorities to stay and work in Sweden.

Our papers of 1936 and 1937 tell that P. E. Smith's method of

* Listed in Acta Endocr. **34,** XXI, 1960, among Westman's publications, Nos: 76, 80, 83–85, 91–96, 106, 111, 115, 124–126, 129, 140, 144, 150, 162.

hypophysectomy in the rat was applied successfully to the rabbit and that the above-mentioned investigation of Westman was extended by studies on hypophysectomized rabbits. Estrogens prolonged the life of corpora lutea even in the absence of the pituitary gland. Our long-term experiments showed, as did those on other species, that ovarian growth, differentiation, and hormonal activities are to a major extent controlled by the pituitary gland even in the rabbit. On this basis experimental enquiries into the control exerted by the midbrain on the pituitary gland could be and were made on rabbits as well as on rats.

During the time this work was performed, Westman, who had been invited to an appointment as university professor and head of the University Clinic for Obstetrics and Gynecology in Lund, moved southward, and I followed. All procedures required for our experiments, even the histological work, were done at a small hospital laboratory, formerly used for routine examinations of urine, blood, and other samples of patients. An old kitchen table served for operations. Elaborate instruments, e.g., an electric drill, were not available. The rabbits were kept in wooden boxes in a cellar at another end of the building, which, because of the long way to the laboratory, caused a loss of valuable minutes when operative procedures had to be done shortly after mating the animals. Gradually our working conditions improved. With support from the Rockefeller Foundation some spare rooms on the ground floor of the clinic were converted into laboratories.

As indicated before, we attempted to and did provide experimental evidence (15 papers, 1937–45) of a control exerted by the brain on the pituitary gland. This holds true especially for the observations on ovulation in rabbits in which the hypophysis was removed or the pituitary stalk cut at various times shortly after mating. Hypophysectomy within 40 to 50 minutes prevented rupture of ovarian follicles, but sectioning the pituitary stalk even at 25 minutes postcoitum did not interfere with follicle maturation. For ovulation to occur normally, the presence of the hypophysis was required during a longer time after mating than an intact pituitary stalk. Regarding the various approaches used, I want to mention a few points concerned with the transection of the pituitary stalk in rats and rabbits and with the transplantation of hypophyseal tissues into the anterior chamber of the eye in rats. I discussed generalities concerned with the techniques and effects of these operations in detail in 1966 (Jacobsohn, 1966). In the present connection, I should like to recall that the results obtained by different workers from experiments with the intricate methods mentioned were not uniform. The causes of discrepancies from the results of others could seldom be revealed, as the possibilities of errors at operation and at the preparation of tissues to be examined are manifold. It was necessary, then, to scrutinize one's own procedures, to pursue the work under a great variety of conditions, and to use reference controls of different types. The material collected from hypophysectomized rabbits, for instance, was most useful with regard to the last point.

The observations made by us (1937–43) clearly and consistently indicated that the anterior pituitary gland was not only intimately connected with, but also controlled by the midbrain, a conclusion which agreed with the results of other workers who approached the problem in a different way, e.g., by nervous stimulation. How the control was transmitted from the brain to the anterior hypophysis remained unclarified, however. When, for instance, the pituitary gland had been separated entirely from the brain without inadvertent trauma, it was still not possible to decide whether the effects were due to an elimination of nerves or to disturbances of the blood flow through the hypophyseal portal vessels, or to both (Westman & Jacobsohn, 1943). The questions of how and where the nervous signal was transformed into hormonal messages remained open.

Around the time when the paper just referred to was concluded, Westman accepted an invitation to become professor and head of the Department of Women's Diseases at the Karolinska Hospital in Stockholm. He left Lund. I remained in the town and started working at the Physiological Institute, which was headed by Prof. Georg Kahlson. As I was still a foreigner without passport and Swedish degree, I could not obtain any post at the university. In order to earn my living and to be able to pay expenses for research (which I did in my spare time, mainly on mammary gland growth and lactation) I performed, among other things, hormonal assays and standardizations for a pharmaceutical firm. In retrospect, I think that the period of work for an industrial body involved a sound reminder of economic responsibilities too often disregarded by those who have never lived outside the sheltered conditions provided by a university. The renewal of my interest in and actions to clarify the neural control of the pituitary gland had to wait until I had obtained Swedish citizenship (1944) and the degree of a Swedish doctor of medicine (1948), which required the presentation of a thesis. The thesis was concerned with mammary growth.

During those five years I followed the literature about the problems Westman and I had been concerned with, and I became more and more interested in the work of G. W. Harris, who at the time was rather unknown. As mentioned earlier, the methods used in studies of the neural control of the anterior pituitary gland were intricate, and they did not lead to uniform results in the hands of different workers. The observations reported on by G. W. Harris were among the very few in agreement with our own. I also thought that his view about the role of the hypophyseal portal system as mediator of the hypothalamic control of the anterior pituitary gland was worth serious consideration.

Small wonder, then, that I was delighted when I was introduced to Harris in 1947 at the International Physiological Congress in Oxford. We talked about the pituitary gland and its control, as well as about methods of study. It was tempting to think of joint work, but I remember a conversation from which I concluded that the economic situation of Harris was approximately the same as mine: Harris asked about getting to Sweden and the possibility of work there. I answered that I was sorry I could tell him only the cheapest way of travel, and, as concerns research, that I used to go into the country on my bicycle to buy rabbits and that I myself collected the greens for the rabbits and the food (table scraps from a restaurant) for the rats. Upon this, he told me that he did the same. It was clear that neither of us had the means necessary for working together in 1947.

In 1949, having obtained the status of a Swedish *Dozent*, I had liberty enough to return to the study of problems left for six years. Thanks to the kind efforts of Professor Kahlson, I obtained a grant from the Medical Faculty of the University of Lund. The door to studies abroad opened. I wrote to G. W. Harris and asked whether I might work with him in Cambridge. His answer was in the affirmative, and I arrived at his laboratory at the Physiological Institute on a morning of June 1949. Harris and another guest worker were just perfusing the head of a rabbit with india ink, and I soon found myself included in the activities at the lab.

It is difficult to write in cool detachment about the work we began in Cambridge and finished in Lund. As time went by, G. W. Harris, his wife, Margaret, and I became united in friendship. What I am going to tell about are efforts to provide experimental evidence of the hypophyseal portal vessels as mediators of the hypothalamic control of the pituitary gland, efforts together with a lifelong friend whom I met for the last time in 1971, a few months before his untimely death.

The story began with a disagreement. Harris had just (1949) concluded an investigation on rats, in which he correlated the effects of sectioning the pituitary stalk with regeneration of hypophyseal portal vessels. To sum up briefly: When regeneration failed, the reproductive organs atrophied. When it occurred, a restoration to normal was seen (Harris, 1950). I had, in Lund, performed similar, but not as ingeniously designed experiments which I never published, because I thought I could not be sure that I had transected the entire pituitary stalk in the rats that appeared normal after operation. I maintained that the result of the operation was necessarily uncertain, because the method does not permit a clear view of the whole pituitary stalk. Harris was confident that he had cut the portal vessels, which then regenerated.

The controversies concerning our views of the value of the method, the transection of the pituitary stalk, created a distressing dilemma which lasted until we agreed that a new avenue of approach to the problem was desirable. We needed a technique which permitted the study of anterior pituitary tissues that had not previously been vascularized by the hypophyseal portal vessels to be examined. Harris suggested hypophyseal transplants placed near the pituitary stalk of hypophysectomized rats, and, needless to add, I was all for it.

Although we started soon with preparing for the experiments planned, it took some time before the necessary equipment was at hand and we had learned to adapt the operative procedures to the special demands of the study. The results obtained when my stay in England was coming to its end clearly showed that a hypophyseal transplant near the pituitary stalk became vascularized by portal vessels. Harris's view of the regenerative capacity of these vessels was confirmed (Harris, 1949), but further work concerning the activity of such grafts was left to be done.

Fortunately, at the time, the head of my department, Prof. Georg Kahlson, happened to visit Professor (later Lord) Adrian, who was the head of the Physiological Laboratory in Cambridge, and we had the opportunity for a demonstration and discussion of our work. The result was that we obtained the support necessary to continue the investigation in Lund. Professor Kahlson's attempts to obtain a grant from the Swedish Medical Research Council for a three-month' stay of G. W. Harris in Lund were successful.

In August 1950 Harris arrived at my laboratory in Sweden. With excellent working facilities and the unfailing support most kindly given by Professor Kahlson, it was possible to realize our plans within the brief period available. The plans we had, and the observations we made, are described in our paper (Harris and Jacobsohn, 1952). We wrote the manuscript in December 1950 in Cambridge, but, well aware of the consequences of our findings, we presented them for the first time on November 6, 1950, in Copenhagen at a meeting of the Danish Endocrinological Society. Before publication, the work was to be presented to the Royal Society and Harris invited me to read the paper. The event took place on November 1, 1951. Unaware of the possibility of being delayed by a fog, I went to London by air. Nothing of the kind happened, but Harris, who was conscious of the weather conditions at that time of the year, had, as he told me afterward, also prepared himself to meet the demands of the occasion.

In spite of our findings supporting the assumptions made by Harris, opposing views continued to be published. One of these was based on observations obtained from experiments with pituitary stalk transections in ferrets, a species in which ovulation does not occur spontaneously. To see, among other things, whether the mechanism of the neural control of the hypophysis differed in reflex ovulators, I studied the problem in rabbits

(Jacobsohn, 1954). The design of the experiments was similar to that used in the previous work by Harris and myself on rats, but the procedures differed in several respects. Nevertheless, the observations made on rabbits agreed with those obtained previously on rats.

The role played by the hypophyseal portal vessels in the neural control of the anterior pituitary gland is now common knowledge. Fortunate are those who, like myself, were able to participate in the search of the secret of this important and beautiful device.

REFERENCES

Corner, G. W. (1938). The sites of formation of estrogenic substances in the animal body. *Physiol Rev.* **18:** 154.

Harris, G. W. (1949). Regeneration of the hypophyseal portal vessels. *Nature* **163:** 70.

Harris, G. W. (1950). Oestrus rhythm. Pseudopregnancy and the pituitary stalk in the rat. *J. Physiol.* **111:** 347.

Harris, G. W., and D. Jacobsohn (1952). Functional grafts of the anterior pituitary gland. *Proc. R. Soc. London, Ser.* B **139:** 263.

Jacobsohn, D. (1954). Regeneration of hypophyseal portal vessels and grafts of anterior pituitary glands in rabbits. *Acta Endocrinol.* (Kbh.) **17:** 187.

Jacobsohn, D. (1966). The techniques and effects of hypophysectomy, pituitary stalk section and pituitary transplantation in experimental animals. Pages 1–21 in G. W. Harris and B. T. Donovan, eds. *The Pituitary Gland,* vol. 2. Butterworth, London.

Westman, A. (1934). Untersuchingen über die Abhängigkeit der Funktion des Corpus luteum von den Ovarialfollikeln und über die Bildungsttätte der Hormone im Ovarium. *Arch. Gynäkol.* **158:** 476.

Westman, A., and D. Jacobsohn, (1943). Über die Wiederherstellung der normalen Vorderlappenstruktur hypophysenstieldurchtrennter Kaninchen durch Oestronzufuhr. *Acta Obstet. Gynecol. Scand.* **12:** 24.

14

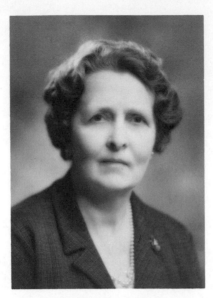

Mary Pickford

Mary Pickford was born in 1902 in Jubbalpore, India. After being educated at Wycombe Abbey School in England, she obtained her Honors B.Sc. degree at Bedford College in London in 1925, and an M.Sc. in the Department of Pharmacology, University College, London, in 1926. Combining research and clinical studies, she qualified in medicine at University College Hospital, London, in 1933, and was a Beit Memorial Fellow in the Department of Pharmacology, University of Cambridge with Prof. E. B. Verney from 1936 to 1939. Mary Pickford then moved to Edinburgh, where she was appointed to a Readership in Physiology in 1952, and to a Personal Chair in 1966. She was awarded the D.Sc. degree in the University of London in 1951 and was elected to Fellowship of The Royal Society in 1966. She retired from the University of Edinburgh in 1971, and is currently part-time Professor of Endocrinology in the Department of Physiology, University of Nottingham.

Stimuli that Release Hormones of the Pars Nervosa

MARY PICKFORD

Forty years on, it is difficult to remember and feel again accurately what it was like in those faraway days of personal ignorance when one was young, newly graduated, and beginning a career in research. Perhaps the effort to remember is comparable with trying to return to the feelings of the first days at boarding school when one was another person in another world. Here follows a summary of my road to neuroendocrinology. It was at the age of about 11 that I decided to become a doctor. None of the family were medical and I have no idea what decided me except an overpowering curiosity in all aspects of living. From the first I was encouraged by an uncle in whose family I was brought up. (My father worked in India so I was left at "home.") A year or so later I decided I wanted to do research, knowing no more about it than that it was a seeking for the why and how. In this ambition I received stimulation of a sort from a family friend, Sir Cooper Perry, who at the time was Superintendent of Guy's Hospital and later became Principal of the University of London. On being told I wanted to do research he said, "Don't think of it. Women are no use at that kind of thing." I said nothing, thought a great deal, and was more than ever determined! When the time came to leave school, there was some opposition to the idea of medicine but physiology was acceptable. This gave me a taste for the subject. But I still felt that medicine was important and would be useful. Later it became possible to work part time in the pharmacology department of University College, London, and part time to learn anatomy and then clinical medicine. The understanding and help of all at both the college and hospital were invaluable and encouraging. The medical students patiently accepted me as both teacher and colleague.

Shortly before this period, E. B. Verney was appointed to the chair of

MARY PICKFORD ● The Hall, Kingsterndale Near Buxton, Derbyshire, England.

pharmacology at University College. He was in every way helpful and kind. He also set an admirable example of how research should be done, with his thoroughness and care for detail. I could not have had a better training. Verney had a habit of never saying why he disapproved of an idea. He would snort or grunt scornfully. This forced me to find out for myself why he thought the foundations of the idea were shaky. Verney obtained a part-time grant for me from the Medical Research Council. During that time the work he did, and I with him, was mainly on the renal circulation. Before Verney moved to pharmacology he had been with E. H. Starling who, by that time, had developed the heart/lung preparation and then, with Verney, the heart/lung/kidney preparation. The heart/lung preparation was the first good method for perfusing an organ with blood. The striking fact about a blood-perfused kidney was the large volume of urine it produced; the rate of flow rose steadily to reach its maximum within about 40 minutes of the beginning of perfusion. Von den Velden had shown that pituitary extract benefited those with diabetes insipidus. Starling and Verney found that the extract also controlled the flow rate from the perfused kidney. Verney went on to show, independently of Starling, that if the intact head of a dog was included in the perfusion circuit, the rate of urine flow never rose, or, if it had already risen, it was reduced when the head was in the circuit. A head from which the pituitary was removed exercised no control over the kidney. At that time Verney used large doses of extract. Later he showed in both man and unanesthetized animals that very low blood concentrations of pituitary extract were antidiuretic, provided that the organism was hydrated.

In the mid-1920s neuroendocrinology did not exist and the term itself was not invented. Some idea of the state of knowledge of the pituitary body, as it was usually called, may be had by looking at the 4th edition of Sir William Bayliss's famous book, *Essentials of Physiology*. This edition was published in 1924. He gave two-thirds of a page to the gland and pointed out that from the combined posterior and intermediate lobes hormones could be obtained that had effects on the kidney and mammary gland and also exerted a strong constrictor effect on the plain muscle of the uterus and blood vessels. It was uncertain how many hormones were concerned. In 1923 Abel had published his unitary hypothesis and in the same year Dudley had separated the pressor and uterine principles. The effects of extracts on the kidney were far from clear. Schafer with Magnus and Herring in 1901 and 1906 had noted that the extract was diuretic in anesthetized animals and caused renal vasodilatation. It was also known that lesions of the posterior lobe led to diabetes insipidus, which could be controlled by pituitary extract. Then, too, in 1920 Camus and Roussy showed that diabetes insipidus followed injury to the tuber cinereum alone. This was a confusing string of facts. Regarding the mammary gland, it was appreciated that pituitary extract could excite "secretion" and this effect was said not to be due to a pressing out of milk. So much for the posterior lobe. Strictly speaking, the following facts are irrelevant, but they deserve mention because they give such an excellent picture of how much physiology has changed since then. First, Bayliss gives two small paragraphs to the anterior lobe of the pituitary which was said to secrete an eosinophil substance alleged to pass into the third ventricle; this lobe might affect growth. The second point is nonendocrinological. At most meetings of the Physiological Society there were hot arguments between Dale and Eccles on the matter of transmission at the neuromuscular junction—was it chemical or electrical?

Shortly after Verney moved to the chair of pharmacology he was joined by Klisiecki of Poland and Rothschild from Germany. The work we did was published in a paper in the *Proceedings of the Royal Society* (*B*) in 1933. This was an important publication and I can say this freely because I was no more than a useful pair of hands. The ideas and the technique were those of Verney. First it was shown that the volume and composition of the urine from one kidney could be taken as control for the other. The rate of absorption of orally given water was determined by noting the volume remaining in the gut at a given time after administration. This volume, plus the loss from the lungs, was subtracted from that given and was the *water load*. It was noticed that the peak water load always preceded the peak rate of urine flow by about 15 min. Another point was that a denervated kidney excreted water in exactly the same way as a normal one. These facts were the foundation for the next step. Mild exercise was found to exert a similar inhibitory effect on both innervated and denervated kidneys, that is, the inhibition could not be ascribed to a renal vasoconstriction, the exercise was too mild to have caused anoxemia, nor could absorption have been delayed since the exercise was undertaken after the time that this was complete. Attainment of the minimal rate of urine flow was gradual and the urinary chloride concentration rose. It had to be concluded that a change in the composition of the blood exerted an effect on the kidney. At that time there were various views as to the site of antidiuretic activity of pituitary extract; it might affect absorption from the gut, or act on the central nervous system or on the kidney. Verney showed more clearly and indisputably than others that the hormone acted independently of the peripheral nerves and that its effect was almost certainly on the renal parenchyma. It was concluded that the pituitary hormone held the kidney in check and that its release was determined by the concentration of water in the blood and tissues and that this affected the central nervous system. At that time the site of the sensory receptors was unknown. The delay between the maximum water load and the maximum rate of urine flow was that needed for the blood concentration of the hormone to fall. The inhibition of mild exercise must have a humoral origin and could be interpreted in terms of an increase in activity of the pituitary body. It was noted in a man with diabetes insipidus that the onset of diuresis after water drinking was earlier than in a normal subject. These conclusions may be compared with previous suggestions that a hormone was absorbed from the digestive tract with the water, that renal nerves were involved, or that the kidney responded directly to an increase in the ratio of water molecules to the total molecules in the plasma. This was not yet neuroendocrinology, but it was an essential preliminary.

Verney first showed the effects of brief exercise on water diuresis in 1933. The experiments were enjoyable for dog and man. The dog stood in a simple Pavlov stand, an affair of rubber-covered string loops hung from an overhead bar and through which the animal's legs were inserted. The dog was given water, and urine was collected from bladder or ureters. When diuresis was established, the dog was quickly removed from the stand and needed little encouragement to chase a ball for a minute or two. After the brief game the dog was returned to the stand and the course of the diuresis was again observed. Experiments such as this needed space and were performed on the roof of the medical school at University College. This meant that the weather must be good, hence part of the enjoyment of the experiments. Incidentally, they offered interest to one or more baboons housed on the roof and belonging to A. S. Parkes. (It was one of these baboons that escaped one day and ran along the parapets of Gower Street peering in at windows and alarming the inmates.) The antidiuresis of exercise was similar to that produced by pituitary extract. Later on Verney built an all-weather indoor treadmill for exercising. This meant, among other things, that the progress of experimentation no longer depended on the weather.

True neuroendocrinology was in the offing. In 1938 an important publication was the monograph by Fisher, Ingram, and Ranson in which, amongst other things, they described the continuity of the hypothalamic-pars nervosa system in cats and monkeys. In 1949 Bargmann showed by means of the Gomori method that a stainable substance could be traced from the paraventricular and supraoptic cells to the pars nervosa. In 1951 Bodian, using the opossum, demonstrated that the branched terminals of the axons in the pars nervosa were cuffed by the stainable matter. Over a number of years the Scharrers had pointed out that in amphibians certain nerve cells were undoubtedly secretory. These were a few of the steps to an understanding of the origin of diabetes insipidus and why it could follow injury to either the pars nervosa or the hypothalamus. Some people were reluctant to accept that nerve cells could transmit impulses and also act as endocrine organs. Personally I found the idea easy to accept, possibly because of ignorance of all the aspects of the problem. But adrenaline circulated in the blood after release from modified nerve cells in the adrenal medulla. And if nerves could produce adrenaline (noradrenaline, as we now know) for local action, they might also make other substances which acted at a distance.

There are many aspects to neurosecretion. Having worked with Verney it was not surprising that I took an interest in the stimulus to secretion. If Verney's hypothesis was correct, that water loss was associated with a decrease in the circulating concentration of antidiuretic hormone (ADH), then the degree of antidiuresis seen when the hormone was injected should relate to the water load of the body. This could be tested by giving the hormone at different times in the course of a water diuresis. At that time vasopressin was not available and the extract perforce used was one assayed in terms of its oxytocic activity. This material was given intravenously to dogs on the rise, plateau, and fall of diuresis, urine was collected separately from the two kidneys and, in some dogs, one kidney was denervated. The results showed that once again normal and denervated kidneys behaved alike and that there was a rough inverse proportionality between water load and percentage inhibition of urine flow when pituitary extract was given. That is, as Verney postulated, somewhere there must be receptors finely appreciative of water load which transmitted information to the pituitary body. The receptors could not be in the pars nervosa itself, as Verney had shown that diuresis was normal when it was removed from dogs.

At this point in time my laboratory work was interrupted by clinical work in hospital and as locum tenens. Undoubtedly it was useful to have had this experience. Certainly it was enjoyable and I could cheerfully have continued in clinical work. But Verney suggested that he support me in an application for a Beit Memorial Fellowship and that if I was awarded one I should again work with him, now in Cambridge. I asked advice of Prof. T. R. Elliott, who was still at University College, whether I could maintain an academic career or whether I ought to stick to clinical medicine. His comment was, "Have you ever heard of a starving physiologist?" That settled it. With Verney's backing I was appointed a Beit Fellow and began three happy years at Cambridge. After that I was appointed to a teaching post in the Department of Physiology in Edinburgh. I stayed there until retirement. I have never regretted throwing in my lot on the academic side.

When Verney was still at University College he was, for a time, joined by a good friend, G. W. Theobald, and they combined in some work. They found that very mild sensory stimuli induced inhibition of water diuresis and that the inhibition appeared to depend on release of the hormone of the pars nervosa. Theobald suggested that the inhibition of exercise might be related to excitement, i.e., to emotion rather than to the exercise *per se*. If emotion could induce antidiuresis, then there must be important nerves concerned in controlling the release of ADH in addition to physical factors such as the state of dilution or concentration of the blood. Thinking about emotional antidiuresis and the by then accepted fact that acetylcholine (ACh) was the transmitter at neuromuscular and preganglionic synapses, it seemed possible that ACh might also transmit to the supraoptic cells in the central nervous system. I was encouraged to test this idea by Dikshit's observation that ACh injected into the cerebral ventricles or hypothalamus led to results similar to those of electrical stimulation of the latter. It was good luck that I tried the supraoptic cells, because they were in fact cholinergic. In addition, as mentioned below, they were reasonably accessible. Again I used dogs, gave them subcutaneous atropine and then ACh injected intravenously during the course of a water diuresis. The first time this was tried the dose of ACh was far too large and, despite the atropine, the blood pressure must have fallen precipitately, as the dog sagged in the Pavlov stand. I was filled with horror and anxiety but the animal recovered quickly and seemed none the worse. Thereafter smaller doses of ACh were used and the only obvious and invariable result was a sigh some 12–15 sec after the injection into the saphenous vein, presumably at the time that the ACh reached the central nervous system. In the hydrated dog, antidiuresis resulted from the injection. The timing and pattern of the inhibition of urine flow was similar to that seen after pituitary extract and not at all like that due to adrenaline. Denervation of the kidneys did not affect the result. It seemed more than probable that ACh acted somewhere in the central nervous system to bring about the release of ADH. The next stage was to try and discover where in the central nervous system the ACh had its action and this was done by injecting it directly amongst the supraoptic cells. In those days no stereotaxic instrument existed for use in dogs, so I used Aschner's old method of splitting the soft palate, chiseling a small hole in the hard palate between the wings of the sphenoid at the site of the penetrating artery, and so exposing the dura under the pituitary. It was then easy to open the dura with a cataract knife and visualize the anterior margin of the pituitary and the posterior margin of the optic chiasma. The operation was done one morning and the observations made the next morning. This meant that the animal had recovered from the effects of the operation, which, in fact, disturbed the dog minimally. It would be lively and willing to eat almost as soon as the effect of the anesthetic had worn off. In chronic experiments the soft palate healed well without being stitched. I had been unfavorably impressed by the after effects of the temporal approach to the pituitary, which was a somewhat damaging operation in any case. This latter approach was necessary for some purposes, but not for mine. On the experimental day the dog was anesthetized with chloralose given with the hydrating dose of water.

This technique meant a slow, smooth onset of anesthesia and an apparently normal diuresis. ACh was injected bilaterally among the supraoptic cells through the hole in the hard palate, by means of a tuberculin syringe to which was attached a long fine needle bent at an obtuse angle at the tip. A small quantity of india ink was added to the injected solution to mark the spot for post mortem examination. By modern standards this injection technique is crude, but it worked. Control injections of normal saline showed the unimportance of any physical damage inflicted on the neurons. The ACh induced an antidiuresis which could be prolonged by the addition of eserine to the solution. No antidiuresis occurred if the posterior lobe had been removed. Once more denervation of the kidneys did not affect the result, and ACh injected amongst other nearby central cells did not lead to antidiuresis. Thus it was certain that ACh was able to stimulate the supraoptic cells and that it could well be the normal transmitter. The conclusions were strengthened when I used the long-acting anticholinesterase, di-isopropylfluorophosphonate (DFP), which had all the effects that might be expected of it. In addition it made it unlikely that ACh acted on the pars nervosa, since this could not have been directly affected by an intrahypothalamic injection, yet no antidiuresis occurred during the period of activity of DFP. Not everyone cared for the idea that ACh was a transmitter to the supraoptic cells, so it was pleasant when corroboration came from some work done by J. H. Burn, who showed that in man both smoking and nicotine injected intravenously inhibited water diuresis and, further, that no inhibition occurred from either stimulus in a subject with diabetes insipidus. In 1966 Lederis demonstrated that although true ACh was present in the pars nervosa its incubation with the lobe did not increase hormone release, whereas ACh incubated with the hypothalamic-neurohypophyseal system did increase the amount of hormone liberated. Much later, it was interesting to read in *Adventures in Physiology,* by Sir Henry Dale, a comment relating to his Harvey lecture of 1936 in which he asked, "Will the concept of transmission by ACh have to be extended even to some central synapses?"

There were, of course, hitches of a technical nature, for instance, in learning to expose the pituitary through the hard palate. I practiced on dead animals and then tried on anesthetized ones. Two died from injury to the Circle of Willis before I discovered that packing and patience would stop the bleeding. After that things went more smoothly. Sometimes there was delay in healing of the skinflap round a carotid loop and the loop would finish up rather short and difficult to use. Then, when inducing diabetes insipidus by section of the supraoptic tracts, the section was on occasion incomplete and, on occasion, the knife went in too deep on one side so that for a while the poor dog tended to move round and round in small circles. I did not discover what tract was sectioned or injured and responsible for this.

This sort of thing delayed progress and was certainly depressing because the experiments were, in any case, slow in giving results and one usually had to wait several months at least for each. So naturally I often felt that I was getting nowhere. Teaching loads were heavy and for years there seemed to be a shortage of staff, so that the unfortunate students had to put up with my efforts to teach them about the special senses and the central nervous system, as well as about subjects on which I was better informed.

When Verney was studying emotional antidiuresis, he found that there were two kinds of inhibitory response, a rapid one that could be abolished by section of the splanchnic nerves and denervation of the kidneys and adrenals, and a slow inhibition due to release of ADH. The slow inhibition could be prevented by the injection of a small amount of adrenaline (i.e., one of the substances released in emotional states) a half minute before the application of the stimulus. Adrenaline did not hinder the renal response to injected posterior lobe extract, so its inhibitory action must be central. Recalling these facts, it seemed worth testing whether adrenaline and noradrenaline could prevent the ACh-induced release of ADH. To this end I again used hydrated dogs and with Helen Duke found that when adrenaline or noradrenaline was given intravenously either shortly before, or with, an injection of ACh, on about half the number of occasions the inhibitory effect of ACh failed to appear. It was not possible to explain the other 50% of results on grounds of dose, timing of the injections, or by the individual dog. When Abrahams and I made injections into an exteriorized carotid artery, we found that we could without fail prevent the ACh inhibition by injecting the adrenaline or noradrenaline 8–40 sec before the ACh. The doses used for carotid injection were far smaller than those used intravenously and this strengthened the belief that both substances were acting in the central nervous system. Small doses of adrenaline were more effective than larger ones, which suggested that their action was unlikely to be a vasoconstrictor one that prevented access of ACh to the supraoptic cells. These results did not tell us the site of action of adrenaline. We noticed that the sigh that always followed the injection of ACh was not interfered with by adrenaline.

Together with Verney's work, this showed the ability of adrenaline and noradrenaline to prevent the release of ACh. But the matter is not altogether as simple as that. Adrenaline can also lead to a prolonged antidiuresis unconnected with changes in measurable renal hemodynamics and which does not appear after destruction of the pars nervosa or the supraoptic tracts, i.e., adrenaline can bring about the release of ADH. This fact was shown by Dearborn and Lasagna. The doses of adrenaline used by them were fairly large, so the conditions were different in the two sets of observations.

Abrahams and I then examined the release of oxytocin in the dog, using the animal's own uterus as a test organ for the presence of oxytocin. We found that this hormone was released by many of the stimuli that released ADH, such as hypertonic saline solutions, ACh, and emotion. Also, in acute experiments under anesthesia we found that the effect of ACh was enhanced by injecting eserine or DFP amongst the supraoptic neurons. Finally, we found that adrenaline could prevent the release of oxytocin just as it did that of ADH.

In diabetes insipidus the preliminary polyuria had been explained as due to transitory paralysis of the output of posterior lobe hormone, and the interphase as depending on an atrophic release. Nothing was known of what happened to oxytocin. Abrahams and I looked at the simultaneous uterine and renal responses after section of the supraoptic tracts in dogs. In addition the observations might tell us whether the two hormones were released in equivalent amounts. It was still not clear whether vasopressin and oxytocin were part of a single molecule or whether they were always independent of each other. The latter seemed the more probable since Harris (1947) had found that electrical stimulation of the pituitary stalk of rabbits led to an increase in uterine activity and inhibition of diuresis which could be matched by injecting 4–10 times as much oxytocin as vasopressin. When Cross compared antidiuresis with milk ejection in rabbits he found an even greater disparity in the amounts of the two hormones released. These findings were difficult to explain at a time when it was not known that there were two kinds of nerves in the pars nervosa, those relating to oxytocin and those to ADH. In our experiments we used dogs, collected urine by means of a self-retaining catheter in the bladder, and recorded uterine contractions from a small balloon inserted into the upper end of one uterine horn brought to the surface of the flank and stitched permanently in place. The dogs were lying down and were totally undisturbed by insertion of the recording balloon. Often they slept throughout the observations. Some of the dogs were provided with exteriorized carotid arteries. Inhibition of water diuresis was induced by the intravenous or intracarotid injection of hypertonic solutions of sodium chloride (NaCl), sucrose, or ACh, and invariably the size and frequency of uterine contractions increased during antidiuresis and declined as diuresis returned. The renal response could be matched by injecting less than 5mu pressor extract and the uterine one by 15–20 times as many milliunits of oxytocic extract. An emotional stimulus also released both hormones. This observation arose in the first place from a botched intracarotid injection. Thereafter the emotional stimulus was no more than making obvious preparations for an injection. In some of the dogs, diabetes insipidus was induced by means of a shallow semicircular incision made between the optic chiasma and the anterior margin of the pars distalis through the usual small hole chiseled in the hard palate. During the preliminary polyuria uterine motility was nil or minimal, during the interphase its activity was considerable, and in the phase of permanent polyuria it faded out and could not be induced to return, any more than could inhibition of water diuresis by the injection of solutions of hypertonic NaCl or ACh. However, the uterus was able to respond to oxytocic extract. The points of interest were the contemporaneous changes in renal and uterine activity and, also, that in dogs the stimuli used appeared to release one part ADH for 15–20 parts oxytocin. There is a third point that was not stressed at the time. In certain of the dogs in this series, as well as in others in later experiments, the ovaries were removed when the uterine fistula was made. It might be expected that this would lead to a rapid decline in uterine activity. However, on the contrary, ovariectomy greatly increased uterine motility as compared with normal animals. This increased activity persisted for up to $2\frac{1}{2}$ months, and thereafter declined.

This last point made us wonder about the still undecided question of the degree of importance to the uterus of the oxytocic factor in stimulating contractions. In the work just described we found that when diabetes insipidus was induced there appeared to be a premature cessation of spontaneous uterine contractions. This suggested that the pars nervosa was responsible for the uterine activity seen in the absence of the ovaries. It was decided to see what happened when diabetes was induced first and the ovaries removed later. Sheila Baird and I found that after section of the supraoptic tracts no uterine activity developed as a result of ovariectomy. When the posterior lobe alone was removed before ovariectomy some uterine activity appeared. But it was weak and faded out prematurely. The interest in the result of posterior lobe removal lies in the fact that, in the dog, there is very little oxytocin in the hypothalamus, though a moderate amount of vasopressin. It would seem then that the pars nervosa and its oxytocin are responsible for the uterine activity. At the time we could suggest no explanation for the "releasing" effect of ovariectomy. Now one asks whether the ovary not only sensitizes the uterus to oxytocin but also, in certain circumstances and in the dog at least, exercises an inhibitory or regulating effect on its release. Without the ovary, the uterine muscle would in time become incapable of response, even to a high concentration of oxytocin.

Then followed a series of experiments that were most enjoyable, though they demanded considerable patience. The object was to use a natural stimulus (suckling) and measure the milk ejection pressure, the weight of milk excreted, and the rate of urine flow, and find out how much oxytocin and vasopressin it was necessary to inject to match the responses. We accustomed pregnant bitches to water diuresis observations. After whelping it was found possible to insert a fine polythene tube into a milk duct in order to record the ejection pressure. After insertion the tube was held in place between finger and thumb; this meant sitting almost immobile for an hour or two. Obviously it was not possible to tie the tube in place as is done in anesthetized rabbits. The weight of milk excreted was measured by weighing the puppy before and after feeding. The rate of urine flow was observed in the usual way. The puppies were delightful and amusing, especially with their hindquarters wrapped in a duster or inserted into little bags (!) so that the weight gain on feeding should not be falsified by loss of urine or feces. The bitches showed great individuality. One would feed one or all her pups at any time, another would feed all her six but never one alone. Yet another refused to suckle in public despite the fact that she was friendly and familiar with the room; she had to be given oxytocin. A comparison of the antidiuretic and milk ejection responses showed that the ratio of vasopressin to oxytocin released was about $1:30$. This was not far from the ratio when an osmotic stimulus was given and the uterus used as the assay organ. We found that ACh and hypertonic NaCl solutions caused milk ejection on intravascular injection and that adrenaline given 10 sec before ACh prevented ejection. Thus the same stimuli caused the release of both vasopressin and oxytocin and the release of both could be prevented by adrenaline and noradrenaline.

We are now fairly certain that vasopressin and oxytocin are made in separate neurons and that it is possible for one to be released without the other. Both hormones are released following an osmotic stimulus or ACh and on suckling. If ACh is the transmitter to both groups of cells, the supraoptic and the paraventricular, it is not surprising that it should bring about the release of both agents. At first sight it seems reasonable that suckling, which induces loss of fluid from the mammary glands, should at the same time reduce loss through the kidneys, though the quantity of vasopressin released is small. Why should an osmotic stimulus liberate both hormones? Is it incidental or are both hormones physiologically necessary in the circumstances? It was this problem that made me begin to take a particular interest in oxytocin. Also intriguing is the fact that it is, apparently, only occasionally useful in the female and, apparently again, never useful in the male. So I turned away from neuroendocrinology in order to examine some of the actions of oxytocin on organs outside the reproductive system. It proved to have a number of unexpected actions and to be a more potent substance than anticipated.

It will have become obvious how much my work owed to that of Verney and that it was an attempt to build on the solid foundation he laid.

To finish, it is perhaps worth asking a question about the difficulty of ensuring a fast rate of urine flow in anesthetized animals and pointing out a loose end that might be of interest to someone. I have already mentioned that water diuresis appeared to be normal in dogs when chloralose was given together with the water. On another occasion the quick-acting barbi-turate, sodium thiopentone, was given during the course of a water diuresis and barely interrupted the rate of excretion of urine. On the other hand, during the recovery phase a considerable antidiuresis appeared and the urine flow rate rose only slowly, just as it does when ADH has been released. During emergence from anesthesia the dog was, of course, regaining con-sciousness. I wondered whether the difficulty of diuresis under anesthesia re-lated to emotional stress and the release of ADH as much as to the anesthetic *per se* and sensory stimulation from operative procedures.

The particular loose end in mind relates to some work published with Dr. F. P. Brooks in 1958 on the subject of the effect of posterior pituitary hormones on electrolyte excretion in dogs. We found that ADH increased the electrolyte excretion when given intravenously during water diuresis and was without this action when smaller doses were injected into the carotid artery. Oxytocin increased electrolyte excretion when the dog was not hydrated and was equally effective whether it was given intravenously or into the carotid artery. The question is, does oxytocin, or a substance like it, exert a central effect of physiological interest?

REFERENCES

Abrahams, V. C., and M. Pickford (1954). Simultaneous observations on the rate of urine flow and spontaneous uterine movements in the dog and their relationship to posterior lobe activity. *J. Physiol.* **126**: 329.

Abrahams, V. C., and M. Pickford (1956). Observations on a central antagonism between adrenaline and acetylcholine. *J. Physiol.* **131**: 712.

Abrahams, V. C., and M. Pickford (1956). The effect of anticholinesterases injected into the supraoptic nuclei of chloralosed dogs on the release of the oxytocic factor of the posterior pituitary. *J. Physiol.* **133**: 330.

Baird, S., and M. Pickford (1958). The simultaneous occurrence of certain changes in uterine and renal activity in dogs, and the role of oxytocin in these phenomena. *J. Physiol.* **144**: 80.

Brooks, F. P., and M. Pickford (1958). The effect of posterior pituitary hormones on the excre-tion of electrolytes, in dogs. *J. Physiol.* **142**: 468.

Duke, H. N., and M. Pickford (1951). Observations on the action of acetylcholine and adrenaline on the hypothalamus. *J. Physiol.* **114**: 325.

Pickford, M. (1945). Control of the secretion of the antidiuretic hormone from the pars nervosa of the pituitary gland. *Physiol. Rev.* **25**: 573.

Pickford, M. (1952). Andiuretic substances. *Pharmacol. Rev.* **4**: 254.

Pickford, M., and J. A. Watt (1951). A comparison of the effect of intravenous and intraca-rotid injections of acetylcholine in the dog. *J. Physiol.* **114**: 333.

15

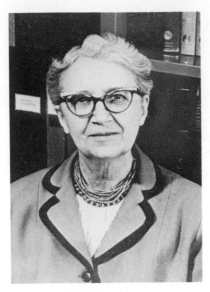

Dorothy Price

Dorothy Price was born on November 12, 1899, in Aurora, Illinois. She received her B.S. (*cum laude*) from the University of Chicago in 1922 and remained there, thereafter receiving the Ph.D. in zoology in 1935. She first worked as an Assistant and later as a Research Associate at the University of Chicago and was appointed Assistant Professor in 1947. She rose to the rank of full Professor of Zoology and remained at Chicago until her retirement in 1965. In 1967–68 she served as Boerhaave Professor at the University of Leiden. She has also been Visiting Professor on several occasions at the University of Puerto Rico and a Visiting Professor at Johns Hopkins University in 1966.

She has served as department editor for the *Encyclopedia Britannica* from 1958–1969 and on the editorial boards of *Physiological Zoology* from 1956 to the present and the *Journal of General and Comparative Endocrinology* from 1961 to 1969.

During her career she has delivered many invited lectures throughout the world. She received the Medal of Honor for Distinguished Service to the University of Leiden in 1967 and the University of Chicago Professional Achievement Award for Alumni, 1971.

Her scientific career has been devoted to the study of the endocrinology of reproduction.

Feedback Control of Gonadal and Hypophyseal Hormones: Evolution of the Concept

DOROTHY PRICE

An invitation to join in the writing of such a book as the editors of this volume visualize offers a challenging opportunity. The contributors can escape from the usual restrictions of scientific jargon, stylized form, and a text liberally larded with references. The mandate as I see it, is to be as candid, honest, and objective as a subjective mind and memory will allow.

In tracing here the steps that led me to enter a field that was to become neuroendocrinology, I must look back 50 years. But my entrance was sudden—practically explosive—one May night in 1930 when I was searching for an explanation for puzzling results of experiments on sex hormone "antagonism." Now I must review past decades in my memory and make these years as vivid for the reader as they still are for me. First of all, I will try to recapture the scientific atmosphere of one of the most exciting periods in the field of endocrinology and physiology of reproduction, the 1920s and 1930s. These years were marked by great discoveries and amazingly rapid advancement, and, toward the end of the period, the birth of neuroendocrinology. I started my scientific studies at the beginning of this time and I lived through it all as a member of the zoology department of the University of Chicago.

SCIENTIFIC LIFE AND TIMES IN THE 1920s AND 1930s

As an undergraduate in the zoology department in 1921 and 1922, I was trained in embryology, histology, vertebrate and invertebrate zoology,

DOROTHY PRICE ● Biology Department, University of Chicago, and Laboratory for Cell Biology and Histology, University of Leiden.

and so on. I was also "indoctrinated" very early in Frank R. Lillie's theory of fetal sex differentiation based upon his famous studies on the bovine freemartin, a sterile female co-twinned with a male. His theory of the causal factor in freemartinism (fetal testicular hormone) and his hypothesis of hormonal factors in normal sex differentiation had enormous impact at the time and have continued to influence scientific thought and research up to the present. When I entered the department as an undergraduate, he was just preparing for publication his 1923 paper on the freemartin. The department was abuzz with it.

Lillie was chairman of our department and a most impressive and awe-inspiring man for undergraduate and graduate students alike. Although he was quiet and reserved to the point of apparent shyness, he was an excellent teacher. Above all, he was a dedicated scientist and a clever administrator. Under his guidance, teaching and research were balanced in the zoology department. Largely because of Lillie's eminence, our laboratory had a stimulating and sophisticated international character, with many foreign visitors and numerous scientists from many countries who wanted to work with him. Of course he attracted large numbers of graduate students who wrote theses under his direction either in Chicago or at the Marine Biological Laboratory in Woods Hole, where he spent every summer as director. Altogether, the zoology department of the 1920s was a wonderful place to be, in my estimation, and I must have continued to be convinced of this, because I remained there until my retirement as a professor in 1965.

When my B.S. degree was granted at the end of 1922, I decided to continue in graduate study and started work on a problem for a master's thesis on intracellular digestion in *Hydra viridis* under B. H. Willier (a former student of Lillie's). I went to work with a will on hydra but they did not always cooperate and my research progressed very slowly. When summer came I left for a vacation at our summer home. There I made a decision and, all unknowingly, shaped my future scientific career. My family had had some financial reverses and I decided that I should stop graduate study and look for a job, probably in teaching. I wrote the news regretfully to a friend in the zoology department and when it was noised about, I got a letter from Willier. He had spoken to Lillie and I was asked to fill an opening as assistant and technician to help in the developing research program of studies on sex. The salary ($1,000 a year) came from a new grant to Lillie from the National Research Council Committee for Research in Problems of Sex (more about this committee later). The position was certainly not an elevated one, but I jumped at the chance to begin in October and had dreams of completing my hydra thesis and taking more graduate courses. However, I never finished that thesis and it was several years before I had any free time for graduate study.

On the first of October I returned to the zoology department in my new capacity and found that I was to start making histological preparations for the research work of several staff members of the department. The prospect was not too appealing. But I was soon appropriated by the young, enthusiastic Carl Moore, who had been a favorite student of Lillie's and had remained his protegé. At this time Moore was an assistant professor but he was well on his way up.

I was quite willing to be "appropriated"; I had studied embryology with Moore and liked and respected him as an enthusiastic and inspiring teacher. Moreover, he was almost unfailingly cheerful and amiable. He worked hard and expected others to do so and I did just that. We got on splendidly and I rapidly became a general factotum. I served as a histological technician, an assistant in operations and in hormone treatments of animals, and a cosupervisor of our animal colonies. In addition, I gradually became a research partner, in a sense, with whom Moore discussed his research problems and their results. I was often asked to read the manuscripts he was preparing for publication and to give my advice on clarity, word usage, and the like. I made corrections but I avoided suggesting drastic changes. Moore was a male chauvinist, and women (with the possible exception of a few including me on *some* occasions) were not really to be considered scientifically equal to men. I think he did not realize the depth of his prejudice. My reaction to this can be imagined but this attitude was (and is) a common characteristic of many men. I chose to disregard it then as much as I could and I accept male chauvinism now with resignation and a certain measure of amusement. Fortunately, not all men by any means are male chauvinists, and many who are, rationalize it or do not admit their prejudices even to themselves. As my former colleague and dear friend Alfred Emerson (the world's greatest expert on termites) explained male chauvinism to me, "Most men really can't help it, Dorothy; it's all that terrible male hormone."

But back to the 1920s: My status and salary lagged far behind my responsibilities, but I was caught up in the excitement of Moore's rapidly developing research in various aspects of the endocrine factors in the physiology of reproduction. I was learning a great deal and meeting many scientists in the great, near-great, or about-to-be-great categories. Moore was at that time a fount of research information for me with my practically nonexistent background. His energy and enthusiasm seemed endless and they were infectious. I was "infected" and considered his research program of great importance, which it was. Early on, he was recognized as an authority on the biology of the testis.

Much of his early work need not concern us here but there was an important thread—tenuous at times—that ran through many of his experiments. That thread was the question of sex hormone antagonism. Soon after Moore had received his Ph.D. degree in 1916, Lillie made a suggestion to him. Lillie was involved at the time in his own studies on the bovine freemartin, a "natural experiment" as he called it. His suggestion was that Moore might try to produce a freemartin by some experimental method. In the bovine freemartin, Lillie had postulated that testicular hormone from the male co-twin crossed through vascular anastomoses in the fetal membranes and masculinized the female by inhibiting the ovary and the female duct system and stimulating the male duct system and male accessory glands. The freemartin ovary sometimes resembled a sterile testis and Lillie considered this an example of inhibition of a fetal ovary by fetal testicular hormone. Whether a fetal ovary might secrete hormones that could inhibit a fetal testis remained an open question. However, such an action was not apparent in Lillie's studies on the testes of males co-twinned with females. In bovine freemartinism there was dominance of fetal testicular hormone (Lillie's explanation of this is not pertinent here) but sex hormone antagonism might exist.

Lillie's suggestion to Moore meant that techniques must be devised whereby male hormone could be introduced into fetal female mammals. Moore began work on this problem at once. Since there were no potent extracts of testes available then (nor for the next 10 years) he must use the testis itself as the source of male hormone. With more determination than luck he tried several methods including transplanting testes into pregnant rats and guinea pigs or directly into developing rat fetuses. These first experiments were abortive in every sense of the word.

Moore then followed a lead provided by the Viennese doctor Eugen Steinach in a series of publications from 1910 to 1913 and again in 1916. Steinach had reported sex gland antagonism when young male and female rats and guinea pigs were implanted with gonads of the opposite sex. Gonad grafts survived in hosts of the opposite sex *only* when these hosts had been gonadectomized before the grafting was done. Here was sex gland antagonism. When gonadectomy was performed before grafting, castrated males were feminized by ovarian grafts and spayed females were masculinized by their testicular grafts. Steinach's claims of sex gland (sex hormone) antagonism and masculinization of females by testicular hormone supported Lillie's later hypothesis on the freemartin. Steinach described the histological structure of the testis grafts he removed as degenerate testis tubules and consistently hypertrophied interstitial cells. This hypertrophy of interstitial cells (already postulated by others to secrete male hormone) suggested to him that these grafts were secreting high levels of male hormone. He then proposed the possibility of using testis grafts as a means of rejuvenating senile male animals and man by the simple expedient of increasing the amount of male hormone.

Moore was not concerned in studying rejuvenation, but some of Steinach's experiments seemed to support Lillie's theory. However, these experiments needed confirmation and Moore was just the man to do it. But, indeed, Moore did *not*! He repeated Steinach's experiments (with modifications) and found no sex gland antagonism in rats and guinea pigs that had received grafts of gonads of the opposite sex. The explanation for much of Moore's early success was not apparent until 1930. He found tubules less degenerate in testis grafts and he did not find consistent hypertrophy of interstitial cells. By the time he published his first results in 1919 and 1920, Moore had effectively disproved sex gland antagonism in postnatal rodents, but he had not advanced an analysis of the freemartin problem.

The subject of male rejuvenation is a digression from the main theme of this paper, but I include it because it furnishes a gaudy background for the scientific atmosphere of the 1920s. Steinach published a startling paper in 1920. His claims were surprising and very important if they were valid. By tying off the vasa deferentia of senile male rats he had been able to effect complete rejuvenation. Vasoligation improved general appearance (even the color of the haircoat), increased vigor, and, importantly, caused the return of interest in the opposite sex. The simple operation of vasoligation, in his hands, resulted in degeneration of the germinal epithelium and increase in interstitial cells in the testis—results similar to those he had reported earlier in testis grafts. He concluded that increase in male hormone was the answer to all the problems of senescence. Steinach was a reputable scientist who believed that he had interpreted his results correctly.

This was a bonanza for clinicians. Vasoligation or vasectomy (removal of a portion of the vasa deferentia) might be the key that would open up marvelous vistas of rejuvenation for men. What could be expected (and what was soon claimed) from vasoligation was nothing less than increased bodily vigor, improved mental faculties, increased longevity, and to top it all, benefits to any number of chronic ailments. Shades of self-rejuvenating treatments by the French physician Brown-Séquard in 1889 with aqueous extracts of dog testes!

The 1920s were ushered in by a wave of so-called Steinach operations that rapidly spread over Europe and to the United States, where hundreds were performed. And all quite uselessly, as Moore was able to show by repeating vasoligation and vasectomy in five species of laboratory mammals. In Moore's experiments, there were varying degrees of degeneration of germinal epithelium but no marked and consistent increase in interstitial cells of Leydig. By objective criteria there was no increase in male hormone production (nor, incidentally, was there any evidence of reduction in testicular hormone).

While Carl Moore was busy disproving Steinach's contentions, new and spectacular claims of rejuvenation appeared. The flamboyant Russian-French surgeon Sergei Voronoff reported astonishing success in rejuvenating sheep, goats, horses, bulls, and even men by means of testis grafts. In 1919 he reported his dramatic success with animals, and in 1922 he proudly presented one of his first rejuvenated human patients before a large audience in Paris. This event practically rocked the world. Almost overnight Voronoff became famous and notorious, a genius and a charlatan. He claimed that testis grafts had completely rejuvenated decrepit old farm animals. By transplanting older testes into young sheep and goats he had caused the precocious development of wool which was of improved quality and quantity (this in French flocks and government flocks in Algeria). He had rejuvenated old men with grafts of monkey testes (which reputedly survived and secreted male hormone for years) and improved mental faculties, memory, and bodily vigor in ways described as entirely satisfactory to the men and to their wives as well.

Voronoff's book *How to Restore Youth and Live Longer*—an English translation in 1928 of the French edition—contained his astonishing claims, and was liberally illustrated with pictures that purported to show rejuvenated men and goats and extrawoolly ewes and rams (sired by testis-grafted rams). Voronoff's claims were certainly incredible, and they were dubious in the opinion of many scientists (including Moore). However, at that time Voronoff was a recognized surgeon and held positions of importance in Paris. He might be a clever and unprincipled fraud but his claims had to be looked into. International delegations of scientists visited him and his flocks in Algeria to see for themselves. According to Sir Alan Parkes in *Sex, Science and Society*, the report of the British delegates to the Ministry of Agriculture after such a visit in 1927 was very cautious. But the Voronoff method for rejuvenating men had fired the imagination of some reputable clinicians (and the cupidity of some dubious characters) who were not so critical and cautious. Fortunately, monkey testes were in short supply but still such operations were done, and even testes of other animals including goats were used.

Voronoff and his claims have long since been relegated to the past, as was the Steinach operation. But the age-old hope of rejuvenating men has not disappeared; it is very much alive today for men *and* women and there are now various ways of "prolonging youth" or rather delaying senescence. None make claims as spectacular as those of Voronoff and Steinach; many, indeed, depend upon administration of gonadal hormones.

I can now return from this long digression, with its stops in Vienna,

Paris, and Algiers, to Chicago in 1923. When I joined Moore's team, he was studying vasoligation and the function of the scrotum as a temperature regulator for the testis. All further plans for experiments on sex hormone antagonism were put aside awaiting the development of potent extracts of testes and ovaries. We had not long to wait!

The story of the astonishingly rapid isolation, identification, purification, and ultimate synthesis of estrogens, androgens, and progestins in the 1920s and 1930s is amply documented in many volumes on library shelves. The names of the biologists and biochemists who shared in all this research read like an international Who's Who of distinguished scientists. To those of us who were working in the field at that time it was exciting and far more important than the spectacular drama of rejuvenation that was being played concurrently.

It all began in 1923 when Edgar Allen and E. A. Doisy succeeded in demonstrating that the follicular fluid from sows' ovaries contained an estrus-producing substance. The estrogens were off to a good start! In a few years, multiple sources of estrogens had been found and a long series of naturally occurring estrogens such as estrone, estriol, and estradiol was known. Their isolation, purification, and crystallization were quickly followed by their synthesis, and research on estrogens flourished.

To complete the female hormone side of the picture, in 1929 George Corner and Willard Allen extracted from corpora lutea of pig ovaries a substance with progestational activity on the uteri of rabbits. Research on progestins followed the course of the estrogens. Rapidly other sources of progestins were discovered and progesterone was very soon isolated, characterized, and synthesized.

The androgens have particular significance for me because I had a part in developing the methods for testing the potency of some of the first testis extracts. The first extracts containing male hormone were prepared from bull testes by Lemuel McGee in F. C. Koch's Department of Physiological Chemistry and Pharmacology at the University of Chicago in 1927. McGee's extracts had androgenic action on capon combs. However, mammalian indicator methods of great sensitivity were desirable and Moore and his group in the zoology department were pressed into service by Lillie and Koch, who arranged the interdepartmental cooperation. T. F. Gallagher replaced McGee in making extracts from bull testes, and Moore shared a part of the project with each of us who worked with him. The prostate of the male rat fell to my lot. I was to study the effects of castration in greater detail than had ever been done and determine whether Tom Gallagher's extracts of testes would repair all of the retrogressive changes (including cytological changes) that occurred following castration.

Gallagher prepared testis extracts as rapidly as possible and we worked frenetically castrating rats, injecting extracts, autopsying, studying slides, and reporting the potency of his preparations. The goal, to speed purification and achieve crystallization of male hormone, depended upon the accuracy and rapidity of our test methods. The ventral lobe of the prostate and the seminal vesicle glands proved to be the most sensitive indicators for male hormone of all those found by Moore's group. However, male hormone from bull testes was not obtained in crystalline form at Chicago after all, but in Amsterdam in 1935 by Laqueur and his collaborators, who chose for it the unfortunate name testosterone. In the same year, testosterone was synthesized simultaneously by two groups of European workers. As with studies on estrogens and progestins, other sources of substances with androgenic potency were then discovered and new androgens were characterized. Androsterone, androstenedione, and many others joined the series of androgens.

I have given only a capsule history of the rapid advance in knowledge of the steroid hormones secreted by testes and ovaries. This advance brought with it not only a better understanding of the effects of gonadal hormones on the reproductive system, and the part that sex hormones might play in the physiology of reproduction, but also the realization that the secretory activity of the gonads could hardly be autonomous and self-regulatory. An extragonadal source of control must exist. The brain and the pituitary had long been suspected of being related to gonad function. Philip Smith had been developing a simplified technique for hypophysectomizing rats. In 1927 Smith, and Smith and Engle, published their exciting findings. Removal of the pituitary gland of mature males and females resulted in dramatic regression in the gonads and accessory reproductive organs; administration of implants (small pieces) of fresh pituitaries to hypophysectomized animals restored these organs to normal. When such implants were put into immature animals, particularly females, they produced startling results—precocious maturity. Zondek and Ascheim also reported in 1927 that precocious maturity could be brought on by administration of anterior pituitary tissue.

These findings were a landmark in the study of the physiology of reproduction and an essential link in the chain of evidence that provided the background for the full emergence of neuroendocrinology. That chain was forged in the 1920s when it was first established that the gonads secreted estrogens, progestins, and androgens and the biological tests for these hormones were developed and refined. The second link was the demonstration that the anterior pituitary gland secreted hormones, gonadotropins, that stimulated the gonads to secrete their specific sex hormones and to ripen germ cells. The impact of the work of Smith and Engle, Zondek and Ascheim, and others was tremendous. The anterior pituitary was called enthusiastically the master gland and the conductor of the endocrine orchestra (an unexpected flight of poetic fancy for a scientist). The anterior pituitary, then, controlled the gonads (as well as other organs). A spate of experiments promptly broke out testing the gonad-stimulating potency of the pituitary under various experimental conditions, including gonadectomy and sex hormone administration.

The discovery of the next important link was inevitable. The anterior pituitary hormones stimulated the gonads to secrete sex hormones and thus controlled sex hormone production, but what controlled the secretion of anterior pituitary hormones and shielded the gonads from overstimulation? How were sex hormones and gonadotropins kept within physiological limits in the systemic circulation?

These questions were not asked just this way at that time nor viewed in broad perspective. Moore and I entered into this aspect in 1929, but we came in backward. Our approach was through a study on sex hormone antagonism—the same old question that had motivated Moore's early research. In the autumn of 1929, Moore began another attack on the concept of sex hormone antagonism. After preliminary experiments in which he injected testis extract directly into the amniotic cavity of developing rats (with disastrous results) he turned to postnatal rats. Now he had available both male and female hormones and could test for direct antagonism of sex hormones on each other and on the gonads. Steinach and Kun had reported in 1926 that treatment of males with estrin resulted in testicular damage and retrogression of accessory reproductive glands. Their interpretation—sex hormone antagonism.

In November of 1929, Moore designed an extensive series of experiments using extracts of bull testes and estrin. Winter of 1930 found us hard at work; by late spring, results were accumulating and some were most unexpected. Male and female hormones had been injected singly or in combination as a mixture into castrated and noncastrated adult male rats, into young intact males, and into spayed adult females. For simplicity I will discuss here only the results in males. The findings in castrated males negated any idea of direct antagonism of the sex hormones themselves; estrin did not interfere with the response of the accessory glands to male hormone. The complicated details of the results on noncastrated males can be reduced to three statements: (1) estrin treatment injured the germinal epithelium and reduced testicular weight in males, in which the accessory reproductive glands (prostates and seminal vesicles) resembled the castrate type in every way; (2) administration of male hormone also had deleterious effects on the germinal epithelium and testicular weight (most conspicuous in delaying development in young males) but the accessory glands were normal; (3) mixtures of the two hormones had the same effect as male hormone alone.

The results were confusing. If the effect of estrin on the testes was sex hormone antagonism, what was the explanation for the effects of male hormone?

Moore prepared study tables and we pored over them together. As his research assistant I had had a hand in every phase of the work and had made an independent study of the slides. But the research was *his*. He had designed the experiments and, more than that, he was counting on his results to scotch once and for all any concept of sex hormone antagonism. He was going to London late in July to present a paper on this research at the Second International Congress for Sex Research. There was great urgency for him to prepare a manuscript, but he could not interpret his findings. One May afternoon late in the month I went into his office when he was studying his work tables and trying to make sense of it all (undoubtedly with the whole idea of sex hormone antagonism and the evidence pro and con going round and round in his head). He said that he must *think* and he wanted me to think too. So far I had left the worrying to him; I had worries enough of my own trying to keep up on histological preparations and begin my doctoral problem (not on sex hormone antagonism).

After dinner that night, I sat down at my desk and thought! I simplified the problem by reducing the results to essentially the three statements that I have given above. Then, quite suddenly a plausible explanation occurred to me. The secretion of male hormone depended upon gonadotropic hormone from the pituitary, and male hormone entered the blood stream and had effects on the accessory reproductive glands that I well knew. If both estrin and male hormone had deleterious effects on testes when injected, there must be a common denominator and the finger pointed to the anterior pituitary. If, in the normal male, the anterior pituitary controlled the secretion of male hormone, and the male hormone, in turn, controlled the secretion of gonadotropin by the anterior pituitary, there would be a splendid scheme for a seesaw balance between production of gonadotropin and production of male hormone and thus, control of their levels in the blood. It would work simply—gonadotropin would stimulate secretion of male hormone and the level would rise in the blood, but when it reached a certain level it would cut off further secretion (or release) of pituitary gonadotropin; falling levels of gonadotropin would reduce secretion of male hormone and when a certain low point was reached, pituitary suppression or inhibition would cease, and up would go gonadotropin levels again in a self-regulating cycle. I did not call this brainchild of mine a theory or a hypophysis and I certainly did not anticipate that it would come to be known as a negative feedback system. I thought it a beautiful and logical scheme and, furthermore, Moore's results fitted in like a dream. Injection of estrin into intact males must act by inhibiting the output of pituitary gonadotropins with resulting deleterious effects on the testes and reduction in male hormone—hence the retrogression of accessory glands. Administration of male hormone (repeated daily) suppressed pituitary gonadotropins, as with estrin, and had deleterious effects on the testis, but any possible evidence of reduction in male hormone levels was masked by the injected male hormone which stimulated the accessory glands directly and kept them normal. It was as simple as that.

I thought of a possible "reciprocal influence," as we eventually called it, between anterior pituitary and gonads and I even considered that the concept would extend to females. I developed this logical scheme before I added some supporting evidence that then came to my excited mind. Gonadectomy had been shown to increase the gonad-stimulating potency of the anterior pituitary; injection of estrin into gonadectomized male and female rats reduced the gonad-stimulating potency of pituitaries. On such slender evidence I hung the Moore-Price theory that night. Of course there was more evidence in favor of my idea, but much of it I did not know.

I pictured the scheme in my mind and drew diagrams—I always do. My mental picture (the original diagrams are lost to posterity) closely resembled Figure 1, but of course I did not then label it in Dutch. Figure 1 is the diagram drawn in 1969 in our laboratory here in Leiden to illustrate the Moore-Price feedback system. It was used in my short talk on Dutch television in a series on models in biological systems. When Professor van der Werff ten Bosch asked me (*urged* me) to give this address, I objected and protested that the theory was outdated as we had proposed it, that any evidence that sex hormones could affect the pituitary directly was thin, and that I was much more interested in our current research on fetal sex differentiation. He, in turn, protested that the Moore-Price theory was the first clear description and demonstration of biological regulation by a negative feedback system, and that it was a cornerstone of neuroendocrinology. Would I cooperate, please? I gave the talk. At his request I autographed the diagram as a souvenir for him. My rewards were roses and a set of silver coffee spoons (the wonderful Dutch!). A more carefully drawn version of Figure 1 was later published in a book on models in hormonal systems (Aafjes, Vreeburg, and van der Werff ten Bosch, 1972).

If the Moore-Price theory was a cornerstone of neuroendocrinology, it crumbled a bit in a few years when the significance of the hypothalamus and the portal system of the pituitary stalk was recognized. Then, it was shown that gonadal hormones control secretion of gonadotropic hormones but not necessarily by influencing the hypophysis directly. A longer route through the brain was demonstrated. Geoffrey Harris and his collaborators were mainly responsible for clarifying these relationships. He more than anyone else brought the new neuroendocrinology into focus in the late 1930s. Figures

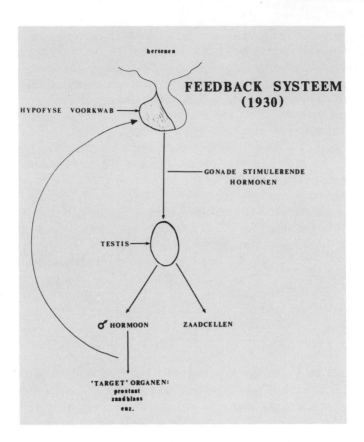

FIGURE 1. Schematic diagram illustrating the Moore-Price negative feedback system between the anterior pituitary and the testis. Figure prepared in Leiden in 1969 (see comments in the text).

2 and 3 are simple diagrams he published later showing that the arrow of the feedback system had shifted upward.

But I am getting far ahead of my story. On that night in May 1930 I had my first taste of the joy of scientific discovery. When morning came I hurried to the zoology department and almost burst into Moore's office to tell him that I thought I had solved the riddle. When I went over my reasoning in detail, he thought for several minutes and then began to warm up; soon he began to consider it a brilliant idea. We hastily began a new series of experiments in which daily implants of fresh pituitary tissue or injections of hebin (gonad-stimulating substance from pregnancy urine) were given in conjunction with injections of estrin or male hormone. The results were just as I had predicted; both male hormone and estrin must have acted to reduce the level of gonadotropic hormone in our earlier experiments; supplements of gonadotropic hormone administered with the sex hormones kept the testes and accessory organs normal. A seesaw, push-pull, or negative feedback, if you like, had been operating. Thus was born the Moore-Price theory of a *Reciprocal Influence between the Gonads and Hypophysis*. That was the way it was.

Moore went happily to London with a new theory, came back promptly and set about writing a short paper (Moore and Price, 1930). This

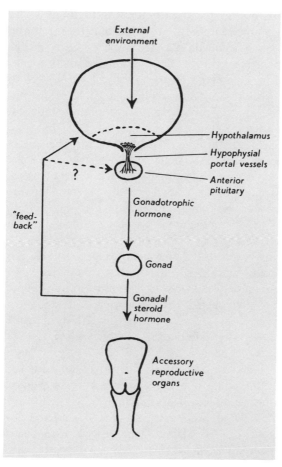

FIGURE 2. From G. W. Harris, *Neural Control of the Pituitary Gland (Monographs of the Physiological Society)*, 1955, Figure 31. Reprinted with the kind permission of Edward Arnold Publishers, Ltd.

was followed by a much longer one (Moore and Price, 1932) giving the details of our experiments and other experiments performed in our laboratory, and marshaling a weight of evidence to support the concept of a reciprocal relation between gonads and anterior hypophysis. This second paper is complicated and somewhat devious in reasoning with overtones of sex hormone antagonism. But everything is there, including speculations that in seasonally breeding animals the gonadotropic secretion of the hypophysis might be found to be low in the period of reproductive quiescence, and that external factors such as light, temperature, and food might be the operative agents acting on the pituitary in some way. We were familiar with the work of Rowan in Canada on the stimulating effects of light on the gonads of juncos in reproductive quiescence and that of Bissonnette on starlings. But these studies in birds gave us no clue as to the importance of the brain as a link in the gonadal-hypophyseal system. The hypophysis was the center of our attention and that of many others with us. Of course there were such animals as the rabbit that ovulate only after coition, and the brain must be involved there. But that was another problem and we were thinking of rats.

However, other workers, among them F. H. A. Marshall, were thinking of the rabbit and the brain and external factors that might affect breeding cycles. In a few years, Marshall published extensive reviews on exteroceptive factors in relation to breeding cycles and investigated the effects of electric shocks applied to the heads of rabbits. He was correct in suggesting to Harris in 1935 that experiments on precisely localized electrical stimuli to various regions of the hypothalamus would be important. Figure 2 is a diagram used by Harris giving his general idea that external factors could act to set off the whole train of events (Harris, 1955). It is noteworthy here that the main arrow leads to the hypothalamus, but a dotted line (plus a question mark) leads directly to the anterior pituitary. He still kept a small question open. It is interesting to watch the accumulation of evidence to show that sex hormones *can* affect the anterior pituitary directly (Bogdanove, 1972). Perhaps an arrow with a thin shaft should still lead to the pituitary.

Moore and I had studied mainly the effects of gonad hormone treatment in males, but while our experiments were in progress, Ihrke and D'Amour, in our laboratory working under Moore's direction, injected male hormone into adult female rats and caused cessation of estrous cycles, which were resumed in three days if injections were stopped; fresh pituitary or hebin administered with male hormone brought cornified vaginal smears in 48 hours. The explanation seemed obvious. In females, the cessation of estrus with male hormone treatment suggested that ovulation had been prevented. Inhibition of ovulation by administration of extracts of the corpus luteum had already been reported for rats, mice, and guinea pigs. It

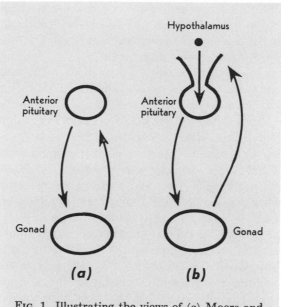

FIG. 1. Illustrating the views of (*a*) Moore and Price, that the rhythmic nature of reproductive cycles is dependent on the reciprocal reaction between the ovary and anterior pituitary, and (*b*) later workers, that sexual rhythm is dependent upon ovarian hormones affecting the anterior pituitary gland through the intermediation of the hypothalamus (from Harris, 1955).

FIGURE 3. From G. W. Harris, Sex hormones, brain development and brain function, *Endocrinology* **75,** 1964 Figure 1. Reprinted with the kind permission of J. B. Lippincott Company.

all seemed to fit into our picture. Male hormone and progestin administration both inhibited ovulation and in the same way, by inhibiting the pituitary and reducing the level of gonadotropin. We did not know it, but in 1930, A. Mahnert, of Graz, published a paper of great interest. He had prevented postcoital ovulation in the rabbit with corpus luteum extracts, and speculated from this that sterilization in animals and *in women* might be achieved by such hormone administration (the italics are mine).

Thereby hangs a rather long tale that is pertinent here. In 1967, seven years after "the Pill" was first approved for prescription use in the United States as a contraceptive measure, Reynolds contributed a letter to *Science* headed "The Pill: Early Breakthrough." He reported that Sturgis, a member of Albright's group at Massachusetts General Hospital, had told him in a letter how he had come to the conclusion that in women injected with estrogens (in a study on dysmenorrhea), ovulation must have been prevented. Sturgis then had the "bright idea" that it might be by inhibition of FSH, but he found to his disappointment that Albright had thought of the same answer the previous week. They published jointly in 1940. Reynolds posed a question of whether there was an "earlier first." Inevitably the letter section soon contained the next instalment under the caption "Rabbits First—Then Humans." This contributor referred to Reynold's claim that Sturgis first discovered the suppression of ovulation with estrogens and pointed out that another group had described the same thing in 1937 in rabbits. (They actually used progestins and progesterone.) The final instalment in *Science* was a broadside from the irrepressible Carl Hartman, entitled "Research Prior to the Pill." With flags flying, he sniped away at Sam Reynolds for calling attention to Sturgis's contribution, and proclaimed that the basic principle of the feedback mechanism had been clearly stated by Moore and Price much earlier. In 1933 he himself had been using amniotin, a mixture of estrogens, in some experiments and he had proposed to a pharmaceutical firm that it might be used in women as a contraceptive (on the basis of a negative feedback system). A letter was then written to a clinician but nothing came of it. After this barrage, Sam Reynolds capitulated and agreed that the Moore and Price paper was probably the earliest breakthrough in principle.

The moral is that "firsts" are very hard to pin down. Sturgis and Albright, independently, concluded that estrogens must be inhibiting ovulation in women (probably by inhibiting FSH) without being aware, apparently, of the volume of earlier work on other species. They certainly did not propose estrogens as a contraceptive measure. Carl Hartman's suggestion in 1933 fell on deaf ears, and he never published it. The unsung and almost unknown hero is Mahnert, who, on the basis of his experiments in rabbits, had the vision to see that progestins might be used for hormonal sterilization in women. But Mahnert and Hartman were far ahead of their times. There is a suitable time, a critical moment, for acceptance and exploitation of ideas, and the 1930s were not *it* for the development of the Pill. When that moment finally came, the names of Pincus, an endocrinologist of broad background, and Rock, a clinician, stand out prominently. The Pill (there are many modifications of the original Pincus Pill) depends for its effectiveness on progestins and estrogens administered together or given sequentially. The rationale for these oral contraceptives is the basic principle of the negative feedback relationship between the ovary and the anterior pituitary. The Pill, which has been such an enormous boon in contraception, must be considered as a triumph for neuroendocrinology.

There is another moral. Moore and I were the first to propose a reciprocal relationship between the gonads and the pituitary in the normal animal (male and female rats) and to visualize how a feedback must be operating to control hormone levels in the blood and effect cyclic events in females. Our theory was based upon our findings in sex hormone-treated animals and supported by research of others. We described the scheme clearly and at length, but of course it was greatly oversimplified and incomplete. While we were spelling it out (mainly from results on males), any number of other workers were probably just on the point of developing a similar scheme for females. Brouha and Simmonet gave a paper at the Second International Congress for Sex Research in 1930 and speculated on what might determine the ovarian cycle. But they ended inconclusively with two possibilities: Folliculine either had a direct antagonistic action on the hormone of the anterior hypophysis or had a depressing action on the function of the anterior lobe.

The concept of a gonad-pituitary feedback mechanism was an inevitable consequence of what had gone on previously in scientific research. It does not matter so much who thought of it first. Ideas, inspirations, logical reasoning, or flashes of intuition, if you like, are rarely the privilege or property of only one person or of a few. Still I am glad that in May 1930 I did not know what was going on in the minds of so many. It would have spoiled part of the fun.

THE 1940s AND WHAT CAME AFTER

As the 1930s came to an end, my own research turned in a different direction. I made, with my collaborators, only two more excursions worth mentioning into neuroendocrinology. One was in 1940, when we began an ambitious study on rats in which we ultimately sacrificed, as the euphemism goes, 1077 male and female rats. We were studying the development of responsiveness to hormones in the reproductive tract, and our criteria were weights and histological structure. We injected standard doses of hormones into intact males and females for 6-day periods beginning on the day of birth, or at 4, 8, 12, 20, 30, or 50 days of age (Price and Ortiz, 1944). The results with androgens and estrogens at the youngest ages are relevant to many current studies and can be summarized briefly. The testis/pituitary axis is already established by 6 to 10 days of age, as shown by reduction of testicular weights with both hormones; estrogen treatment resulted in reduction of male hormone secretion. The ovary/pituitary axis is not definitely established until 14 to 18 days, as judged by reduction of weight with

androgen and estrogen and the histological findings of reduction of inter-
stitium and theca and decrease in size and number of large follicles.

The other venture was a short excursion into the branch of
neuroendocrinology that is concerned with hormones and behavior. It was a
by-product of our studies on sex differentiation in fetal guinea pigs and the
inception of hormone secretion by fetal gonads. In 1959 I was writing a
chapter with H. G. Williams-Ashman for the new edition of *Sex and
Internal Secretions*. The editor, W. C. Young, was an old friend from our
graduate days in the zoology department at Chicago and on his frequent
trips through Chicago we discussed his research and mine and the progress
of my chapter. He and his collaborators, Phoenix, Goy, and Gerall, were
just publishing a paper that year on the effects of androgens on fetal female
guinea pigs with respect to postnatal masculinization of behavior and
production of hermaphroditism. I, with Ortiz and Pannabecker, had been
testing the androgenic secretion of fetal guinea pig testes by culturing them
with rat Wolffian ducts. I told Bill that at 32 days of fetal age (the only age
we had tested so far) the testes were normally secreting androgens and the
ovaries were not. He was greatly interested in our findings and I assured
him that we were going to extend the work. This was not possible until
1963, when J. J. P. Zaaijer came to Chicago on leave from the University of
Leiden and we were joined by E. Ortiz (then at the University of Puerto
Rico). Together we forged ahead, first in Chicago and, after my retirement,
at Leiden. As part of our own program we extended the range of ages of the
fetuses, and I continued to keep Bill Young up to date. These reports had a
special point. He and Goy and Bridson had discovered that there was a
critical period of maximum susceptibility to prenatal androgens in the female fetus in relation to masculinization of postnatal behavior. We were
able to say by 1964 that at the period of greatest female susceptibility, the
30th to the 35th day, the fetal ovary was not secreting androgens but testes
were highly androgenic. These findings suggested that the organization of
the neural pathways mediating patterns of male behavior might normally
be controlled by fetal testicular androgens (Price, Ortiz, and Zaaijer,
1967).

In 1965, Young was organizing a Symposium on Hormones in Behavior to be held in Puerto Rico in June, 1966, and he invited me to present
our work. In the spring of 1965, just before I went to Leiden, he was due in
Chicago and we had made an appointment for luncheon, but he became
very ill and did not come. He did not live to attend the meeting that he had
organized so carefully.

To bring my autobiographical account up to the moment, my current
research is on fetal sex differentiation and secretory activity of fetal gonads,
adrenals, and the placenta. That story does not belong here.

THE SOURCE OF FUNDS FOR BIOLOGICAL RESEARCH ON SEX

The funding of early research in the United States on so-called problems of sex has an interesting history which is fortunately well documented (Aberle and Corner, 1953). In 1921, when European laboratories were trying to recover from the tragedy and disorganization caused by the First World War, many laboratories in the United States were active and preparing to embark on new phases of research. Sex had been a subject that was taboo for open and frank discussion (incredible as that seems now) in the United States and as for research on any aspect relating to sex—that was impossible! In 1921 the Committee for Research on Problems of Sex, of the National Research Council (an agency of the National Academy of Sciences) was organized. Its primary purpose was the promotion of studies on human sex behavior but its scope was immediately extended far beyond that. Lillie was one of the five members of the original committee and represented the biological field. His masterly *Classification of Subjects in the Biology of Sex* coupled with the wise allocation of funds in the 1920s–1950s had much to do with the rapid advance of biological research that has been recounted in this paper (there was also great progress in psychological and behavioristic fields). The American contribution to the great surge of findings from 1923 to 1935 in the knowledge of pituitary and gonadal function and the characterization of sex hormones is largely attributable to the way the committee operated in distributing the funds that were made available to them. But the funds, the basic element in the whole scientific advance, depended upon the vision, dedication, and social consciousness of philanthropists. The funding originally came from the Bureau of Social Hygiene, Inc. (Rockefeller-sponsored). From 1933 on, the Rockefeller Foundation provided yearly grants (substantial at that time) that were administered by the committee and covered far-ranging research. Subsequently, the Rockefeller Foundation financed directly the programs of Lillie (Chicago), Evans (University of California), Hisaw (Wisconsin), P. E. Smith (Columbia), Stockard (Cornell University Medical School), and through them, their collaborators and co-workers. To mention only a few of the pertinent names of those who received financial aid from the committee in the first twenty-five years: Moore, E. Allen, Doisy, Corner, W. Allen, P. E. Smith, Engle, Koch, Hisaw, Leonard, Meyer, Greep, Evans and Simpson, Albright and Sturgis, and Hartman. The committee not only dispensed funds for much of the early research in the United States but it sponsored the publication of a book, *Sex and Internal Secretions,* in 1932, to gather together the important findings in the past ten years. This book was immensely successful. Scientific progress was so rapid that a second edition was published in 1939. These two have remained classical source books.

By 1950, the large Federal granting agencies of the National Science Foundation and the National Institutes of Health of the U.S. Public Health Service had taken over much of the major funding and Moore and I received our main support from them. But for 1922–23, Lillie was granted $1,500 by the Committee for Research on Problems of Sex and that was how it all began for me.

REFERENCES

Aafjes, J. H., J. T. M. Vreeburg, and J. J. van der Werff ten Bosch (1972). *Modellen van het hormonale stelsel.* Wetenschappelijke Uitgeverij, Amsterdam.

Aberle, S. D., and G. W. Corner (1953). *Twenty-five years of sex research. History of the National Research Council Committee for Research in Problems of Sex. 1922–1947.* W. B. Saunders, Philadelphia.

Bogdanove, E. M. (1972). Hypothalamic-hypophyseal interrelationships: Basic aspects, Pages 5–70. *in* H. Balin and S. Glasser, eds. *Reproductive Biology,* Excerpta Med., Amsterdam.

Harris, G. W. (1955). *Neural Control of the Pituitary Gland,* Arnold, London.

Harris, G. W. (1964). Sex hormones, brain development and brain function. *Endocrinology* **75:** 627.

Moore, C. R., and D. Price (1930). The question of sex hormone antagonism. *Proc. Soc. Exp. Biol. Med.* **28:** 38.

Moore, C. R., and D. Price (1932). Gonad hormone functions, and the reciprocal influence between gonads and hypophysis with its bearing on the problem of sex hormone antagonism. *Am. J. Anat.* **50:** 13.

Price, D., and E. Ortiz (1944). The relation of age to reactivity in the reproductive system of the rat. *Endocrinology* **34:** 215.

Price, D., E. Ortiz, and J. J. P. Zaaijer (1967). Organ culture studies of hormone secretion in endocrine glands of fetal guinea pigs. III. The relation of testicular hormone to sex differentiation of the reproductive ducts. *Anat. Rec.* **157:** 27.

16

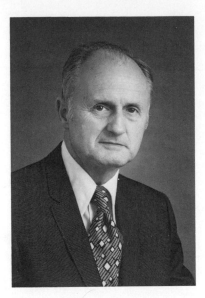

Charles H. Sawyer

Charles H. Sawyer, affectionately known as "Tom," was born on January 24, 1915, in Ludlow, Vermont. He received his A.B. from Middlebury College in Vermont in 1937 and then spent a year as Dutton Traveling Fellow at Cambridge University in England. He returned to the United States and received his Ph.D. in Zoology from Yale University in 1941. He served as an Instructor in Anatomy at Stanford University from 1941 to 1943 and then moved to the new medical school at Duke University in North Carolina where he rose from Associate to Professor of Anatomy. In 1951 he moved to the new medical school at UCLA as Professor of Anatomy and served as Chairman of Anatomy there from 1955 to 1963. He was also Acting Chairman in 1968.

Dr. Sawyer is a member of many societies which include the American Association of Anatomists, the American Physiological Society, the American Society of Zoologists, the Endocrine Society, the Histochemical Society, the International Brain Research Organization, the Association for the Psychophysiological Study of Sleep, the International Society of Neuroendocrinology, the Society for the Study of Reproduction, and the Society for Experimental Biology and Medicine. He has served on the editorial board of the *American Journal of Physiology* from 1972 to 1974, and on the Board of *Endocrinology* from 1955 to 1959. He was a member of the editorial board of the *Proceedings of the Society of Experimental Biology and Medicine* from 1959 to 1962. Since 1965 he has been coeditor of *Experimental Brain Research.*

He has served on many national and international committees. He was on the Anatomy Panel of the National Board of Medical Examiners and its chairman in 1964. He has been on the council of the Endocrine Society from 1968 to 1970 and a member of the National Membership Committee for the Society of Experimental Biology and Medicine. From 1969 to 1971 he was a member of the board of directors of the Society for the Study of Reproduction. He has served the Public Health Service as a member of the Fellowship Review Board in Pharmacology and Endocrinology and as a member of the Neurology Study Section A from 1963 to 1967. He is a council member of the International Society of Neuroendocrinology.

Twenty-Five Years in Neuroendocrinology of Reproduction (1945–1970)

CHARLES H. SAWYER

Born and raised in Vermont, I graduated from Middlebury College in 1937 with an A.B. in biology and an interest in enzymes and hormones. Actually I had gone to college to major in music but had switched majors after a month in Longwell's course in general biology. The interest in enzymes and hormones had been stimulated by Barney, the other member of Middlebury's two-man biology department. On graduation I was lucky enough to win Middlebury's Dutton Traveling Fellowship, which provided for a year's study abroad, and I registered in physiology and biochemistry at Cambridge University. Two years before the start of World War II, British physiology was very excited about acetylcholine, cholinesterase, and neurohumoral transmission, and Dale and Loewi had just received the Nobel Prize for their research on humoral mediation of the nerve impulse. In England Dale, Feldberg, Gaddum, and Vogt were advancing neurohumoral concepts, and Adrian in his first year as professor of physiology at Cambridge was transmitting them sympathetically, although he was himself a Nobel Laureate in electrophysiology. Marshall (of *Physiology of Reproduction* fame) lectured to us about sex behavior in cats, and steroid hormones were stressed in biochemistry. By further good fortune I met two Americans in Cambridge who were influential in my career plans: Donald Barron and Edgar Boell. Barron, a popular lecturer in neuroanatomy and former Yale zoologist, helped me obtain a teaching assistantship at his alma mater and remained a trusted advisor. Boell was a visiting investigator in Joseph

CHARLES H. SAWYER ● Department of Anatomy and Brain Research Institute, UCLA, Los Angeles, California 90024.

Research in the author's laboratory has been supported largely by grants from the National Institutes of Health and The Ford Foundation.

Needham's biochemistry laboratory, measuring respiration in the developing amphibian embryo. He had accepted an instructorship in zoology at Yale, and we were destined to arrive at New Haven simultaneously although neither of us knew the other's plans. One person whom I failed to meet in Cambridge in 1937–38, because he was in London that year, was Geoffrey Harris, who had already induced ovulation in the rabbit by electrical stimulation of the hypothalamus and pituitary. Fond memories of Europe including skiing in the Austrian Alps, a visit to Vienna three months before Hitler's *Anschluss,* and bicycling along the Rhine, where I spent the summer of 1938 learning enough German to pass my Ph.D. language requirement on arrival at Yale.

Influenced by America's leading experimental embryologist, Ross G. Harrison, almost all of the vertebrate zoologists at Yale's Osborn Laboratory worked on amphibian embryos. Harrison had retired just before my arrival but he was still active in research, as were also such famous zoologists as Petrunkevitch, Woodruff, Coe, Hutchinson, and Nicholas. Under the direction of Boell and Nicholas, I undertook as my doctoral thesis a microchemical study of the ontogeny of the enzyme cholinesterase in salamander embryos, correlating its growth with Coghill's physiological stages of developing motility. The sharpest rise in enzyme content occurred with the onset of rapid swimming movements. Innervated muscle at this stage became rich in cholinesterase, but nerveless muscle, produced by surgically removing the developing spinal cord, failed to show the rise in enzyme concentration. The onset of motility could be delayed by culturing the embryos in cholinesterase inhibitors such as physostigmine. Even more exciting was the observation that they turned black from maximal expansion of their melanophores. Was this due to the direct action of acetylcholine or to the activation of secretion of melanophore stimulating hormone from the pituitary gland? In a report of these experiments published some years later (1947) I was able to show that the latter was true—a neurohumoral transmitter activated the release of a pituitary hormone. Meanwhile my interest in neuroendocrinology had been kindled.

In the summer of 1941 I received my Ph.D. in Zoology from Yale, married Ruth Schaeffer, whom I had first met in the biology laboratory at Middlebury College, and accepted an instructorship in anatomy at Stanford University. We drove west on our honeymoon shortly before Pearl Harbor was to plunge the United States into World War II. At that time the Stanford anatomy department had a strong tradition in endocrinology: C. H. Danforth had coedited the 1939 edition of *Sex and Internal Secretions,* J. E. Markee was an authority on the endocrinology of menstruation, and Hadley Kirkman was an expert in pituitary cytology. Some years earlier Hinsey and Markee had proposed that the secretion of anterior pituitary hormones might be stimulated by a humoral mechanism. I discussed with Markee the possibility of collaboration in a study of nervous control of ovulation in the rabbit, a species with which he was working. However, the heavy teaching schedule imposed by the war effort prevented expansion of my research program beyond some cholinesterase studies on mammalian neuromuscular junctions and regenerating nerve fibers.

At the end of 1943 Markee accepted the chair in anatomy at Duke University and invited us to accompany him to North Carolina to implement the proposed collaborative research. We were reluctant to leave Stanford but the offer was too good to refuse, so in January 1944 we drove back across the country to Durham under difficult wartime gasoline rationing conditions. The teaching schedule at Duke was lighter than at Stanford and by summer we had research projects under way, not only with Markee, but also with Henry Hollinshead and Jack Everett. Hollinshead was especially interested in the autonomic nervous system and chemoreceptors, and Everett was already an authority on reproductive cycles in the rat. He had also taken a Yale Ph.D. under Nicholas at Osborn Zoological Laboratory some years before me, but we had never met until I arrived in Durham. At first we worked jointly on hormonal control of serum cholinesterase in the rat and found that estrogen stimulated enzyme production in the liver via a pituitary hormone. With Markee and Hollinshead we started electrical stimulation of the rabbit's cervical sympathetic chain and vagus nerve to see if either would induce ovulation. The results were negative, so we proceeded to apply the stimuli directly to the hypothalamus and to the pituitary gland. Threading a curved electrode through the superior orbital fissure into the basal hypothalamus we found that electrical stimulation induced the release of pituitary ovulating hormone at parameters which were ineffective when applied with the same electrode directly to the pituitary gland approached parapharyngeally (Markee, Sawyer, and Hollinshead, 1946). Only when the electrical stimulus to the pituitary was increased to a level which gave definite signs of spread of current to the hypothalamus was this stimulus effective. This finding was counter to the earlier reports of Harris, and it suggested that the hypothalamic stimulus was effective by a humoral rather than a nerve-fiber link. Wislocki and King had earlier inferred that blood in the hypophyseal portal system must flow downward from median eminence to pituitary rather than vice versa as its discoverers, Popa and Fielding, had proposed. We interpreted our results in terms of a portal system neurohumoral hypothesis. Simultaneously, in England, Green and Harris were demonstrating the direction of blood flow in the hypophyseal portal system by infusion experiments, but we were unaware of their work until their 1947 paper appeared. They adopted our finding that the anterior pituitary was essentially inexcitable electrically as a strong argument for the neurohumoral hypothesis (see Harris, 1955, for other references).

In the mid-1940s the recognized neurohumoral transmitters were acetylcholine (ACh) and epinephrine. Could either of these be the agent responsible for releasing pituitary ovulating hormone? With Markee and Hollinshead (see references in Markee, Everett, and Sawyer, 1952) we tested this hypothesis by injecting them intravenously and into a carotid artery of estrous rabbits with negative results. Even when infused directly into the pituitary gland via a parapharyngeal approach, ACh failed to induce ovulation, but to our delight intrapituitary infusions of Parke-Davis adrenalin resulted in ovulation in a significant number of animals. At that time the potent adrenergic blocking agent, Dibenamine, was being introduced to pharmacological research, and we found that a rapid postcoital injection of this adrenolytic agent would block copulation-induced ovulation. This was confirmatory evidence that an adrenergic mechanism might be involved in the natural reflexogenous activation of release of pituitary ovulating hormone in the rabbit. A cholinergic component was also indicated when we found that very rapid injections of atropine (less than 30 sec postcoitum) would block the ovulatory stimulus (Sawyer, Markee, and Townsend, 1949). Later experiments revealed that intraventricular injections of epinephrine and norepinephrine were as stimulatory as intrapituitary infusions, and electrical changes in the brain coincident with intraventricular norepinephrine's induction of release of ovulating hormone suggested an action at central synapses rather than at the pituitary level (references in Sawyer, 1962).

Unlike the reflexly ovulating rabbit, the rat ovulates cyclicly in a *spontaneous* manner on the night of proestrus. With Everett we tested Dibenamine and atropine as blockers of ovulation in this species, first the estrogen-induced ovulation on days 4–6 of pregnancy (Sawyer, Everett, and Markee, 1949) and then cyclic ovulation by treating with the drug on the morning of proestrus (see Everett, 1960). The blocking drugs were found effective when given as late as 1400 h but not when withheld until 1600 h at proestrus, thus defining a *critical period* of neurogenous stimulation of the pituitary. Treatment with pentobarbital at 1400 h of proestrus blocked ovulation and revealed a 24-hr rhythmicity in the LH-control mechanism (see Everett, 1960), and Everett has expanded on this finding in his chapter of this book.

In 1951 Dr. H. W. Magoun invited me to join his new Department of Anatomy at UCLA. Magoun had become a leading authority on the hypothalamus, brain stem inhibitory and activation systems, and sleep and wakefulness while in Ranson's Neurological Institute at Northwestern

University, and that laboratory had pioneered in studies on neurohypophyseal control of water metabolism and the effects of hypothalamic lesions on pituitary-gonad function. Magoun was already thinking of establishing a similar institute at UCLA, and the prospect of working with him in such a group in California was so great that I accepted the invitation without hesitation.

Magoun encouraged us to make the transit from Durham to Los Angeles by way of a Ciba Foundation Conference on neuroendocrinology in London, a meeting (Wolstenholme, 1952) in which John Green discussed the comparative anatomy of the pituitary portal system, Harris and Jacobsohn reported that pituitary transplants under the median eminence became functional as portal vessels reached them, and Everett described our joint experiments on hypothalamic control of ovulation in the rat. Here also, Harris, Jacobsohn, and Kahlson reported data suggesting that histamine might be a neurohumoral transmitter to the adenohypophysis, a suggestion which led us to experiments at UCLA revealing that intraventricular histamine synergized with pentobarbital as a central nervous stimulant of the release of pituitary ovulating hormone in the rabbit. Later that year (1951) the Duke collaborators reviewed their preceding six years' research at the Laurentian Hormone Conference (Markee, Everett, and Sawyer, 1952).

I was so impressed with the work of John Green that I recommended to Magoun that we recruit him to our young UCLA Department of Anatomy and incipient Brain Research Institute. We were successful, and in the summer of 1952 Green arrived in Los Angeles to start two new phases of his illustrious career: electron microscopy of brain-pituitary structure and electrophysiology of the rhinencephalon. That same summer, Everett visited our Long Beach VA Hospital Laboratories, where our research facilities were located until UCLA built its new medical center, and we mapped a stereotaxic atlas of the rabbit brain, for which Green designed a head holder (Sawyer, Everett, and Green, 1954), and we began stereotaxic electrical stimulation and recording experiments.

In 1953 Charles Barraclough came to UCLA as a postdoctoral fellow and we collaborated on the effects of morphine, reserpine, and chlorpromazine on the rat estrous cycle, ovulation, pseudopregnancy, and thresholds of electroencephalographic (EEG) arousal. In the electrical recording experiments we were aided by my graduate student, Vaughn Critchlow, who was later to be the first to induce ovulation in the rat by electrical stimulation of the hypothalamus. On his own, Barraclough maintained and expanded a program started with Leathem at Rutgers: Early androgen treatment of the female mouse results in sterility. Shifting to the rat, Barraclough and his graduate student Roger Gorski observed that the androgen-sterilized female could be made to ovulate with appropriate hormonal priming and electrical stimulation of the hypothalamus but she never ran estrous cycles. It was as if her brain had been masculinized. Barraclough and Gorski found that the converse was true: Removing the testes from the newborn male rat resulted in the brain's developing female type cyclicity that would induce ovulation in transplanted ovaries. It appears that the rat brain is female type at birth, and it remains as such if not subjected to the action of natural or exogenous sex steroids during the critical first five days. The mechanisms by which gonadal hormones exert this "organizing" action are a major area of current neuroendocrine research (see Sawyer and Gorski, 1971).

In the mid-1950s we became interested in osmoreceptor function, and with the aid of such visiting investigators as Bo Gernandt, Robert Holland, and Barry Cross we explored the rabbit brain with recording electrodes for areas responsive to intracarotid injections of hypertonic solutions capable of triggering release of the neurohypophyseal hormones, vasopressin and oxytocin. Dramatic EEG changes were recorded in the olfactory bulb and its projections and we suggested that the elusive osmoreceptors might reside in the bulb. We had to abandon this idea, however, when with John Sundsten we found that a basal island of preoptic-hypothalamic tissue was all that was needed to induce a milk-ejecting discharge of oxytocin in response to an intracarotid injection of hypertonic saline. Meanwhile, down the hall, Cross and Green had made the first unit recordings of supraoptic neurons firing in response to the hypertonic stimulus; however, this was done in the intact brain, making it impossible to localize the receptor site (see Beyer and Sawyer, 1969; Sawyer, 1970).

In his book *Hormones and Behavior*, Beach (1948) proposed that hormones exert their influence on behavior by raising or lowering thresholds of activity in the central and peripheral nervous systems. With access to electrophysiological equipment in the mid-1950s we decided to test this hypothesis relative to sex hormonal effects on hypothalamopituitary gonad function on the one hand and sex behavior on the other. We had observed in experiments at Duke University that in the estrous rabbit progesterone initially heightens the degree of estrous behavior and facilitates the induction of ovulation and later promotes anestrus and inhibits ovulation—biphasic effects in both instances.

Two regions of the brain with close structural and functional relations to the hypothalamus are the reticular activating system (RAS) and the rhinencephalon or limbic system. The two systems exert complementary influences. Magoun and Moruzzi had shown a few years earlier that the RAS could be stimulated directly to induce a state of EEG arousal in the cerebral cortex. Since this response could be stimulated electrically, its threshold could be measured and the influence of hormones on the threshold assessed. With Kawakami, who joined us first in 1956, we found that low-frequency stimulation of rhinencephalic-hypothalamic projections induced a phenomenon which we called an *EEG-afterreaction*. It consisted of a period of slow wave sleep followed by what is now recognized as paradoxical sleep—a sequence occurring naturally only postcoitally in female rabbits under our recording conditions; hence the name of EEG-afterreaction. Since it could be induced by electrical stimulation, it provided another response for threshold investigation. Testing the effects of progestins on these thresholds we found that during the initial facilitation period both EEG arousal and afterreaction thresholds dropped and during the inhibitory stage they rose to heights far above normal—parallel biphasic effects (see Sawyer, Kawakami, Markee, and Everett, 1959).

Long acting derivatives of progesterone were found to extend both phases of the threshold curves, i.e., the initial lowering and the secondary elevation. During the first phase the release of pituitary LH is readily induced but during the second the rabbit will not ovulate even if she mates. Interestingly, two of the longest acting progesterone esters, 17 α-OH-progesterone caproate and dihydroxy progesterone acetophenide, have been used in women as long-acting antifertility agents—a single injection per month replacing daily ingestion of pills. A second series of antifertility steroids comprised nortestosterone derivatives, widely used in contraceptive pills. These steroids, like testosterone, elevate the EEG afterreaction threshold without initially lowering it and they do not change the EEG arousal threshold. Treated rabbits will mate but not ovulate. From these and other data it appears that the EEG afterreaction threshold mirrors the threshold of pituitary activation and that antifertility steroids act on the brain to the extent that they elevate the threshold of rhinencephalic-hypothalamic activation. The EEG arousal threshold, on the other hand, does not seem closely concerned with pituitary secretion but rather with estrus—the appetitive phase of sexual behavior. The hormones, then, facilitate and inhibit pituitary activation and estrous behavior while lowering and raising brain thresholds (see Sawyer and Kawakami, 1961; Sawyer, Kawakami, and Kanematsu, 1966; Kawakami and Sawyer, 1967).

The discovery that the postcoital EEG afterreaction in the female rabbit contained a phase of paradoxical sleep (PS) led to studies on hormones and sleep. Kawakami found that the whole afterreaction sequence of slow wave sleep and PS could be conditioned to occur in response to a tone if the rabbit was primed with estrogen. Spies later demonstrated that the presence of the pituitary gland was necessary to initiate the postcoital phase of PS. Kawamura noted that brain temperature rose during PS, a change later found by Baker and Hayward to be due to increased blood flow to the preoptic region. Khazan discovered that rabbits deprived of PS by subjecting them to a "white" noise rapidly compensated for the loss when the noise was turned off. Malven studied sleep cycles in the female guinea pig and noted a reduction in both phases of sleep at estrus. In the female rat Lisk discovered that PS could be triggered by simply turning off the lights. Johnson later observed that in artificially short days produced by controlled lighting all of the rats' PS occurred in the dark. However, under normal conditions of 14 hr of light per day this nocturnal species sleeps less at night, and Colvin found that during the night of proestrus when she is behaviorally in heat the female rat shows practically no paradoxical sleep at all. Large doses of progesterone induce slow wave sleep, and a related steroid, hydroxydione, has been developed to serve as an anesthetic. The basic mechanisms underlying the effects of hormones on sleep are unknown but they may well involve alterations in sensitivity of *receptors* to cerebral monoamines. The importance of the amines to sleep mechanisms has been recognized for some time (see Sawyer, 1969*b*).

Starting in 1960 the technique of implanting crystalline hormones directly into the brain was widely applied in studies of feedback action of target organ hormones on hypothalamopituitary function. Previously Flerko and Szentágothai in Hungary had implanted ovarian tissue into the rat brain and pituitary gland, and Harris and Michael had described behavioral effects of large implants of diethyl-stilbestrol in the hypothalamus of the ovariectomized cat. The first stereotaxically localized implants of crystalline estradiol and testosterone were placed in the rat brain by Robert Lisk while he was still a graduate student with Hisaw at Harvard. Lisk differentiated a basal hypothalamic area where the steroids induced gonadal atrophy from a more rostral preoptic region where they influenced sex behavior. In our laboratory Julian Davidson studied the effects of estrogen implants in the female rabbit's hypothalamus and pituitary and testosterone in the male dog's brain and hypophysis. In the basal hypothalamus, but not in the pituitary or other parts of the brain, the steroids induced gonadal atrophy. In the rabbit hypothalamus the estrogen-effective area differed from the site in which, with Peter Smelik, we found that cortisol implants blocked adrenocortical function—the stress-induced release of adrenal steroids. The effective site of estrogen action was the same as that in which, in earlier experiments, we had found that electrical stimulation induced ovulation and lesions caused ovarian atrophy (see Sawyer, 1963, 1969*a*).

On Davidson's departure Shigeto Kanematsu continued experimentation with estrogen implants and found that intrapituitary estrogen did exert an effect: activation of mammary glands, implying the release of prolactin, but no ovarian or uterine atrophy. This led him to measure LH and prolactin in the pituitary, using the bioassay methods available in those days, the

Parlow ovarian ascorbic acid depletion assay for LH and the pigeon crop sac method for prolactin. Intrahypothalamic estrogen appeared to interfere with synthesis and release of pituitary LH while intrapituitary estrogen implantation resulted in release and depletion of pituitary prolactin. We also found that intrapituitary implants of norethindrone did not block copulation-induced ovulation whereas, without interfering with LH synthesis, intrahypothalamic implants were effective in blocking its release for 5–7 weeks. The results suggested that the effective ovulation blocking action by the steroid occurred at the hypothalamic level. Kanematsu reached a similar conclusion on the basis of pituitary cytological studies in rabbits, in which intrahypothalamic estrogen implants prevented the castration-induced hypertrophy of gonadotrophic cells, whereas intrapituitary implants did not. Unfortunately the editor of *Endocrinology* reversed the legends in our $500 color plate in the December, 1963, issue, and this key illustration appeared to support Bogdanove's "implantation paradox" theory published adjacently in the same number of the journal. Bogdanove proposed that intrahypothalamic estrogen may act directly on pituitary cells to which it is carried by the portal system and that the median eminence is the optimal site for steroid implants to exert a direct influence on adenohypophyseal cells. Whereas Kanematsu's rabbit data did not support the direct action hypothesis, we had to admit that Bogdanove's proposal had some merit when Palka and Ramirez in our laboratory discovered that radioactive estrogen appeared to move from median eminence to pituitary in the rat. Palka also showed that estrogen placed in the ventromedial hypothalamic nucleus—implants which did not affect the pituitary gland—maintained estrous behavior in ovariectomized rabbits (see Sawyer *et al.,* 1966; Sawyer, 1967).

Confirmatory evidence for a direct action of steroids on the pituitary gland also came from rabbit experiments. Hilliard, Endröczi, and their associates found that progestin output from the ovary could be used as a measure of LH release from the pituitary. Intrapituitary infusions of rabbit median eminence extract containing LH-releasing factor (LRF) caused a rapid release of LH, but systemic pretreatment with norethindrone blocked LH release and subsequent ovulation. The blockade by norethindrone could be partially reversed by simultaneous subcutaneous injection of estrogen, suggesting that both steroids exert at least part of their influence on hypothalamopituitary function by a direct action on the hypophysis (see Hilliard, Spies, and Sawyer, 1969).

Mention was made before of Sundsten's hypothalamic islands which supported neurohypophyseal function. In the early 1960s a much improved chronic method of *deafferenting* the hypothalamus, i.e., partially or totally separating it from the rest of the brain with a stereotaxic knife, was devised by the Hungarian anatomist, Bela Halász. Halász spent a year (1964–65) at

UCLA working with Gorski, and they made a thorough study of changes in pituitary secretion induced by deafferenting the hypothalamus in the rat. They found that cyclic nervous influences on ACTH and gonadotrophic secretion were missing, eliminating the typical diurnal changes in levels of adrenal steroids and cyclic ovulation. Important extrahypothalamic influences were shown by partial cuts to enter the *hypophysiotrophic* area from the rostral or preoptic end. The deafferentation technique has been widely applied in experiments on many species over the past ten years (see Sawyer and Gorski, 1971).

One of the goals of our Brain Research Institute laboratory has been to obtain electrophysiological correlates of hypothalamopituitary function and the feedback actions of pituitary and target organ hormones on the brain—influencing behavior and pituitary secretion. Earlier EEG studies on the effects of progestins and antifertility steroids on EEG thresholds have already been mentioned. Our first hypothalamic unit studies with Ramirez on the effects of progesterone left us in some interpretational disagreement with Cross and Barraclough, who had proposed that intravenous injection of progesterone, in propylene glycol to rats under urethane anesthesia, exerted specific effects on hypothalamic neurons. We monitored cortical EEG simultaneously and observed that the intravenous injection of progesterone induced a sleeplike EEG change coincident with the slowing in unit firing and we concluded that this effect of the steroid was a generalized response of the brain. This was confirmed in experiments with Beyer, who introduced the multiunit recording method to neuroendocrine research while visiting our laboratory, and in further studies with Komisaruk and his colleagues. On the other hand, Terasawa recorded multiunit activity in the median eminence while injecting progesterone subcutaneously in oil, and she observed what appeared to be stimulatory and inhibitory effects of the steroid independent of the EEG changes. She had previously noted elevated multiunit activity in the basal hypothalamus following electrochemical stimulation of the preoptic region, stimuli that released LH as evidenced by ovulation (see Beyer and Sawyer, 1969; Sawyer, 1970).

In the absence of the target organs pituitary trophic hormones can still influence hypothalamic activity, an effect possibly related to a short-loop or internal feedback action of the trophins. Examples of these effects observed in our laboratory include a slowing of unit activity in the ventromedial area (Ramirez) and a lessening of multiunit activity (MUA) in the preoptic area (Terasawa) together with elevated MUA in the median eminence following systemic administration of LH. The latter was eliminated by anterior deafferentation (Terasawa). In the adrenalectomized rat ACTH raised the MUA in the median eminence while dexamethasone depressed it—Sawyer *et al.* findings confirmed by Steiner *et al.* with their elegant micro-iontophoretic system (see Beyer and Sawyer, 1969; Sawyer, 1970).

In the 1960s interest returned to the effects of brain catecholamines on neuroendocrine function. Fuxe and his associates in Sweden had mapped the localization of norepinephrine and dopamine in the brainstem with a fluorescence method, and new drugs permitted control of the synthesis and breakdown of the amines (citations in this paragraph may be found in Weiner, Gorski, and Sawyer, 1972). Dopamine was recognized as a functional agent in its own right as well as a precursor of norepinephrine, and dopamine was plentiful in a nigrostriatal system as well as in the tuberoinfundibular region. On the basis of staining characteristics, Fuxe proposed that dopamine was inhibitory to gonadotrophic secretion. However, publications of Schneider and McCann and Kamberi and his associates reported stimulatory effects of this amine on LH release. Meanwhile we had observed that reserpine, which depletes hypothalamic catecholamines, stimulates lactation in the rabbit and pseudopregnancy in the rat as well as blocking ovulation in that species. Bengt Meyerson noted that monoaminoxidase inhibitors partially restored ovulation in reserpine-blocked rats. Confirming this finding, Lydia Rubinstein tested the effects of intraventricular infusions of catecholamines on ovulation in the pentobarbital-blocked rat and found dopamine quite ineffective in triggering the process. Epinephrine was most effective and norepinephrine gave partial success. Weiner and others observed that intraventricular epinephrine or norepinephrine induced a biphasic elevation and depression of multiunit activity in the median eminence of the proestrous rat, but dopamine was also ineffective in this regard. More recently we have repeated these experiments in estrogen-primed rabbits, and we find that intraventricular dopamine not only fails to stimulate LH release, it actually inhibits release by a subsequent injection of norepinephrine. Moreover the blocking effect of a large dosage of dopamine may last for several weeks (Sawyer, Hilliard, Kanematsu, Scaramuzzi, and Blake, 1974).

The advent of radioimmunossay to our laboratory in 1970, with Bruce Goldman, Charles Blake, Rex Scaramuzzi, and David Whitmoyer largely responsible for instituting the Midgley-Niswender-Parlow methods, has resulted in an explosive productivity that would require another chapter to document. The availability of purified LHRH, and later the synthetic hormone from Schally's laboratory, has also stimulated many studies. The voluminous research of our recent postdoctoral fellows and graduate students cannot be summarized here and must await another review of the *Recent Advances* type. The same is true of the recent contributions of our colleagues, earlier graduate students and visiting investigators now active in their own laboratories—these include Drs. Adler, Barraclough, Beyer, Clemens, Critchlow, Cross, Croxatto, Davidson, Endröczi, Flerko, Gallo, Gorski, Halász, Haun, Hayward, Hilliard, Holland, Kalra, Kanematsu, Kawakami, Kawamura, Khazan, Komisaruk, Kordon, Lawton, Lisk, Malven, Meyerson, Palka, Radford, Ramirez, Smelik, Spies, Sundsten, Taylor, Terasawa, Tindal, Traczyk, Yokoyama, and Zimmermann. Fortunately, relatively recent research of a large number of these investigators was presented in a symposium on *Steroid Hormones and Brain Function* which Gorski and I organized for the UCLA Medical Forum in 1970 (Sawyer and Gorski, 1971) and the interested reader is referred to that volume.

REFERENCES

Beach, F. A. (1948). *Hormones and Behavior*. Hoeber, New York.

Beyer, C., and C. H. Sawyer (1969). Hypothalamic unit activity related to control of the pituitary gland. Pages 255–287 *in* L. Martini and W. F. Ganong, eds. *Frontiers in Neuroendocrinology 1969*. Oxford University Press, Oxford, England.

Everett, J. W. (1960). The mammalian female reproductive cycle and its controlling mechanisms. Pages 495–555 *in* W. C. Young, ed. *Sex and Internal Secretions*. Williams and Wilkins, Baltimore.

Harris, G. W. (1955). *Neural Control of the Pituitary Gland*. Edward Arnold, London.

Hilliard, J., H. G. Spies, and C. H. Sawyer (1969). Hormonal factors regulating ovarian cholesterol mobilization and progestin secretion in intact and hypophysectomized rabbits. Pages 55–92 *in* K. W. McKerns, ed. *The Gonads*. Appleton, Century-Crofts, New York.

Kawakami, M. and C. H. Sawyer (1967). Effects of sex hormones and antifertility steroids on brain thresholds in the rabbit. *Endocrinology* **80:** 857.

Markee, J. E., J. W. Everett, and C. H. Sawyer (1952). The relationship of the nervous system to the release of gonadotrophin and the regulation of the sex cycle. Pages 139–163 *in* G. Pincus, ed. *Recent Progress in Hormone Research,* Vol. 7. Academic Press, New York.

Markee, J. E., C. H. Sawyer, and W. H. Hollinshead (1946). Activation of the anterior hypophysis by electrical stimulation in the rabbit. *Endocrinology* **38:** 345.

Sawyer, C. H. (1947). Cholinergic stimulation of the release of melanophore hormone by the hypophysis in salamander larvae. *J. Exp. Zool.* **106:** 145.

Sawyer, C. H. (1959). Nervous control of ovulation. Pages 1–20 *in* C. W. Lloyd, ed. *Recent Progress in the Endocrinology of Reproduction*. Academic Press, New York.

Sawyer, C. H. (1962). Mechanisms by which drugs and hormones activate and block release of pituitary gonadotropins. Pages 27–46 *in* R. Guillemin, ed. *Proceedings of the First International Pharmacological Meeting,* vol. 1. Pergamon Press, New York.

Sawyer, C. H. (1963). Neuroendocrine blocking agents and gonadotropin release. Pages 444–459 *in* A. V. Nalbandov, ed. *Advances in Neuroendocrinology*. University of Illinois Press, Urbana.

Sawyer, C. H. (1967). Effects of hormonal steroids on certain mechanisms in the adult brain. *Proceedings of the Second International Symposium on Hormonal Steroids*. Excerpta Medica, Int. Congr. Series No. 132, p. 763.

Sawyer, C. H. (1969a). Regulatory mechanisms of secretion of gonadotrophic hormones. Pages 389–422 *in* W. Anderson, W. Haymaker, and W. J. H. Nauta, eds. *The Hypothalamus.* Charles C Thomas, Fort Lauderdale, Florida.

Sawyer, C. H. (1969b). Some effects of hormones on sleep. *Exp. Med. Surg.* **27:** 177.

Sawyer, C. H. (1970). Some endocrine applications of electrophysiology. Pages 389–430 *in* L. Martini, M. Motta, and F. Fraschini, eds. *The Hypothalamus.* Academic Press, New York.

Sawyer, C. H., J. W. Everett, and J. D. Green (1954). The rabbit diencephalon in stereotaxic coordinates. *J. Comp. Neurol.* **101:** 801.

Sawyer, C. H., J. W. Everett, and J. E. Markee (1949). A neural factor in the mechanism by which estrogen induces the release of luteinizing hormone in the rat. *Endocrinology* **41:** 218.

Sawyer, C. H., and R. A. Gorski, eds. (1971). *Steroid Hormones and Brain Function.* UCLA Forum Medical Sciences No. 15, University of California Press, Los Angeles.

Sawyer, C. H., J. Hilliard, S. Kanematsu, R. Scaramuzzi, and C. A. Blake (1974). Effects of intraventricular infusions of norepinephrine and dopamine on LH release and ovulation in the rabbit. *Neuroendocrinology* **15:** 328.

Sawyer, C. H., and M. Kawakami (1961). Interactions between the central nervous system and hormones influencing ovulation. Pages 79–100 *in* C. A. Villee, ed. *Control of Ovulation.* Pergamon Press, New York.

Sawyer, C. H., M. Kawakami, and S. Kanematsu (1966). Neuroendocrine aspects of reproduction. Pages 43, 59–85 in *Endocrines and the Central Nervous System. Res. Publ. Assoc. Res. Nerv. Ment. Dis.* Chap. 4.

Sawyer, C. H., M. Kawakami, J. E. Markee, and J. W. Everett (1959). Physiological studies on some interactions between the brain and the pituitary-gonad axis in the rabbit. *Endocrinology* **65:** 614–688 (five papers).

Sawyer, C. H., J. E. Markee, and B. F. Townsend (1949). Cholinergic and adrenergic components in the neurohumoral control of the release of LH in the rabbit. *Endocrinology* **44:** 18.

Weiner, R. I., R. A. Gorski, and C. H. Sawyer (1972). Hypothalamic catecholamines and pituitary gonadotrophic function. Pages 236–244 *in* K. M. Knigge, D. E. Scott, and A. Weindl, eds. *Brain-Endocrine Interaction, Median Eminence: Structure and Function.* S. Karger, AG, Basel.

Wolstenholme, G. E. W., ed. (1952). *Anterior Pituitary Secretion. Ciba Foundation Colloquia on Endocrinology,* vol. 4. J & A Churchill, London.

17

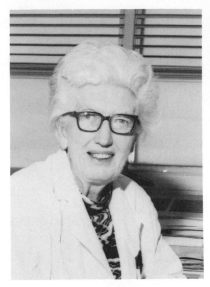

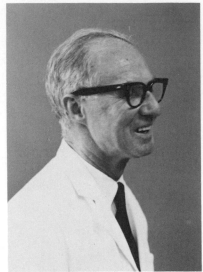

Berta Scharrer   Ernst Scharrer

Berta Scharrer was born in Munich, Germany, on December 1, 1906. She received a Ph.D. from the University of Munich in 1930. She held the following positions: Research Associate, Research Institute of Psychiatry, Munich, 1931–1934; Research Associate, Neurological Institute, Frankfurt am Main, 1934–1937; Research Associate, Department of Anatomy, University of Chicago, 1937–1938; Research Associate, Rockefeller Institute for Medical Research, New York, 1938–1940; Instructor and Fellow, Department of Anatomy, Western Reserve University, Cleveland; John Simon Guggenheim Fellow, Department of Anatomy, University of Colorado School of Medicine, Denver, 1947–1948; Special Research Fellow, USPHS, Department of Anatomy, University of Colorado School of Medicine, 1948–1950; Assistant Professor (Research), Department of Anatomy, University of Colorado School of Medicine, 1950–1955; Professor of Anatomy, Albert Einstein College of Medicine, New York, 1955–present, and Acting Chairman, 1965–1966; 1974–present.

She is a member of the National Academy of Sciences, American Academy of Arts and Sciences, *Deutsche Akademie der Naturforscher Leopoldina*, American Society of Zoologists, American Association of Anatomists; Corporation, Marine Biological Laboratory, Woods Hole; European Society for Comparative Endocrinology (honorary); and International Society for Neuroendocrinology (council member).

Ernst Scharrer was born August 1, 1905, in Munich, Germany. He received a Ph.D. in 1927 and an M.D. in 1933, both from the University of Munich. He received a Dr. honoris causa from the University of Marseille, France. The positions he held include Assistant, Department of Zoology, University of Munich, 1928–1929; Sterling Fellow, Osborn Zoological Laboratory, Yale University, 1929–1930; Assistant Professor, Department of Zoology, University of Vienna, 1930–1931; Investigator, Research Institute of Psychiatry, Munich, 1931–1933; In charge of Neurological Institute, University of Frankfurt am Main, 1933–1937; Rockefeller Fellow, Department of Anatomy (Neuroanatomy), University of Chicago, 1937–1938; Fellow, Rockefeller Institute for Medical Research, New York, 1938–1940; Assistant Professor of Anatomy, Western Reserve University School of Medicine, Cleveland, 1940–1946; Associate Professor of Anatomy, University of Colorado School of Medicine, Denver, 1946–1954; Professor of Anatomy and Chairman of the Department, Albert Einstein College of Medicine, New York, 1955–1965. He died on April 29, 1965.

Neurosecretion and Its Role in Neuroendocrine Regulation*

BERTA SCHARRER

The leitmotiv of this retrospective survey is the phenomenon of neurosecretion. The gradual evolution of our current views on its place in neuroendocrinology will be discussed in terms not of one research career but of two, a husband-and-wife team that ended, after 30 years, with the death of Ernst Scharrer in 1965. As happens so often, the foundations for this investigative work were laid during student days, and its course was shaped by many events unforeseen at the time.

Ernst Scharrer was a student working for his Ph.D. degree when he made his discovery that certain hypothalamic neurons specialize in secretory activity to a degree comparable to that of endocrine gland cells. In 1928, when these results were published, I was a fellow student in the same institute, the Department of Zoology of the University of Munich, headed by Karl von Frisch.

In recapturing the excitement of those early years, one must recall that German students, after their graduation from the very strict *Gymnasium*, suddenly found themselves in an atmosphere of almost complete academic freedom. I remember my rising fascination with this new world of the intellect opening up before me, the spell cast by an outstanding group of academic teachers and investigators.

High standards of scholarship prevailed in the science faculty at that time, and the laboratory in which we undertook our first steps in biological research was no exception. Richard Hertwig was still at work at the old Zoological Institute, housed in a converted 17th-century monastery, our beloved *Alte Akademie*. Sensory physiology was the keynote of the depart-

* This text has appeared in somewhat different form in: *The Neurosciences: Paths of Discovery* (F. Worden, ed.), M.I.T. Press, Boston.

BERTA SCHARRER ● Department of Anatomy, Albert Einstein College of Medicine, Bronx, New York 10461.

mental research program, and the honeybee was the experimental animal that yielded the most spectacular results and brought von Frisch worldwide acclaim. The most decisive imprint we received in those days was that of the heuristic value of a broad comparative approach.

Those were happy, almost carefree days. Our love for and commitment to scientific research were firmly established by the time we received the *Doctor Hut*.

But what was in store for us next? In the early thirties, prospects for an academic career in Germany were bleak and, for a woman, virtually nonexistent. Ernst decided to acquire an additional degree, in medicine, and I to obtain a certificate for teaching in a German *Gymnasium*. During those years we managed to keep laboratory fires burning, both of us having found working space at the Research Institute of Psychiatry in Munich, then under the inspired directorship of Walther Spielmeyer.

After our marriage in 1934, following Ernst's research appointment at the Edinger Institute of Neurology in Frankfurt am Main, the road seemed open for a joint effort to probe into the role of neurosecretion. We decided to divide the animal kingdom; Ernst would continue his studies on vertebrates, and I would set out to search for comparable phenomena among invertebrates. Several sojourns at the Stazione Zoologica, Naples, and a collecting trip around Africa yielded a wealth of material, as did the fauna of the Marine Biological Laboratory, Woods Hole, Massachusetts, at a later time.

Newcomers to the academic scene of the medical faculty of Frankfurt, we were warmly received and encouraged in our work by Albrecht Bethe, who was then codirector of the Neurological Institute, a man of boundless curiosity and youthful enthusiasm for new ideas. Other contacts that developed into lifelong friendships were with Tilly Edinger, daughter of Ludwig and a renowned paleoneurologist, and with Wolfgang Bargmann who, in later years, was to contribute so much to the solution of the problem of neurosecretion.

The institute was well equipped, and work progressed beautifully in this deceptively sheltered milieu, but the political climate in Germany was becoming increasingly intolerable and the outlook was grim.

When Ernst was granted a Rockefeller Fellowship in 1937, we set out for the University of Chicago in high spirits and, having had to leave behind all our scientific material, prepared for a new start. His sponsor was C. Judson Herrick, Ludwig Edinger's American counterpart in comparative neurology, and also an early proponent of the concept of structure/function relationship. We both benefited greatly from our contacts with him as with other members of the anatomy department (George Bartelmez, William

Bloom, Robert Bensley, David Bodian), and of the zoology department next door (Paul Weiss, Carl Moore).

Then followed two years at the Rockefeller Institute (now Rockefeller University) in New York, under an arrangement made by Charles Stockard (Cornell University Medical School) who had taken a great interest in neurosecretion. Unfortunately, his untimely death cut short a collaborative study envisioned to become part of his overall program with purebred dogs. Subsequent moves took us to Ernst's first teaching position at Western Reserve University, Cleveland, Ohio, and then, in 1946, to the University of Colorado Medical School at Denver.

In 1955, we again shipped our growing collection of slides, books, and reprints, this time to the newly opening Albert Einstein College of Medicine, New York, where Ernst had accepted the chairmanship of the Department of Anatomy. It was here, no longer subject to the rule of nepotism, that I received my first regular academic appointment. This and other manifestations of the pioneering spirit of this fledgling institution provided us with a tremendous impetus.

Yet, conditions that might appear to have been restrictive for me during the two preceding decades had their positive side. It was a privileged existence; free from official duties and other pressures and much encouraged by my husband, I was allowed to develop and pursue my research program. The fact that much of it was carried out on a lowly laboratory animal, the cockroach, a choice originally dictated by the limited facilities available to a "guest investigator," likewise turned into an asset.

It is tempting to speculate on the variety of factors determining the gradual elucidation of the phenomenon of neurosecretion which, in spite of various side excursions, has remained our central interest throughout the years. The road was long and arduous, and for many years rather lonely. There was much uncertainty, but never any real doubt about the final outcome. In retrospect, there is every reason to be satisfied with the course of events that brought triumph during Ernst's lifetime.

It is quite remarkable that, from the very beginning, the sights set for this course of investigation had pointed in the right direction. The two initial propositions made by Ernst Scharrer (1928) in his first study on a teleost fish, *Phoxinus laevis*, turned out to be correct, i.e., the endocrine nature of special hypothalamic neurons, and their relationship with hypophyseal function. This was a bold concept that did not fit into any existing mold, and it is not surprising that it was received with skepticism. Why should members of a class of cells as readily defined as neurons be capable of functioning as glands of internal secretion?

What is less understandable, however, is the almost universal rejection by the scientific community of the validity of cytological evidence for the existence of a secretory process. I vividly remember Ernst's disappointment after an eagerly anticipated discussion with Professor Ranson in 1937 that was intended to correlate and interpret their respective results. As stated by another prestigious investigator, H. B. van Dyke (1939): "The evidence that such cells secrete colloid and are to be considered a 'diencephalic gland' is morphological and does not deserve acceptance at this time."

Clearly, a more convincing approach, such as the search for the functional role of neurosecretory centers by classical endocrinological methods, was now called for. But, for a number of reasons, early attempts in this direction were unrewarding. Would this work have progressed more satisfactorily had the resources of Stockard's program not ended all too soon?

One of the recurrent criticisms, according to which the cytological characteristics of neurosecretory cells were judged to be nothing more than manifestations of postmortem changes or pathological processes, had to be countered by demonstrating the very wide occurrence of such neurons in the animal kingdom. A search in the literature had yielded information on "glandlike" nerve cells in the spinal cord of skates, described and correctly interpreted by Speidel, and on comparable cellular elements in various other animal phyla, reported by Hanström. Ernst's studies soon encompassed representatives from all classes of vertebrates, and my own early contributions among invertebrates ranged from opisthobranch snails and annelids to arthropods. This broadly based search for cytophysiological correlates revealed a remarkable degree of analogy (Scharrer and Scharrer, 1944) and presented us not only with a wide choice of experimental animals, but with insights that could not have been obtained from mammalian material alone.

It is a matter of record that the first evidence for neurohormonal activities was the result of studies in invertebrates. As early as 1917, transplantation experiments in caterpillars had led the Polish biologist Kopeć to the conclusion that their brain furnishes a *pupation hormone*. Many years had to pass before the localization of this endocrine factor in implants of the dorsomedial cerebral area by Wigglesworth put the spotlight on a group of neurosecretory cells, first demonstrated by Weyer in the same part of the insect brain. Circumstantial evidence of this kind was highly welcome, but much still stood in the way of the primary goal, which was to elucidate mammalian hypothalamic function. Both the design and interpretation of comparable experiments among vertebrates were handicapped by the greater structural complexity of their neurosecretory centers and by the inadequacy of the histological methods then available for their visualization.

A lucky break occurred when Bargmann (see Chapter 3) and his collaborators experimented with procedures originally designed by Gomori for the demonstration of the secretory product of pancreatic beta cells. By selectively staining the material elaborated in the perikarya of neurosecretory cells, these and comparable methods permitted its being traced throughout the entire neuron. In other words, a marker had been found that linked the cells of origin with special storage and release sites for their distinctive products. Examples of such structures are the neurohypophysis of vertebrates and the analogous corpus cardiacum of insects.

The functional implications of these spatial relationships became increasingly apparent and gave rise to the concept of *neurosecretory systems* as structural and functional units, whose prototype is the hypothalamic-hypophyseal system of vertebrates.

The key to the correct interpretation of such systems was the realization that the terminals of the neurosecretory neurons forming the hypothalamo-neurohypophyseal tract fail to establish synaptic contact with other neurons or nonneural effector cells. The redundancy of this nerve supply to the posterior lobe, long a source of puzzlement, and the close affiliation of the axon terminals with the vascular bed, suddenly made sense. Such an arrangement is designed for the discharge of special neurochemical messengers destined to become blood-borne in amounts appropriate for control of multiple effector cells at some distance from the storage and release sites. Expressed in different terms, the stainable secretory material found in abundance within the neurohypophysis was now judged to be of hypothalamic origin and, more specifically, to be manufactured in the perikarya of the nuclei supraopticus and paraventricularis and their homologues.

Vasopressin and oxytocin, contained within this visible substance, thus became prototypes of a new class of neurochemical mediators, for which the designation of *neurohormones* is appropriate.

The posterior pituitary had lost its rank of an endocrine gland in its own right, and was now demoted to that of a storage depot (Bargmann and Scharrer, 1951). The term *neurohemal organs*, introduced by Knowles, gained wide acceptance, especially when analogous structures were identified in various arthropods. Interestingly, the best known among them, the corpus cardiacum of insects, harbors not only neurosecretory material of cerebral origin, but additional hormonal principles produced by intrinsic parenchymal cells.

The time had come for the *neurosecretory neuron* to be accepted as a new and distinctive cell type with dual properties, i.e., neural and glandular. The major criterion for the separation of this special neuron from its conventional counterparts was that, instead of engaging in synaptic chemical transmission, it manufactures peptidergic neurohormones in substantial amounts, in a manner comparable to that observed in classical protein-secreting cells.

But this new insight, important as it was, did not provide an answer to the central question of why neurons should deviate so profoundly from the norm, if all they accomplish thereby is the dispatch of hormonal signals to terminal target cells, such as those of the kidney, the mammary gland, or the integument. As Ernst Scharrer postulated in 1952, the *raison d'être* for the neurosecretory neuron with its highly specialized dual properties lies in the need for effective communication between the neural and the endocrine regulatory centers, each of which operates in its own way. This important conceptual step marked the emergence of a new phase in neuroendocrine research, placing the main emphasis on the mechanism of control over the first way station of the endocrine apparatus, the adenohypophysis of vertebrates, and analogous structures in invertebrates. As will become apparent, the mechanisms this *final common path* comprises turned out to be more complex than originally anticipated.

By this time, a respectable number of investigators here and abroad had developed an interest in neurosecretory phenomena but, in part due to the Second World War, exchange of information and personal contacts were limited. A most auspicious occasion for an overview of the entire field, encompassing invertebrates and vertebrates, was the First International Symposium on Neurosecretion held at the Stazione Zoologica, Naples, in 1953. Its 20th anniversary was recently commemorated by the Sixth Symposium in London, the intervening conferences having taken place at approximately four-year intervals in Lund, Bristol, Strasbourg, and Kiel.

The proceedings of these symposia constitute a record of the history of progress in this field (Anon., 1954; Bargmann, Hanström, and Scharrer, 1958; Heller and Clark, 1962; Stutinsky, 1967; Bargmann and Scharrer, 1970). The topics featured in consecutive programs reflect an ever-growing spectrum of information as well as shifts in focal areas that have been sparked by conceptual and methodological advances. It is quite evident that substantial progress has accrued from a combination of biochemical, neurophysiological, and pharmacological approaches. Work along these lines is reviewed in other chapters of this volume.

What should be stressed here is that throughout this modern period of investigation morphological studies continue to hold their own. This is due primarily to the wealth of information derived from electron microscopy and, more recently, from fluorescence and immunoenzyme cytochemistry as well as the cobalt/axonal iontophoresis method.

What have we learned from all this about the mode of operation of the hypothalamic-adenohypophyseal axis?

Perhaps the most impressive insight concerns the diversity of the mechanisms that are available for the dispatch of neural signals to the endocrine apparatus (see B. Scharrer, 1970, 1972). The neurochemical messengers in operation range from neurohormonal to neurohumoral (not blood-borne) and include conventional synaptic transmitters as well as neurosecretory mediators that are released in more or less close proximity to their endocrine effector cells.

Are some of these variants adaptive modulations that permit every nuance in the orchestration of neuroendocrine activity, or are they signs of redundancy? Be this as it may, their detection required a modification of the characterization of the neurosecretory neuron, since one of its originally conceived criteria, namely the dispatch of neurohormones, no longer universally applied.

The phenomenon of neurosecretion found its proper place within the larger framework of neuroendocrine communication which, in turn, became the central feature of the new discipline of neuroendocrinology (Scharrer and Scharrer, 1963; E. Scharrer, 1966). Neurology and endocrinology, having long followed their separate ways, had to take notice. The programs of neurobiological meetings of the past decade reflect a growing interest in this affiliation. The same holds for endocrinology, in that 1953 marks the first appearance of *neurosecretion* in the annals of the Laurentian Hormone Conference.

Recognition of the diverse modes of operation of neurosecretory neurons has elucidated the relationship of these cells to more conventional types. It has also directed attention to comparable modulations within the range of conventional neurons and has thus clarified the entire scope of neurochemical mediation, which may be viewed as follows:

Since all neurons share the capacity to synthesize and release distinctive chemical mediators, the existing dichotomy should be viewed as a matter of degree. It derives from the fact that, in the course of phylogeny, the classical *neurosecretory neuron* has developed its secretory activity to the point where it takes precedence over all of the cell's other functions. This specialization enables the nervous system to communicate by means of neurohormonal as well as neurohumoral signals, and the class of neurosecretory neurons takes its place on one side of a spectrum, the other of which is occupied by conventional neurons. Furthermore, the different levels of specialization within the class seem to hold unequal rank in terms of functional significance as well as of frequency.

The position at the nonconventional end is taken up by the first-order systems in which neurohormonal commands reach terminal target cells directly via the general circulation. In higher animals the existence of this relatively primitive mechanism can be interpreted as a carryover from an early state in the evolution of the endocrine system.

Next in line is the group of neurosecretory neurons that have risen to a key position commensurate with their dual capacities, i.e., that of serving as *final common path* by which the nervous system accomplishes its liaison with the endocrine apparatus. The availability of multiple neurochemical, especially neurosecretory, pathways appears to fulfill the complex requirements of the neuroendocrine axis.

An examination of the "conventional" side of the range reveals structural and functional digressions from the pattern of orthodox neural transmission which, although less prominent, parallel some of those first recognized within the group of neurosecretory neurons. Thus, the two sides of the neurochemical spectrum are neither rigidly uniform nor separated by as clear-cut a line of demarcation as originally conceived. Instead, there is an intermediate zone where one neuron type gradually blends into another. The striking features distinguishing classical neurosecretory from conventional neurons have now become "part of a whole" and serve to underscore not merely the existence but the remarkable degree of flexibility inherent in neurochemical communication.

The classical neurosecretory cell retains its special position within this spectrum as a neuron that engages in secretory activity to a degree above and beyond that of other, i.e., more conventional, neurons. The concept of neurosecretion, once considered heretical, has reached its golden age. It has attained respectability and, in the process of entering the domain of modern biological thought, it is now approaching anonymity.

REFERENCES

Anon. (1954). Convegno sulla Neurosecrezione (Riassunti). Proc. Ist Internat. Symposium on Neurosecretion, Naples, Italy, 1953. Pubbl. Staz. Zool. Napoli **24**: (Suppl.): P. 98.

Bargmann, W., B. Hanström, B. Scharrer, and E. Scharrer, eds. (1958). *Zweites Internationales Symposium über Neurosekretion (Lund, Sweden, 1957)*. Springer-Verlag, Berlin/Göttingen/Heidelberg. P.125.

Bargmann, W., and B. Scharrer, eds. (1970). *Aspects of Neuroendocrinology. Proceed. Vth Internat. Symposium on Neurosecretion*. Springer-Verlag, Berlin/Heidelberg/New York. P. 380.

Bargmann, W., and E. Scharrer (1951). The site of origin of the hormones of the posterior pituitary. *Am. Sci.* **39**: 255.

Heller, H., and R. B. Clark, eds. (1962). *Neurosecretion. Proceed. IIIrd Internat. Symp. on Neurosecretion. Mem. Soc. Endocr.* vol. 12. Academic Press, London/New York. P. 455.

Knowles, F. and L. Vollrath, eds. (1974). *Neurosecretion—The Final Neuroendocrine Pathway. VIth Internat. Symposium on Neurosecretion, London 1973*. Springer-Verlag, Berlin/Heidelberg/New York. P. 345.

Scharrer, B. (1970). General principles of neuroendocrine communication. Pages 519–529 *in* F. O. Schmitt, ed. *The Neurosciences: Second Study Program*. The Rockefeller University Press, New York.

Scharrer, B. (1972). Neuroendocrine communication (neurohormonal, neurohumoral, and intermediate). Pages 7–18 *in* J. Ariëns Kappers and J. P. Schadé, eds. *Progress in Brain Research*, vol. 38. Elsevier Company, Amsterdam/London/New York.

Scharrer, B., and E. Scharrer (1944). Neurosecretion. VI. A comparison between the inter-cerebralis-cardiacum-allatum system of the insects and the hypothalamo-hypophyseal system of the vertebrates. *Biol. Bull.* (Woods Hole, Mass.) **87:** 242.

Scharrer, E. (1928). Die Lichtempfindlichkeit blinder Elritzen (Untersuchungen über das Zwischenhirn der Fische. I.). *Z. Vgl. Physiol.* **7:** 1.

Scharrer, E. (1952). The general significance of the neurosecretory cell. *Scientia* (Milan) **46:** 177.

Scharrer, E. (1966). Principles of neuroendocrine integration. Chap. 1 *in Endocrines and the Central Nervous System. Res. Publ. Assoc. Res. Nerv. Ment. Dis.* **43:** 1.

Scharrer, E., and B. Scharrer (1963). *Neuroendocrinology.* Columbia University Press, New York and London. P. 289.

Stutinsky, F., ed. (1967). *Neurosecretion. Proceed IVth Internat. Symp. on Neurosecretion.* Springer-Verlag, Berlin/Heidelberg/New York. P. 253.

Van Dyke, H. B. (1939). The physiology and pharmacology of the pituitary body. II. University of Chicago Press.

18

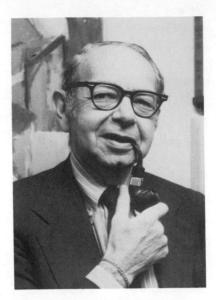

M. C. Shelesnyak

Moses Chaim Shelesnyak was born on June 6, 1909, in Chicago, Illinois. He received a B.A. degree in Zoology (with Honors) in 1930 from the University of Wisconsin, and a Ph.D. in Anatomy in 1933 from Columbia University. While at Columbia University, he was a University Fellow in Medicine in 1932–1933, and a General Education Board Fellow in Child Study in 1936–1938. He was a University Research Fellow at Birmingham University, England, in 1957–1958, and at the same time, a Sir Simon Marks Fellow, UK.

Positions held include the following: Instructor in Physiology and Pharmacology, Chicago Medical School, 1935–1936; Lecturer in Human Growth, New College, New York, 1936–1937; Dean of Boys, Hebrew Orphan Asylum, New York, 1938–1940; Research Associate, Beth Israel Hospital, New York, 1940–1942; Head, Environmental Physiology and Ecology Branch, U.S. Office of Naval Research, 1946–1949; Lecturer in Ecology, The Johns Hopkins University, 1949–1950; Weizmann Institute of Science, Rehovoth, Israel, Senior Scientist, 1950–1958, Associate Professor, 1958–1959, Professor, 1959–1967, Head, Department of Biodynamics, 1960–1968; Associate Director, Interdisciplinary Communications Program, Smithsonian Institution and The New York Academy of Sciences, 1967–1968; Executive Secretary, Council on Communications, Smithsonian Institution, 1968–present; Director, Interdisciplinary Communications Program, Office of Assistant Secretary (Science), Smithsonian Institution, 1968; Director, International Program for Population Analysis, 1972–present. He served as Lieutenant Commander in the United States Naval Reserve, Active Duty, 1942–1946.

Some of the societies of which he is a member include: American Chemical Society, American Physiological Society, the Endocrine Society, Endocrine Society of Israel, New York Academy of Sciences, Sigma Xi, Society for Experimental Biology and Medicine, and the Society for the Study of Fertility (London). He is a corresponding editor of the *Journal of Reproduction and Fertility* (London) and a member of the editorial board of *Contraception*. He has published more than 160 scientific publications and is author of the book *Across the Top of the World* (1946) and editor of *Ovum-Implantation*, 1969 and *Growth of Population*, 1969. He was awarded the Oliver Bird Prize (1958) for Research in Reproduction Physiology.

Comments

M. C. SHELESNYAK

The invitation to submit some "... personal and idiosyncratic accounts of the steps taken and the drive and motivation that led workers like yourself to interest themselves in the relationship between the brain and endocrine system," was difficult to turn down. Of course, my action immediately reveals an important element in the research worker's character (shared by most everyone else); namely, seeking self-satisfaction and nuturing one's ego. My second reaction, however, was curiosity about why I was asked, since direct and straightforward investigations of problems in neuroendocrinology did not cover much of my published work. But thinking about the matter (the invitation was too attractive to refuse, yet I had to demonstrate substantive involvement in the development of neuroendocrinology), I discovered a good deal of work, mostly by indirection and by relationship to some other research problem. Some work was actually by serendipity. Nonetheless, these incursions into areas of neuroendocrinology were not random; they resulted from a philosophical and conceptual approach to research that I have developed over the years.

Two principles which have guided my research and that of my students have been, first, to explore "mechanisms of action." In fact "... for me, the challenge and excitement of scientific research is fulfilled only when investigations are formulated for, and focused on the exploration of mechanisms of action" (Shelesnyak, 1963). The second principle was to employ "multidisciplinary approaches" to study of mechanisms of action of biological or societal problems. With regard to reproduction specifically, I wrote in 1964:

> Reproduction, (however) does not concern only the sum of those primary and secondary acts and actions which are involved in successful conception, in the production of a healthy offspring. Indeed reproduction must be viewed in the full ecological sense; and thus assessment of reproductive capacity involves more than its biological and physio-

M. C. SHELESNYAK ● Interdisciplinary Communications Program, Office of Assistant Secretary (Science), Smithsonian Institution, Washington, D.C. 20036.

logical performance. It involves demographic, social, cultural and anthropological aspects.

However, it would be going beyond good sense to expect the endocrinologist who is studying reproductive processes and means for control of fertility, to explore all the environmental aspects: those cultural, social and anthropological factors; the class differences, social and economic differences, religious tabus, rituals, fertility rites, and the host of other peripheral factors which play a role in modifying basic biological reproductive capacity. Nevertheless, it must constantly be borne in mind, whether we study the human or other animal, that fertility, itself, is a manifestation of an extremely complex constellation of various biological, physical and social factors (Shelesnyak, 1964).

The idea to institutionalize this concept was expressed as follows:

Clearly there are a number of effective means of fertility control, but for global use, each has certain disadvantages. It can be accepted as fact that there will not be a single universally accepted method. The more fundamental and extensive our knowledge of the biodynamics, the greater the probability of devising methods.

At least three tasks confront us: to establish a synthesis in the field of enquiry into reproduction to permit the development of centres uniquely concerned with the reproductive function and the formation of cadres of specialists; to carry out concerted, inter- and multi-disciplinary attacks on selected events or phases in reproduction to elucidate the underlying mechanisms of action and means of regulation; and to play a role in training people, especially from emerging countries, so that they can serve as leaders in their homeland for the establishment of centres for the study of reproduction and application to local problems. As a closing reflection, it should be realized that the writer's concepts of biodynamics, of the nature, organization, and operation of the Institute of Biodynamics are under test, an experiment, the results of which will be available for scrutiny in the course of the next ten to fifteen years (Shelesnyak, 1966).

My suggestion for developing a corps of investigators to carry out research in reproduction along these lines has not materialized. The idea of *biodynamics* (Shelesnyak, 1966) as a field, and *biodynamists* as practitioners in that field, appears not to have achieved any real acceptance.

As for the beginnings of my interest and work in science, it was my good fortune to have parents who encouraged my interests in science, in research, rather than in the pursuit of medicine, law, or the business world. Reflecting on the past, I see that my high school teachers—especially of sciences—were all remarkable and each played unforgettable roles in encouraging me in biology, chemistry, and physics. (Astronomy and geology were added by my physics teacher.) They offered me opportunities to carry on special experiments, field trips, and even to give lectures and demonstrations to classes. As a freshman at the University of Wisconsin, I had the opportunity to work and learn in the laboratory of Professor Roebuck (low temperature physics). Mr. Ehlman, my high school physics teacher, was a classmate of Roebuck's and made the arrangements. The excitement of research touched me early.

Yet it was only in my senior year at Wisconsin, when I stopped wandering through physics, chemistry, math, and the humanities that I concentrated on zoology. Registering for courses that year, I was confronted with the news that I had the (mandatory) privilege of doing a research project or thesis for the bachelor's degree, as a result of the fact that I was in the upper something-or-other of the class. And with remarkable luck I came into Professor Hisaw's group at the beginning of the golden age of modern endocrinology of reproduction. Rollie Meyer, Whitey Fevold, Kip Weichert, Sam Leonard, Chris Hamre were instructors and graduate students. Roy Hertz and I, as best I can recall, were the only two undergraduates doing endocrine research.

Chris Hamre was assigned to be my mentor. His study of thyroid growth and development in *Salmo fario* (Brown trout) afforded me the opportunity of collecting fry of various ages. My first "official" venture into research was a study of *The post-embryonic differentiation of the hypophysis cerebri of* Salmo fario (*Brown trout*). My introduction to endocrinology was via the pituitary, and the research immersed me into microscopic avenues. I recall what seemed miles of paraffin ribbons six and seven micra thick of longitudinal and transverse sections of brains of the fish fry. Then there were the hundreds of slides which I prepared and examined and described in the thesis. I dug up the only copy of the thesis a few days ago and, frankly, I was impressed and pleased with the workmanship. The review of literature was extensive. Though only two investigators, Haller in 1896 and Boeke in 1902, looked at *Salmo fario*, 64 references to other species of fish were read and reported in the study (13 in English, 18 in French, and 31 in German!). The discussion of endodermal versus ectodermal origin of the hypophysis was still popular, but increasing evidence of dual-layer origin was beginning to appear.

That final year at the University of Wisconsin moved me from special interest to deep commitment to the biology and physiology of reproduction. Roy Hertz and I applied to Columbia University for admission to the Department of Anatomy, to study for doctorates under Philip E. Smith and E. T. Engle. I spent the summer of 1930 poring over, page by page, the second edition of Marshall's *Physiology of Reproduction* (1922). It was a wonderful summer.

Earl Theron Engle was my teacher and mentor; to him I owe a great deal. He stimulated me to look far beyond the limits of my Ph.D. project. In fact, he made me aware of the relation of science to society and the importance of the holistic nature of nontrivial problems in science and in society.

The first day in the laboratory, he gave me six female rats, two males, some cages, and said: "Breed your own colony; no one should try to do research in endocrinology of reproduction without knowing how to breed and care for an animal colony, and all the basic facts of the colony"—cycle-regularity of the females, litter size, sex distribution, rates of growth and development. . . . Professor Engle also told me: "You are not here to help me with my research or for me to exploit you; I am here to help you. Think about problems of interest and we'll discuss them." What a far cry from the situation today!

The first published study of my researches relate the nervous system to endocrinological responses: the induction of pseudopregnancy in the rat by electrical stimulation of the cervix (Shelesnyak, 1931). The reason for the work was to develop a more effective means of preparing pseudopregnant rats for my studies of decidualization.

The problem with which I was confronted was to develop an effective method by which pseudopregnancy could be induced in the rat and which could be timed precisely. The use of the vasectomized male was almost 100% effective, but time of stimulation was not under the experimenter's control. Moreover, it was an extremely difficult technique for use with immature rats in which precocious puberty was produced by hypophyseal implants or by extracts of the urine of pregnant women. The use of a glass rod to stimulate the cervix, which was described by Long and Evans in their classical work, *The oestrus cycle in the rat and associated phenomena* (1922, Mem. U. Calif. **6**.) although effective, was so in only about 68% of the trials.

The success of the vasectomized male could be attributed to many factors, even the probability of the reaction in the female to sterile coition being a "learned" response. The glass rod may have acted as a mechanical substitute for the copulation plug, as suggested by Long and Evans, or for the penis, and so simulated the male, or as a simple nervous stimulus. R. K. Meyer, S. L. Leonard, F. L. Hisaw (1929, PSEBM **27**:340) reported that stimulation of anesthetized rats with a glass rod was only half as effective as it was in the unanesthetized female. At that time a neurohumoral pathway was unsuspected. But added to the fact that the response to mechanical stimulation was poor, control over the degree and extent or spread of stimulation was very limited. Thus, the attempt to induce pseudopregnancy by electrical stimulation had some attractive features: precise localization of the electrodes, control of the intensity and waveform of the electrical current, and control over exact time during the cycle when stimulus was applied. These appeared to offer some leads to understanding the mechanism of action.

Neither elegant stimulators nor CROs were available at that time. I made electrodes by fusing a pair of copper wires in a glass tube, which served as the handle. (The standard electrodes, made with wires set in hard rubber or Bakelite, which were available in every physiology department, were too large.) The copper wires were connected to the secondary coil of a primitive "Inductorium." With the use of a small nasal speculum and head mirror, placement of the electrodes at the os cervix was possible; and, of course, moving the secondary altered the output. Two 6-V dry cells served as the power source.

The method, tested on females in various stages of the normal four-day estrous cycles, proved to be effective, provided it was applied during the estrogen predominant state, and was most effective (92%) when applied during the few hours of proestrus. Thus, the time of maximal sensitivity to stimulation was determined. The proof that it was the electrical stimulus which was effective was evidenced by the fact that placing and holding "cold" electrodes did not produce any mechanical stimulus to provoke pseudopregnancy.

Since the work I carried on in the next few years at Columbia was on decidualization of the uterus of the immature rat, I did not use the electrical method of inducing pseudopregnancy. (It was rediscovered in 1938 by Greep and Hisaw [PSEBM **39**:359].) But it was used extensively years later in our studies at the Weizmann Institute. A more sophisticated stimulator permitted refined control of application of controlled wave form and discharge intensity, as well as interval of stimulation. These modifications resulted in greater than 98% effectiveness in over 5000 trials.

Although I did not continue to explore this pseudopregnancy-related nervous mechanism, I remained much intrigued. After publishing the report on these experiments, I chanced across the work of W. Blotevogel (Sympathetikus und Sexualzyklus. II. Das Ganglion Cervicale Uteri des Kastrierten Tieres. *Z. f. Mikr. Anat. Forsch.* 1928, **13**:625) on chromaffin granule fluctuations of the ganglionic regions of the rat cervix with variations on estrogen and progesterone status. The work fascinated me; I volunteered and gave a departmental seminar on his work. It left a lasting impression.

These studies were reported in my first published work (Shelesnyak, 1931). I recall my excited reactions to the response of some readers. First of all, in those days (before printed reprint request cards, for two copies! were sent out by departmental secretaries) most reprints were requested in brief notes, with comments regarding the writer's interest. It is difficult to convey the feelings of a new graduate student who received notes from George Corner, Edgar Allen, Herbert McLean Evans, Carl Hartman—with encouraging words. But perhaps the most exciting was a letter from England. Some chap from Oxford, Geoffrey W. Harris, asked for greater details, and my suggestions for stimulating the rhesus pituitary! With audacity of youth, I suggested the idea of a large induction coil as a primary coil to be incorporated as part of the animal cage, and a small coil as the secondary to be implanted under the skin, with leads to the hypophyseal region. Years later, visiting Jeff in London and reminiscing, I talked with him about that idea. Since I can't recall that the method was successful (I know he tried it), I assumed it was not.*

During my days at Columbia, Prof. Philip Smith taught me his original surgical method for hypophysectomy, but I never did that surgery in any of my research. I did work with him on the response of the ferret estrous pattern to changes in light cycles. He had an emotional block to eye surgery, so I transected optic nerves. (The work was never published.)

The next episode, which may be of interest to the neuroendocrinologist, was my work probing nonolfactory relations between nasal regions and reproductive activity. At the turn of the century, Fliess (an otologist with many interests) described his success in treating menstrual disorders by applying silver nitrate to selected regions of the nasal mucosa. Sam Rosen, M.D. of the E.N.T. Department of Mount Sinai Hospital of New York, invited my attention to the problem and offered facilities to explore "a nasogenital relationship." A large basement room as a laboratory and a small animal room (where we started a rat colony) were made available. It was very good fortune that, soon after my arrival, Prof. S. L. Loewe (of Dorpat) came to the United States as a refugee from Germany and shared the laboratory at Mt. Sinai with me. A pioneer in endocrinology, a pharmacologist, a highly cultured gentleman, he became friend and teacher. He introduced me to the idea of using pharmacological substances as tools for research.

The investigations of the nasogenital relationship in rats revealed that the application of silver nitrate to the mucosa of the conchae induced pseudopregnancy. It was a true progestational uterus which responded to trauma to form deciduomata (Shelesnyak and Rosen, 1938). That action was due to an anesthetization, rather than irritation, since local application of nupercaine also induced the progestational condition of the uterus but oleum sinapsis did not alter the estrous cycle. This led to seeking some neuromechanism. The anatomy suggested possible nervous spread to the pituitary. Collaborative work with L. R. Zacharias led to exploring the role of the sphenopalatine ganglia, which supplies the major portion of the innervation of the nasal mucosa. Extirpation of the sphenopalatine ganglia induced pseudopregnancy (Shelesnyak *et al.,* 1940). The possibility that the hypophysis was involved was proposed at that time, although the matter was not pursued. However, an extensive study of sexual function of the female rat (adult and infantile) deprived of the sphenopalatine ganglia revealed that the

---

* Harris actually made excellent use of this suggestion to develop the technique of remote control stimulation of the hypothalamus in the rabbit rather than in the rhesus monkey. [EDITOR'S NOTE]

establishment of vaginal cornification, reproducing capabilities, induction of pseudopregnancy by cervical stimulation, all remained normal in the absence of the ganglia. The pseudopregnancy response to removal of the ganglia was a response to removal rather than to its absence (Rosen *et al.*, 1940).

During that time I began to study the effect of various drugs—mainly those acting as, or on, autonomic nerves: sympathetic and parasympathetic, lytic and mimetic. Unfortunately the work was incomplete when I left to serve in the U.S. Navy (World War II) and all the protocols of those experiments were lost in moving from the laboratory. However, my awareness of the potential use of pharmacological agents in the study of endocrine-reproductive process was already ingrained, and a decade later when I returned to the laboratory, I began the use of drugs as instruments for exploring mechanisms of action.

In the autumn of 1950, I joined the newly formed Department of Experimental Biology at the Weizmann Institute of Science in Rehovoth, Israel. Once again, an animal colony was to be created. I planned to tackle a question which troubled me for years: *the mechanism of ovum-implantation or nidation*. The initial approach was to explore the nature of the stimulus which provokes the progestational endometrium of the pseudopregnant rat to decidualize and develop deciduomata.

During the first year at the Weizmann, the late Alan Guttmacher, a friend for many years and at the time still associated with the Johns Hopkins at Baltimore, visited Israel. He brought me the news of the then newly organized Population Council of New York, and of possible support for my research. Guttmacher's visit and his interest in my research led to a visit by Warren Nelson, the first director of the Medical Division of the Population Council. The support of the Population Council and later of the Ford Foundation was generous from those early days onward.

Evidence was accumulated, from the inhibition of decidua formation by antihistamines, to support a hypothesis of histamine activation of the endometrium to decidualize. In the course of analyzing the mechanism by which antagonists to histamine prevented decidualization, the ergotoxine complex was used (ergotoxine effectively prevented decidual development and also interrupted pregnancy). Particularly the effectiveness of subcutaneous injections of these ergot drugs in inhibiting decidual formation and pregnancy resulted in initiating an extensive series of studies to understand the mechanism of ergot action (Shelesnyak, 1957). Early in those studies (in 1954) it was stated: "The assumption appears sound that the action of ergotoxine in suppressing the decidual reaction is by disturbance of the estrogen-progesterone balance mediated by the ergotoxine stimulation [*sic*] of the hypothalamus which in turn disturbs anterior hypophysis secretions" (Shelesnyak, 1954).

During the period beginning in 1953 and throughout my activity in the laboratory (I left the institute in August 1967), we carried on many investigations of the actions of ergotoxine drugs, particularly of ergocornine, as they affected interruption of progestation in the rat. Eldad S. Kisch M.D., studied for his doctorate of philosophy with me. He made extensive investigations of the mechanism of ergocornine action in the interruption of progestation of the rat. His thesis (Kisch, 1967) is a source of a great deal of experimental evidence to support specific action of the drug on hypothalamic activity related to prolactin. However, a great deal is yet to be learned about the metabolic actions of these drugs and some recently synthesized related compounds. (See work of Meites.)

The accumulating evidence of ergocornine-hypothalamus interrelationships led to some intriguing experiments which were carried out during a fortnight visit in the summer of 1966 to Cambridge, England. Ian Silver, working in Barry Cross's laboratory, joined me and actually did most of the experimental work. From that lab we learned that the unit firing rates in the hypothalamus of the rat are precisely correlated with its estrogen or, as the case may be, its progesterone status. We had amply shown that pseudopregnancy (as well as progestation) in the rat can be terminated by a single dose of ergocornine, and that termination is followed with the appearance of estrus within 24 hours. It was therefore of interest to investigate the action of ergocornine on the unit firing patterns of the hypothalamus of the pseudopregnant rat. Within minutes after the injection of ergocornine into the pseudopregnant rat, the unit firing pattern was altered from the moderate and slow progesterone pattern to the rapid firing estrous type. Administration of progesterone (which "reverses" the ergocornine action with respect to decidual inhibition) reversed the firing pattern. A subsequent administration of ergocornine did not change the effect of the progesterone action. Unfortunately the results of these experiments remain unpublished.

It should not escape notice that our involvement in these investigations of neuroendocrine phenomena resulted from our exploring the mechanism of nidation. Similarly the doctoral research of my former student, Dr. Ayalla Barnea, on the sympathetic nervous system and reproductive patterns in the rat (Barnea, 1966) incorporated significant findings on catecholamine content of uterus during estrus and progestation. However, neither an intact sympathetic nervous system nor cervical ganglion were essential to achievement of estrous periodicity or nidation.

Puttipongse Varavuhdi, from Bangkok, helped in understanding the mechanism of nidation and contributed to investigating the interrelationship between the CNS, the adenohypophysis, and ovary. His Ph.D. thesis contains a wealth of interesting data (Varavuhdi, 1965).

G. Zeilmaker spent a short while with me at the Weizmann before he went on to take his doctoral degree in The Netherlands. His early work with us led to his pursuing an interest in ergocornine action, and to his proposing the hypothalamus as the site of action.

The ergocornine story has an informative history and some lessons to teach. It is an example of how the pursuit of a mechanism of action by multidisciplinary means can lead to new interests—beyond helping to elucidate the "target" physiological process, in this case, nidation. Not too long after I first observed the intriguing action of ergotoxine drugs on pseudopregnancy, early pregnancy, nidation, and decidualization, Professor Meites came to the Weizmann to spend his sabbatical in our department. (At the time, I was in experimental biology. Other than my work in biodynamics, carcinogenesis was the main subject.) Meites's interest was shared, and we did some things together—he taught us to bioassay prolactin. (That dates us.) He and I actually did some extensive studies on lactation suppression in the rat by ergocornine. That work did not get published; actually it was never completed to our mutual satisfaction. It is fitting that one of the editors of this book (J. Meites) is in the best position to reveal one of the branches which developed from the ergocornine story—its role in prolactin secretion.

In retrospect, although the nasogenital studies may have foretold the action of external stimuli on the hypothalamus, with resulting modifications of hormonally controlled behavior (perhaps even pheromones?), our work did not generate any further directly derived research.

In the course of writing these notes, I looked again and again at the mandate given me. Closing these remarks can be made fitting only by expressing my deep appreciation for the valuable contributions of teachers, students, and colleagues; each person is a mix of the three. It is also gratifying to be able to thank those who helped support research—the Population Council, Ford Foundation, Sandoz, Ciba,—and individuals of those and other institutions.

Of course, achievement of understanding and discovery are satisfying. But beyond that and including the failures, the dead ends, the frustrations, the sometime pettiness of destructive competitiveness—truly, the real satisfaction to me in my scientific work, was the company I kept. The stimulation and excitement of dedicated people—some were just plain devoted and hard working, many were exceptional, some were very imaginative and creative and brilliant. This was the company I kept.

Warren O. Nelson, and later Sheldon J. Segal of the Population Council, O. Harkavy of Ford Foundation, New York, and A. Cerletti and A. Fanchamps of Sandoz, Basel, were particularly helpful. And among my staff of the Biodynamics Department of the Weizmann Institute, Drs. P. F. Kraicer, G. J. Marcus, and H. R. Lindner, and Mr. Shalom Joseph, animal caretaker and senior technician, are among those to whom I shall always be indebted.

REFERENCES

Barnea, A. (1966). The sympathetic nervous system and reproductive patterns: Analyses of uterine catecholamines during oestrus and progestation. Doctoral thesis, Weizmann Institute. Rehovoth, Israel.

Kisch, E. S. (1967). Analysis of the interruption of progestation in the rat by the ergot alkaloid, ergocornine: A contribution to the understanding of the mechanism of nidation. Doctoral thesis, Weizmann Institute. Rehovoth, Israel.

Rosen, S., M. C. Shelesnyak, and L. R. Zacharias (1940). Naso-genital relationship: II. Pseudopregnancy following extirpation of the sphenopalatine ganglion in the rat. *Endocrinology* **27:** 463–468.

Shelesnyak, M. C. (1931). The induction of pseudopregnancy in the rat by means of electrical stimulation (1931). *Anat. Rec.* **49:** 179.

Shelesnyak, M. C. (1954). Ergotoxine inhibition of deciduoma formation and its reversal by progesterone. *Am. J. Physiol.* **179:** 301.

Shelesnyak, M. C. (1957). Some experimental studies on the mechanism of ova-implantation in the rat. *Rec. Progr. Hormone Res.* **13:** 269–322.

Shelesnyak, M. C. (1963). Interdisciplinary approaches to the endocrinology of reproduction. Pages 231–243 *in* P. Eckstein and F. Knowles, eds., *Techniques in Endocrine Research.* Academic Press, London.

Shelesnyak, M. C. (1964). Exploration of biological bases for fertility control. *Proceedings of the IInd International Congress of Endocrinology.* Excerpta Medica, Amsterdam. P. 1365.

Shelesnyak, M. C. (1966). Biodynamics and the population explosion. *Ariel,* No. 13: 21. (A review of the Arts of Sciences in Israel) Ministry of Foreign Affairs, Jerusalem.

Shelesnyak, M. C. and S. Rosen, (1938). Naso-genital relationship: The induction of pseudopregnancy in rat by nasal treatment. *Endocrinology* **23:** 58.

Shelesnyak, M. C., S. Rosen, and L. R. Zacharias (1940). Naso-genital relationship: III. Some aspects of sexual function in female rats deprived of sphenopalatine ganglia. *Proc. Soc. Exper. Biol. Med.* **45:** 449–451.

Varavudhi, P. (1965). Studies on the mechanism of nidation and interrelationship between the CNS, the adenohypophysis and the ovary. Doctoral thesis, Weizmann Institute. Rehovoth, Israel.

19

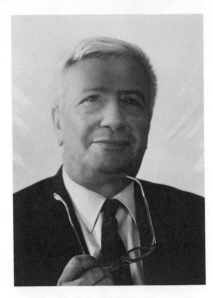

F. S. Stutinsky

F. S. Stutinsky was born in Creutzwald (Moselle), France, on March 8, 1909. He received a Baccalaureate in 1928; M.D., with Silver Medal for his doctoral thesis at the Faculty of Medicine, Paris, 1939; B.S., 1941, Doctor of Science, Paris, 1955. The positions he has held include the following: Demonstrator of Experimental Biology, Faculty of Science, Paris, 1934; Lecturer in Physiology, Institute of Physical Training, 1946–1947; Chief Demonstrator of Animal Biology, PCB, Faculty of Science, Paris, 1949–1956; Chief Demonstrator of Comparative Physiology, Faculty of Science, Paris, 1956–1957. Since 1957 he has been Professor of General Physiology, Faculty of Science, Strasbourg.

He is a member of the Association of French Anatomists, Society of Endocrinology, Association of French Physiologists, French Society for Experimental Neuroendocrinology, Royal Society of Medicine (affiliate member), International Society for the Study of Reproduction, French National Committee for Physiological Sciences, Commission on Neuroendocrinology of the International Union of Physiological Sciences. He has been an invited speaker at many meetings, including the first Symposium on Neurosecretion, Naples, 1953; Symposium on the Diencephalon, Milan, 1956; First International Congress of Endocrinology, Copenhagen, 1960.

F. S. Stutinsky was president of the Fourth International Symposium for Neurosecretion, Strasbourg, 1965, and president of the 43rd Congress of French Physiologists, Dijon, 1975. He was a Laureate of the Academy of Science, Paris, 1957 and 1969. His decorations include Croix de Guerre, 1939–1940, and Officier de l'Instruction Publique.

How I Did Not Discover Neurosecretion

F. S. STUTINSKY

It was in 1931, while training at Hôtel-Dieu as a second-year medical student in the department of an endocrinologist, Dr. Paul Saintoin, of the Hôpitaux de Paris, that I had the opportunity of meeting the assistant to Prof. Et. Rabaud, Professor of Experimental Biology at the Sorbonne. Already a Doctor of Science, she sought to perfect her training as a biologist. She had told me that she was doing research work and I occasionally asked her how her work was progressing. I also expressed interest in her director's numerous publications and the general ideas which he put forward. For reasons unknown to me, but which at the time struck me as flattering, she told Et. Rabaud about these conversations, and one day passed on an invitation for me to come and talk with him. Very flattered, I made an appointment to see him, and went to his office feeling rather nervous. His office, like all the rooms of that historic monument, the Sorbonne, had a very high ceiling and was enormous, furnished with tables draped in green felt and covered with books and papers, and a high wall bookcase. On the other side of the light-colored oak desk I saw a small man in a white coat, with interesting features: a high forehead, a large aquiline nose, his complexion set off by a crown of white hair and a great grey walrus moustache. He was wearing round, metal-rimmed glasses, and the very thick lenses readily betrayed his acute shortsightedness, of which I was later to have ample repeated confirmation. But there were clear eyes below those thick white eyebrows, and a shy smile stretched out his thin lips. I no longer recall what were the terms of our discussion, but after three-quarters of an hour, I was offered a post in the laboratory, to carry out research—on tissue cultures. Tissue cultures, indeed!—for at the time, nothing could have been further

F. S. STUTINSKY ● Laboratoire de Physiologie générale, Université Louis-Pasteur, 67000 Strasbourg, France.

from my mind than neuroendocrinology; I was fascinated by the problem of cancer, which I hoped to study by *in vitro* culture of cancerous tissues.

Looking back today, I am quite sure that neither myself (and I can plead my inexperience at the time) nor my director (I was subsequently to see in this one of his inadequacies) was really aware of the technical and theoretical knowledge such a project involved, nor of the working conditions it required. Neither were available, but it took me some time to realize this. Morever, Professor Rabaud was no ordinary French biologist: He was an opponent of Morganian genetics, and also delighted in denying morphological adaptation, and attempted to review the "useless" and even harmful organs. His pet theory was that there existed a "complex" between the organism and environment, an idea which bore the marks of a faithful disciple of Lamarck. Once stripped of its polemical content, the idea of the influence which its surroundings have on an organism was in fact quite interesting. My director also convinced me that one had to have two research projects: one which would give immediate results, and the other, long-term results; for this advice, I remain indebted to him. For all the optimism with which he greeted my proposal "to study cancer," he was not pinning his hopes on my finding a solution to the problem overnight.

Just at this time, I happened to come across a paper by Zondek and Krohn on the pars intermedia. This new finding fascinated me, and I set about trying to confirm these authors' results in *Phoxinus laevis* and the frog. Straightaway I made a "discovery". Apart from the extracts of the *neurointermediate lobe* of the ox, a whole series of extracts of acetone powder produced in the two animals, respectively, an erythrophoro- and a melanophoro-dilatation (Stutinsky 1934*a,b*). Whether it was a question of the absence of specificity, as Rabaud believed, or, as my future director, R. Collin suggested, a question of *hormonopexia* on the peripheral glands of a substance of hypophyseal origin, I cannot say; I myself have not tried to solve this problem (although it would be well worth taking up). However, this discovery had this to its credit: On the one hand, it pleased my director, who abhorred "specificity" and "tests" and on the other hand, it put me in contact with Prof. R. Collin, of the Medical Faculty at Nancy. He, along with Drouet, had just proposed a test to examine the pituitary basis of Basedow's disease by seeking erythrophoro- or melanophorodilatations induced by injections of urine from these patients. A short controversy ensued which delighted Rabaud, who throughout his entire scientific career believed that one had to be *against* someone. This controversy did not last, but it had repercussions to which I shall return.

Handling frogs with their pigmentary reactions and the necessity of adapting the frogs to the white background led me to investigate the conditions of melanokinesis and, thereby, to study the effects of incident light and reflected light on an organism. This new orientation again delighted my director, especially when he realized that this provided a spectacular and slightly less speculative way of studying the influence of an environmental factor on an organism. This was of crucial importance for me, since I realized that light could only act on an organism through its nervous system, and through the pituitary gland. This hypothesis was borne out in the first place by examining the results of Hogben and Winton, of Houssay, and by a personal histological study of frog pituitary under various lighting conditions (Stutinsky, 1936). Unfortunately, I knew nothing about hypophyseal cytology, nor did I know anyone, even in Paris, who did. Those who can recall what histological techniques were like in 1934–35, and the divergent and uncertain results they produced, can imagine the confusion of a beginner faced with the motley aspect of a section of the pituitary gland. Everything I came across raised problems for me, and the experimental structural variations which I thought I observed were not always reproducible. I was marking time. Luckily, my military service, which was postponed till the age of 27 for medical students, was imminent.

In October 1935 I left for Lyons, where all the medical sections of every military zone in France were assembled. After three months of training, I was posted to Metz to the 61st R.A.D. (divisionary artillery regiment) as the deputy doctor, with the rank of company sergeant-major. My duties consisted of helping the doctor, a captain, or replacing him, but practically speaking, my afternoons were free. Since Metz was only an hour's train ride from Nancy, I decided to go and see R. Collin in his laboratory, which he had just named Neuroendocrinology Laboratory. In 1936, it was the first laboratory in the world to carry this name. I had, by way of a letter of introduction, the little scientific controversy which had brought us to loggerheads a couple of years earlier.

I met a very friendly man, dressed in a high, white collar, a black jacket, and pinstripe trousers—very much in the old French tradition, or in any case, that of the old Lorraine bourgeoisie. His accent, lingering on the end of the syllables, left no doubt about it. He looked at me squarely through his pince-nez, which he adjusted frequently. I explained the problem to him and my hypothesis, namely that, in the course of time, light must modify the structure of the pituitary. He was of the same opinion, and that is how I came to join R. Collin's laboratory first, on a part-time basis, and then, after my military service, on a full-time basis for six months.

I have wonderful memories of that time. First, I met a remarkable, cultured man, with wide interests, artistic, enthusiastic, modest, and forever kindly. I met P. Florentin, who held the title of *agrégé*, and who took great interest in me, since he too was interested in hypophyseal cytology of batrachians and fishes. We worked a great deal, but under no constraint. I met D. Picard (Marseille) there too, and much later, E. Legait, who was to succeed R. Collin and with whom I had taken physics and chemistry at Nancy. Still later, once R. Collin and I had become friends, he invited me to his home, where I met his wife, his only daughter, and numerous sons—all of whom made up a very pleasant family indeed—and finally, his future son-in-law, Professor Barry (now in Lille), who has made a significant contribution to our knowledge of the structure of the hypothalamus.

Professor Collin, who was renowned as a hypothalamopituitary histologist, had originally propounded the theory of *neurocrinie,* that is to say, he described a pituitary *colloid* in the neural lobe originating in the lysis of invaded glandular cells and its secretion in the *tuber,* i.e. the infundibulum. He channeled the colloid up along the nerve fibers as far as the hypothalamic neurons, where it was absorbed. In other words, he had the colloid take the opposite direction to that which Scharrer—who had already described at length a *diencephalic gland*—had made it take.

I think it is worth rereading today, in full, Collin's criticism of Scharrer's findings, if only to illustrate how one can argue very logically from incorrect data, and that physiological conclusions drawn from purely morphological observations should always be subject to caution. Says Collin*:

Finally, Scharrer feels that the nerve elements of certain tuberal nuclei are capable of secretion, suggesting a diencephalic nerve gland, and thus he feels justified in using the word "neurocrinie" to describe the activity of this nervous gland.

What is opposing the two theories of "neurocrinie" is clear: the first, which I have no reason whatever to abandon, is based on the oft-repeated observation of secretion in the diencephalic nerve tissue of a colloidal substance produced outside it, by the pituitary gland. The second theory, that of Scharrer, is based on the observation of secretory phenomena of the nerve cells of the hypothalamus, and curiously enough it splits up nervous activity into two functions: the glandular function, and the nervous function proper, which are somehow mysteriously associated. The "neurocrinie" which I have observed is heterogeneous, bringing to the vegetative zones of the hypothalamus functional elements which are foreign to it. According to Scharrer, "neurocrinie" is homogeneous or localised, representing a glandular activity of the same nerve elements which furthermore exercise a regulating function on the phenomena of vegetative life.

The differences between these two conceptions do not seem to me irreconcilable. I have been fortunate enough to have been able to study Scharrer's preparations, and I feel that I may draw from them certain points which, far from modifying my own opinion, are in fact complementary to it.

Let us note firstly that the data of "neurocrinie" which I have described have not been invalidated, and that Scharrer himself does not reject them. We ought, then, as good scientists, to take them into account and integrate them into an appropriate

---

* This discussion was published in *Annales de Thérapie biologique,* ed. by the Laboratoires du Docteur François Debat 15 avril 1934 p. 503–521, a journal now defunct. A summary of this discussion can be found in R. Collin and F. Stutinsky, *Les problèmes posés par la neurohypophyse,* J. Physiologie, Paris, 1949, **41:** 7–118.

theory. Now it seems that Scharrer, whose attention was naturally focussed on the cytology of tuberal nuclei, particularly since his material, namely the brains of lower Vertebrates, would favour this point of view, did not take sufficient account of the pituitary gland's activity, which should not be isolated from that of the vegetative centers.

On the contrary, I think we should try to explain Scharrer's pictures by comparing them with my own. On these grounds, my observations today would be as follows:

1. As regards Mammals, no doubt remains as to the pituitary origins of the colloid and its upward transfer, suggesting the notion of a glandulo-neural or hypothalamo-hypophysial functional complex. In the species studied, there is always more colloid in the posterior lobe than in the hypothalamus: in other words, the whole of the pituitary gland's interstitial colloid does not get as far as the hypothalamus, either it passes into the vessels ("hemocrinie"), or it makes its way out into the ventricular fluid ("hydroencephalocrinie"). Now, either the presence of the interstitial colloid in contact with cells from the tuberal nuclei has no functional importance whatever—which seems absurd—or it may indicate action upon the vegetative neurons. Thus, it must be useable by these neurons, thanks to a special physico-chemical constitution of their cytoplasm and their nucleus, and to a particular secretory structure. However, our knowledge of the cytology of the tuberal nuclei in Mammals has not yet enabled decisive proof of this utilisation. On the other hand, the results of examining tuberal nuclei of Teleostei, whose nerve cells possess some of the clearest secretory characteristics, seem subject to further data being available, to comply with the hypothesis of an absorption by the components of these cells nuclei of the colloidal substance produced by the pituitary gland. I have in fact observed in the Teleost specimens of Scharrer, or of my colleague P. Florentin, a curious disproportion in the colloid content of neural lobe of the hypophysis and that of the tuberal region. If the tuberal nuclei produced the colloid, it would be found accumulated around them in a much higher proportion than elsewhere in the neurohypophysis. However, as is the case for Mammals, the opposite is observed: the colloid is undeniably supplied by the pituitary gland and thus we are naturally led to believe that the secretory pictures, which the tuberal nerve cells furnish, correspond to images of absorption of the hypophysial colloid. Undoubtedly there are still gaps in this interpretation as regards microscopic observations and further proof is needed, but in my opinion, it should be carefully considered if we are to arrive at a definitive theory of "neurocrinie".

2. Scharrer's argument, drawn from Trendelenburg's experiments, must be weighed up carefully. Trendelenburg, who did apply a histological check to the infundibulum of the hypophysectomized dogs, does not fail to report on Ramirez Corria's work, which describes a considerable hypertrophy in *pars tuberalis* in six hypophysectomized dogs, and on the similar results obtained by Koster.

Trendelenburg adds that it is likely that this hypertrophied epithelium of the *pars tuberalis* produces the hormone under discussion (the antidiuretic hormone found in the infundibulum of hypophysectomized dogs).

In 1924, I, for my part, had noted the difficulty in separating the *pars tuberalis* from the infundibulum without injuring the latter. To perform a hypophysectomy without injuring the tuberal region, a portion of the *pars tuberalis* must be left in place and the outgrowth of this fragment in the infundibulum is then feasible.

The outcome of this information is that before explaining the results of Trendelenburg's experiments by an increase in the glandular capacity of the tuberal nerve cells, we should eliminate once and for all any attribution of this function to the remaining *pars tuberalis*.

3. With respect to the scientific disagreement which puts me at variance with

Scharrer, it would be well to handle with great precision the very terms employed, if we are to reach a final agreement. All histologists agree on the distinction between the secretory property, common to all cells of the organism, and the glandular function, which attribute is confined to very few. In the picturesque terms of Auguste Prenant, a secretory cell consumes, but does not export. On the other hand, a glandular cell exports a product necessary for the activity of other cells. I am quite prepared to believe that within the functional couple made up by the pituitary gland and certain vegetative nuclei of the hypothalamus, it is the pituitary gland which exports, and the nerve cells which receive.

According to my interpretation, the latter use the product exported by the pituitary gland, and the undeniable secretory phenomena, which these nerve cells display, represent the various phases of use of these products. Indeed, it is noteworthy that Scharrer's thesis does not explain clearly the destination of the products supposedly formed by the nerve cells. He nevertheless admits that they empty into the third ventricle or into the blood vessels. But we know that the pituitary colloid also has as outlets the ventricular fluid ("hydroencephalocrinie") and general circulation ("hemocrinie"). It seems difficult to believe that the pituitary gland should be duplicated by a diencephalic gland which would at the same time take on important nerve functions, whereas to recognize that a hormone can act upon a nerve cell for example by modifying its excitability, is in line with a whole series of general biological data. I am quite aware of the danger, especially in biology, of making use of theoretical arguments, whose rational edifice can be demolished by experimental facts. But in the present state of affairs, the theory has only a very limited application: to determine, from a cytological viewpoint, how the hypophysial colloid is used by the nerve cells, and here I seek to bridge the gap between Scharrer and myself.

4. As far as I am in a position to judge from the preparations I have been able to observe, it is not certain that all the pictures observed by Scharrer correspond to legitimate secretory phenomena. Several of these seem to depict degeneration; Scharrer himself notes sclerosed nerve cells in the Perch.

5. Restricting ourselves to secretory phenomena displayed by nerve cells, Scharrer remarks that these phenomena are not limited to the diencephalic gland. He points out the existence of a mesencephalic gland in the area of the tegmentum for some Cyprinides (Minnow, Tench). Recalling the existence of secretory figures in the spinal chord of Selacians and bony fish, he concludes, with Parker, that the nervous system seems to play a by no means unimportant role in the humoral regulation of certain functions.

Without denying the existence of secretory structures in the nervous system, we wonder if, at the level of certain neurons, the neural regulations themselves do not presuppose a secretory structure receptive to hormonal substances. In fact, in order to play their role of regulators, the central vegetative neurons must either react to the relevant neural impressions, triggered by mechanical, thermal, or chemical stimuli, or else they must be modified directly by the humours. In both cases, they respond to a change in the organic balance: this does not lead us away from classical physiology. On the contrary, according to Scharrer, these vegetative neurons are able to modify glandularly the humoral balance of the organism, and would thus embrace within their cellular entity a twofold operational function: a chemical and a neural function. Here again, any *ex cathedra* attempt to settle the question would go beyond the limits of our experimental data: with these few thoughts, I simply wished to point out the scope of the problems which would be raised by the attribution of a glandular (and not merely secretory) role to the nerve cells, if this role were legitimately proven.

At the time, neither Scharrer nor Collin had at their disposal the technical resources to settle the problem once and for all. However, I can vouch for how close Collin came to discovering neurosecretion, missing it only because of a detail in the use of the histological staining technique. I am all the more sensitive to this failure since, during my stay in Nancy while preparing my doctoral thesis, the same misadventure—the use of this inadequate technique—stopped me from discovering neurosecretion. In fact, under the influence of prolonged exposure of a frog to light, with a black background, one can observe, with a trichromatic technique (hemalum, erythrosin, light green, as advocated by P. Florentin) paths of colloid going from the hypophysis to the preoptic region. However, the use of a better fixative than the picric acid in Bouin's fluid (an osmic fixative or chromium fixation) with a toluidine blue-erythrosin stain would have clearly shown—as I discovered after 1949—that these colloidal traces were nerve fibers of the neurosecretory pathway. This is obvious from certain figures in my doctoral thesis in Medicine of 1939 (Stutinsky, 1939*a*) and in an article which appeared in 1939 (Stutinsky, 1939*b*) which the war totally buried and forgot. Unfortunately still obsessed by the theory of *neurocrinie,* I sought the origins of the colloid in the pars intermedia, which does, moreover, produce certain colloidal transformations under these conditions.

During the same period, my efforts to defend *neurocrinie* brought me into a brief disagreement with E. Scharrer. The section of optic nerves in *Rana temporaria* enabled me to observe, in some mesencephalic neurons, protoplasmic inclusions which were stained by eosin or fuchsin (Stutinsky, 1937*b*). The pictures obtained looked very much like the figures already described by Scharrer. However, since I saw them especially after section of the optic nerves, I interpreted them as figures of degeneration; it will be remembered that Collin tended to interpret certain pictures of the *diencephalic gland* as being ones of degeneration, and he agreed with this interpretation. This research was important to me in that it put me in direct contact with Professor Scharrer. While writing the present article, I came across his request for reprints of this work, written from Chicago and dated September 7, 1937 and which I received in Paris after my return to the Biology Laboratory there. Scharrer's reply to my sending him the reprint came soon afterwards. I have looked for it, and cannot find it, but I have read and reread it so often that I remember whole sentences of the letter: "Do not put too much faith in Collin's ideas," he wrote. "Since I have come to know, through P. Florentin [who had done a training period in Scharrer's laboratory in Frankfurt], the techniques used in his laboratory, I, along with many other research workers no longer bother about his conclusions. On the other hand, I am always ready to accept results based on experimental work, and in this respect, I think your observations concerning neurons of the frog mesencephalon are of importance." I did not study the problem further, for I was busy with writing up my thesis on the optopituitary reflex in the frog; moreover, the international political climate was becoming increasingly stormy. The manuscript was completed in the spring of 1938, and it was printed by the end of 1938. In February 1939, I defended my thesis, which was awarded the Silver Medal of the Faculty of Medicine of Paris.

By September 1939, war had broken out. I covered the entire campaign in Lorraine in front of the Maginot Line with a reconnaissance group. Taken prisoner in June 1940, I was kept on as a doctor in camps in France until August 1941. Then, the German occupation of Paris, and what went with it, prevented me from staying there, and after many adventures, I fled to the south of France. While it deprived me of any possibility of experimental work, this enforced resting period did nevertheless allow me to ponder over certain problems. That is how I came to plan a reflectometer for live frog's skin to record the influence of external and hormonal conditions on the degree of expansion of the melanocytes. After the war, I carried out this experiment upon returning to Paris, and for some months I took reflectometric measurements on frog's skin (Stutinsky, 1945). This did not get me very far, but rather showed me that cutaneous reactions, which expressed modifications in the functioning of the pars intermedia, constituted a simple reaction, but of complex origin. Most important, I corroborated the findings I had published in my doctoral thesis, namely, that these reactions disappeared under two conditions: section of the optic nerves, which produced an average expansion of the melanocytes; and section of the infundibulum, which induced permanent dilatation associated with a hypertrophy of the pars intermedia which, as it has been shown later, exists also in mammals.

After consideration of the optopituitary reflex, I concluded that no progress could be made in this field without a better understanding of the innervation of the pars intermedia and of the pituitary gland in general. It would prove a difficult study since the capriciousness of the silver impregnation is discouraging for the experimenter. I obtained the best results with specimens under freezing conditions. As this proved to be difficult with my laboratory material, I tried bovine hypophysis and in the year 1945–46 I obtained an interesting result which once again put me at odds with my former director, Professor Collin.

Silver impregnation of the ox pituitary revealed dilatations along the nerve fibers, bulb endings, such as Tello had described in 1912 in man. He interpreted these as due to degeneration since his material came from autopsies, and for a long time afterwards, Stöhr, Hagen, and, in general, many German histologists, accepted this theory. Being under the influence of Collin, I did not venture explicitly to relate these bulbs to the colloid or even better to the Herring bodies, but I emphasized that my technique did not enable me to observe the colloid and that, apart from the bulbs and nerve fibers, there was no visible colloid other than pericapillary granulations (Stutinsky, 1946, 1947, 1950a).

Soon another technique was to confirm my doubts about the cellular origins of the Herring bodies. With Altman's method for detecting mitochondria on frozen slides, fixed with chromium mixtures and having undergone postchromation, long ribbons of nerve fibers with irregular disposed bulbs could be observed, which could only be nerve dilatations, i.e., the Herring bodies. Morever, these bulbs contained chondriocontes, whose presence inside the nerve fiber was very much disputed at the time. I do not know exactly how Professor Bargmann heard about this work, but he referred to it when sending me his first reprints on neurosecretion. A reading of Bargmann's findings rid me of any remaining hesitation and I, in turn, tried the Gomori method. Now, I had been familiar with this method for almost two years, but my luck was such that I missed, for the second time, discovering neurosecretion. In fact, I encountered the Gomori method in 1947, at the meeting in Paris of the French anatomists, where a young South American histologist demonstrated this method on various tissues. The production of chromic haematoxylin was not difficult, but at that time in France, it was impossible to get hold of phloxine. I thought phloxine was an indispensable dye—which, as everyone knows today, is not the case—and I did not use the chromic haematoxylin until I received Dr. Bargmann's letter. From this point on, interesting results began to accumulate. The early fifties were years of intensive work. Applying concurrently the Hortega method for the pituicytes, and the Gomori or Bodian methods for the nerve fibers to the same specimen, I demonstrated that the Herring bodies belonged to the nerve fibers and that the pituicyte behaved essentially like a satellite cell. I revealed the accumulation of neurosecretion in the infundibulum after hypophysectomy, in the rat, the presence of a "regeneration" of the neural lobe in the hypophysectomized animal, and showed that three months after operation, significant quantities of antidiuretic hormone, even higher than normal, remained in the hypothalamus.

In 1951, at the meeting of French-speaking anatomists in Nancy, R. Collin gave a paper on hypophyseal *neurocrinie* in which he still maintained the duality of the colloid origins, while at the same time leaving plenty of leeway for my interpretation of the Herring bodies. I had written to tell him that I would be bringing as yet unpublished arguments, and that my new findings impelled me to accept the hypothesis of neurosecretion. After having observed pictures of accumulation of neurosecretion after hypophysectomy, I had published a brief note on the subject for the Biological Society in Paris (Stutinsky, 1950*b*, 1951*a*), but R. Collin had not yet heard about this. In my paper at Nancy, I described these results which were accompanied by good color slides and the impact it made was such that the end of colloidal *neurocrinie* could be dated from this meeting (Stutinsky, 1951*b*).

For France, at any rate, my findings constituted the starting point for the neurosecretion vogue and also for the application for the Gomori technique to invertebrates (Stutinsky, 1951*c*). But perhaps it was in my own circle that I encountered the greatest skepticism and resistance at the time. An old friend, a distinguished neurohistologist, urged me strongly to fix the brains more adequately, and he maintained, not without reason, that Bouin's fluid was a very poor fixative for nervous tissue. He maintained, as did particularly some American histologists, that the Herring bodies and the deformations of nerve fibers were essentially artifacts. From time to time, people would also come to counsel me to "change subjects," to drop a question which could only cause me problems.

There were others too, such as Gabe, who was working, like myself, at the time, in the Laboratory of Comparative Anatomy headed by Professor M. Prenant. After a seminar, in which I had presented before the whole laboratory the state of my research and proposed applying the Gomori method to the study of the pars intercerebralis-corpora cardiaca complex, he declared that this method represented no superiority and no improvement over classical histological methods, which he was using for the same purpose. As we know, he ended up by changing his mind.

In 1946, I started part-time work in an industrial laboratory for therapeutic products, a start which, on one hand, placed at my disposal the resources of a slaughterhouse, and, on the other, enabled me to take part in the purification of certain hormones, and at that time, in particular, of adrenocorticotrophic hormone (ACTH). I had to administer several doses of ACTH according to the old Sayers method, i.e., to detect the drop in ascorbic acid of the adrenal glands. In 1951, I attempted to escape the tyranny of the hypophysectomized rat by giving doses of ACTH to normal animals. I was reprimanded several times for this. If the principle proved to be poor, it nevertheless afforded some interesting observations (Stutinsky, Schneider, and Denoyelle, 1952):

1. Vasopressin is capable of inducing a significant drop in ascorbic acid in the adrenal gland, whereas oxytocin is not.
2. This process requires the presence of the hypophysis.
3. The activity of vasopressin on the adrenals is synergistic with ACTH.
4. All ACTH extracts, even the American standard ones, contain vasopressin.

In the conclusions, I stated (p. 649) that "vasopressin or more generally, neurohypophyseal substances, could constitute the mysterious neurohormonal stimulus capable of triggering off ACTH secretion, despite the section of hypothalamohypophyseal pathways (Bonvallet *et al.*, 1951)." In the same conclusions, I also suggested the use of vasopressin for examining the hypophysioadrenal axis and more particularly the corticotrophic function of the hypophysis. This study, and especially the conclusions, are rarely cited. Above all, it brought me vigorous methodological criticism, notably from Guillemin; however, I may venture to add that at the time no one had yet spoken of a *releasing factor.*

I believe it was in 1952 that I met the Scharrers while they were passing through Paris, but it was only for a short visit of my laboratory, and an exchange of views.

It was in 1953 that the great family reunion of "neurosecretionists" took place at the first symposium in Naples. Everything came together at once—the sun of southern Italy, the beauty of the Bay of Naples, and most important, the rapid discovery of real human warmth, of an intellectual collusion. We owe this discovery to Ernst and Berta Scharrer.

It was there too, that I met Bargmann, Hanström, Sir Solly Zuckerman, Sir Francis Knowles, and many others, for the first time. This meeting will remain important for all those who took part in it, and their team spirit has been evident in subsequent symposia. Although the neurosecretionists were quickly and quite naturally absorbed by neuroendocrinology, the symposia on neurosecretion continued to be held every four years. The sixth one took place in September 1973 under the chairmanship of Sir Francis Knowles. It was at the same time the 20th anniversary of the Naples meeting.

After 1953, the notion of neurosecretion gained the support of the majority of neuroendocrinologists, but not of all. Sir Solly Zuckerman remained an opponent of it for a long time, and especially G. W. Harris, who is among those who have done the most to explain the relationship between the hypothalamus and the hypophysis. His objections are still clearly set out in his 1955 book on neural control of the pituitary gland; in particular, he found the idea of a regeneration of neurosecretory fibers hard to swallow. He made this clear at the Bristol meeting in 1956, and at the time, his opinion, along with other commentaries, did me great harm in the minds of certain Parisian directors whose veto then excluded me from the Paris Science Faculty.

I held nothing against Harris, and several years later in 1968, I proposed that he be made Doctor Honoris Causa at the Faculty of Science in Strasbourg. Owing to the 1968 "incidents," his visit to Strasbourg was not as spectacular as such academic ceremonies usually are, for there was a fear of student interference. However, everything went off well; he was highly appreciative of his diploma and of the Alsatian cuisine and wine. He deserved to be better known, and I think our esteem was soon mutual.

Reviewing the various stages in my scientific career, I find that they amount to a long series of failures and near-misses, often due to unimportant things, usually in the order of technical inadequacies or maladjustments, whose vital importance I slowly became aware of later. What positive contributions I have been able to make have generally brought me much criticism, which in at least one case has temporarily halted my career and set it off in a different direction.

In spite of all this, on one or two occasions I really had the feeling of having seen something new for the first time and even if in the year 2000, neuroendocrinologists do not credit me with these firsts, their unwillingness to do so will in no way subtract from the exultation which overtook me during the first years of neurosecretion, nor from the memory of the joy of colleagues meeting, sharing common problems—this powerful and exhilarating feeling of having played a useful part in a common task.

REFERENCES

Bonvallet, M., E. Morel, and P. Benda (1951). Sur le mécanisme de la transmission à l'hypophyse des stimuli provoquant la décharge émotionnelle d'hormone corticotrope, chez le Chien. *C. R. Soc. Biol.* **145**: 1055.

Stutinsky, F. (1934a). Expansion des erythrophores chez *Phoxinus laevis* par des produits non hypophysaires. *C. R. Soc. Biol.* **115**: 241.

Stutinsky, F. (1934b). Déterminisme expérimental de l'expansion des chromatophores. *C. R. Soc. Biol.* **116**: 284.

Stutinsky, F. (1936). Effets de l'illumination continue sur la structure de la glande pituitaire de la Grenouille. *C. R. Soc. Biol.* **123**: 421.

Stutinsky, F. (1937a). Modifications histologiques de l'hypophyse de la Grenouille après lésion infundibulaire. *C. R. Assoc. Anat.* (Marseille) **32**: 396.

Stutinsky, F. (1937b). Inclusions cytoplasmiques dans certains neurones du mésencéphale de la Grenouille aveuglée. *C. R. Soc. Biol.* **124**: 137.

Stutinsky, F. (1939a). *Contribution à la physiologie hypophysaire des Batraciens.* Thése de Médecine, Paris, 1 vol., 224 pp., 29 fig. G. Thomas, ed., Nancy, 1939.

Stutinsky, F. (1939b). Le "réflexe opto pituitaire" chez la Grenouille. *Bull. Biol. Fr. Belg.* **73**: 385.

Stutinsky, F. (1945). Etude de la mélanocinèe chez la Grenouille à l'aide d'une cellule photoélectrique. Action de l'intermédine chez la Grenouille normale. *C. R. Acad. Sci.* **221**: 153.

Stutinsky, F. (1946). Sur certaines terminaisons nerveuses de la neurohypophyse des Mammifères. *Ann. Endocrinol.* **7**: 231.

Stutinsky, F. (1947). Sur l'aspect morphologique de certaines terminaisons nerveuses dans la neurohypophyse du Boeuf. *Bull. Assoc. Anat.* **52**: 452.

Stutinsky, F. (1950*a*). Sur la signification des "corps de Herring" de la neurohypophyse. *Assoc. des Anatomistes,* Louvain, 493.

Stutinsky, F. (1950*b*). Colloide, corps de Herring et substance Gomori-positive de la neurohypophyse. *C. R. Soc. Biol.* **144:** 1357.

Stutinsky, F. (1951*a*). Sur l'origine de la substance Gomori-positive de la neurohypophyse. *C. R. Soc. Biol.* **145:** 367.

Stutinsky, F. (1951*b*). Répartition et origine de la substance Gomori-positive chez le Rat. *Assoc. des Anatomistes,* Nancy, 942.

Stutinsky, F. (1951*c*). Etude de l'innervation du complexe rétro-cérébral chez *Periplaneta americana,* à l'aide de l'hématoxyline de Gomori. *Bull. Soc. Zool. Fr.* **76:** 307.

Stutinsky, F. (1952). Sur l'origine diencéphalique des hormones dites "posthypophysaires." *C. R. Soc. Biol.* **146:** 1691.

Stutinsky, F. (1957*a*). Recherches expérimentales sur le complexe hypothalamo-neurohypophysaire. *Arch. Anat. Microsc. et Morphol. Exp.* **46,** no. 1.

Stutinsky, F. (1957*b*). Recherches morphologiques sur le complexe hypothalamo-neurohypophysaire. *Bull. Microsc. Appl. Mémoire hors série* No. 2.

Stutinsky, F., M. Bonvallet, and Morel (1951). Réponses éosinopéniques d'origine émotionnelle chez le Chien. *J. de Physiol.* **43:** 661.

Stutinsky, F., J. Schneider, and P. Denoyelle (1952). Dosage de l'ACTH sur le Rat normal et influence de la présence des principes posthypophysaires. *Ann. Endocrinol.* **13:** 641.

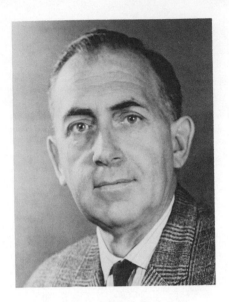

János Szentágothai

János Szentágothai was born in Budapest, Hungary, in 1912, and received his M.D. from the University of Budapest in 1936, after which he joined the medical school faculty. In 1947 he became Professor of Anatomy and Chairman of the Department at Pécs University Medical School. In 1963 he moved back to Budapest as Professor and Head of the First Anatomy Department of the Semmelweis University Medical School. Dr. Szentágothai's neuroanatomical studies cover a wide field, from the functional anatomy of synapses to the analysis and functional interpretation of neuron networks. His main interests were initially the spinal cord; later he became involved in hypothalamic studies and eventually shifted to the study of the cerebellum and lately to the cerebral cortex. He is a member of the Hungarian Academy of Sciences, Belgian Royal Academy of Medicine, National Academy of Sciences (Washington), and the American Academy of Arts and Sciences (Boston).

Under the Spell of
Hypothalamic Feedback

JÁNOS SZENTÁGOTHAI

If it were not for its insignificance, my relation to neuroendocrinology could be best characterized by the Hungarian saying, "He enters [into the story] like Pontius Pilate into the Apostolic Creed." As I was educated as a neuroanatomist during the mid-thirties, my knowledge of endocrine mechanisms was on the (lower) level of the contemporary German textbooks of physiology. About the hypothalamus I knew that it might have something to do with the control of visceral and metabolic functions, and how to demonstrate to the students its gross anatomy in our routine practical course of brain dissection. My interests were focused in those years—at the First Anatomy Department of Budapest University and during the last years—and shortly after the retirement of my teacher, Michael von Lenhossék—upon the structure of peripheral vegetative innervation.* Understandably, I soon became interested in the question of the central origin of preganglionic fibers and their supranuclear connections. Very little, apart from the rather vague classical data, was known at that time of the question. Laruelle (1936), the famous Belgian neurologist, was the only scientist particularly engaged then in the study of the vegetative nuclei of the spinal cord, and a short visit to his laboratory during the summer of 1939 impressed me with the potentialities of this field. So that when I built my first stereotaxic instruments in 1940—a polar coordinate instrument for cats (illustrated cursorily in a paper in 1942, Szentágothai, 1942a), a smaller instrument for rats assembled from old microscope stages (Figure 1A), and a special instrument for the spinal cord (Figure 1B, mentioned in a publica-

---

* I have told the story of my early adventures with the defense of the neuron theory and the use of axonal degeneration methods quite recently in a chapter of the book entitled *Paths of Discovery*. F. W. Worden, ed., MIT Press, Boston.

JÁNOS SZENTÁGOTHAI • First Department of Anatomy, Semmelweis University Medical School, Budapest IX, Hungary.

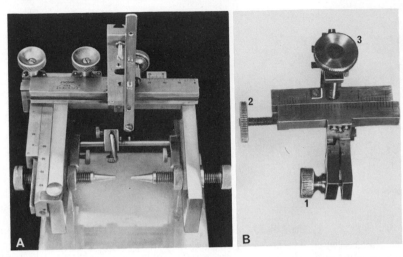

FIGURE 1. A Stereotaxic instrument assembled from two microscope stages. Such an instrument for rats was built first in the Budapest anatomy department around 1941. This instrument is a later version, although without major change, because the first model was lost during the end of World War II. B Stereotaxic instrument made for operation on the spinal cord. 1 = brackets and screw for fixation of the instrument on a spinous process; 2 = wheel for horizontal movement; and 3 = for vertical movement, the electrode carrier is concealed from sight at upper part of the photograph. No movement in the sagittal direction was necessary for work on the spinal cord. This apparatus was also lost during the siege of Budapest but the next, slightly modified, version was described later (Szentágothai, 1951).

tion only much later in 1951)—I ventured into the study of the vegetative nuclei giving rise to the preganglionic fibers of the parasympathetic system. The results were not very encouraging so that my original plans to trace their descending connections stepwise backwards ended in frustration. I published only one paper on the neuronal links of the light reflex pathway of the pupil (Szentágothai, 1942*b*) and much later another on the localization of the parasympathetic lower brain stem nuclei (Szentágothai, 1952). The situation was probably premature for such an enterprise: Even with the powerful techniques of today, notably electron microscopy, and the important knowledge of and the technical approach to monoaminergic pathways, this job is not an easy one and will need the concerted efforts of various laboratories. My first attempts to break into the hypothalamus over the descending pathways were thus defeated.

Already as early as 1939–40 my attention was called to the findings of Ernst and Berta Scharrer on neurosecretion by my department chief F. Kiss—the successor of M. von Lenhossék—who always had a special inclination for unorthodox and unaccepted concepts (which neurosecretion then undoubtedly was). We made, therefore, lesions in the hypothalamus, particularly in the supraoptic nucleus, in order to trace the neurosecretory pathway. However, again the axonal and synapse degeneration—which worked so nicely in the central fibers of primary afferents and in descending spinal pathways—did not yield tangible results in the neurohypophysis. So this second attempt became another failure, for which I do not even have the consolation of the first, where at least I can persuade myself that the situation was premature technically. Had I not confined myself to a single method—the tracing of axons to their synaptic terminals by experimental degeneration—I could have easily reached a major breakthrough then. However, conceited as one can only be in one's late twenties, I thought the cumbersome application of the Bielschowsky silver stain* to degenerated pathways and synapses or terminals as the only and ultimate tool in neuroanatomy, which would solve all conceivable problems (and if not, so much the worse for the problems). I was well aware at the time of the studies by S. W. Ranson and co-workers at Northwestern University in Chicago and have to be really ashamed for not having understood the implications and not made the appropriate conclusions to hang on tenaciously and try to use other techniques. Still another experiment we did with a co-worker of mine, Louis Bakay, Jr. (now Professor of Neurosurgery at Buffalo General Hospital), was to destroy stereotaxically the pineal gland in male puppies and to look for their expected precocious sexual maturation—a further naïve approach that ended in failure, although we tried to work out a quantitative technique for the evaluation of the intensity of spermiogenesis. Eventually my interests became increasingly absorbed by the oculomotor system and its labyrinthine connections, which appeared to me vastly superior in elegance and clinical significance (a view emphatically endorsed by the leading figures of neurology and internal medicine in Hungary) to the wishy-washy data on the neural relations of endocrine mechanisms.

All this ended rather abruptly with the terminal phase of World War II in the inferno of the extermination of some, and uprooting of other, segments of the population. After returning in early 1946 from brief military service and some months as prisoner of war, I had to take over the chair of anatomy at Pécs University in the southwest of Hungary, which was not only vacant but literally empty: not a single teaching staff member being available. In the first months I managed with a small enthusiastic group of third- and fourth-year medical students who helped me with running the dissections and histology courses, and among whom I had the good fortune to encounter Béla Flerkó. Very luckily, some of my stereotaxic instruments were preserved in Budapest, so that I could start immediately with my work

* I have told the early story of the application of silver stains to experimentally induced degeneration of synapses in the article mentioned in my first footnote.

on the vestibulo-ocular and on the monosynaptic reflex arcs. I had not the slightest intention to return to the problem of the hypothalamus.

New teaching staff positions being made available around the end of 1946 and the beginning of 1947, I was glad to receive an offer from a young M.D. whom I had taught anatomy at the beginning of his studies and of whom I had lost sight since: Nicholas Stephen Halmi, who had just finished his studies at another university. I knew Dr. Halmi as a young man of exceptional mental capacities but was hardly prepared to get a young postdoctoral fellow who knew everything about hypothalamohypophyseal relationships that was known in 1947. He somehow had managed to get hold of the relevant western literature of this field, while the circulation of scientific periodicals and the subscriptions by universities were still little better than at a complete standstill. He knew that I had stereotaxic instruments and came with a ready program of experiments with hypothalamic lesions. Stereotaxic lesions placed into the tuberal region of rabbits yielded a number of impressive endocrine syndromes, but Dr. Halmi did know so much more about this field—and also my own studies on the labyrinthine reflexes were then at their climax—that I remained an interested outsider. Soon afterward Dr. Halmi left for the United States, where his early studies on pituitary cytology contributed very significantly to the development of this field.

According to the natural course of events one should have expected that this line of research would soon be abandoned in our department. However, Dr. Halmi's successful, albeit brief, activity exercised a lasting influence on the younger members of the staff—still partly medical students—notably Béla Flerkó, Béla Mess, and Béla Hálasz. Although I tried my very best to get everybody in the department engaged in some "nice legitimate" neurohistological work, most of my co-workers wanted to do endocrinology, with some hypothalamic experiments as the ultimate, but "the less neurohistology the better." (I still cannot get rid of the suspicion that my dear young friends—in spite of all their devotion—regarded my neurohistology as something of a devilry or witchcraft, because "how in the world could one infer anything from such inconspicuous silver-stained fragments in the thicket of the neuropil?" Actually I cannot blame them, because very few could have then predicted the spectacular later development in neurohistology that was to emerge from the suppressive silver stains, from electron microscopy, and from the renaissance of the Golgi method.) For the time being I persuaded Béla Flerkó to study the life cycle of the ciliary epithelium of the fallopian tube, a subject known to me since my early apprenticeship at the Budapest First Department of Anatomy. The development of cilia had fascinated M. v. Lenhossék (1898) and later a pupil of his, my immediate laboratory chief, P. v. Mihálik, whose pioneering studies

(1934–35) on the intravacuolar development of the cilia still did not gain the attention they deserve. Although Flerkó did very well in these studies (1951) and I already had great hopes in gaining leverage for the study of the then obscure replacement mechanisms of one-layered epithelia,* he soon became interested in the hormonal background of the cyclic epithelial changes and in 1950–51 we were back at the hypothalamus. My interest was still halfhearted in the beginning but Flerkó, an exceptionally thorough and tenacious worker, came up soon with indications from the literature (Hohlweg and Junkmann, 1932; Dey, 1941, 1943; Hillarp, 1949) and his own observations (1954) of the feedback control of gonadotrophic functions of the pituitary by peripheral hormone actions on the hypothalamus. This was finally a concept that appealed to my romantic nature and we all came for some years under the spell of this central idea. Actually we were not the only research group in Pécs who worked in this line of research, parallel studies being conducted in the physiology department under K. Lissák (Endröczi, Lissák, and Tekeres, 1961), and we were in fruitful collaboration with the Department of Pathophysiology headed by Sz. Donhoffer, where the food selection, metabolism, and temperature regulation of many of our animals bearing diencephalic lesions were studied.

It is now very strange to look back upon the many naïve and even bizarre traits of our work during the early fifties. Apart from certain limitations in equipment and chemicals and lack of standardized animal food caused by the postwar difficulties, most of this was due to my own inexperience, the lack of proper schooling and tradition in this line of research, and virtually no possibility for the direct exchange of ideas (by means of visits, participation in international meetings, fellowships for the younger co-workers, for example) with the international scientific community engaged in the research of this field. Having practically nothing—besides stereotaxic instruments, general operative facilities, and conventional histological equipment (which was, in fact, quite good in the anatomy departments of Hungary)—we had to rely almost exclusively on histological methods. There was also little hope for a rapid improvement in experimental facilities. We were a traditional type of anatomy department, after all, and if gradually funds became available for the purchase of modern postwar type equipment, the truly experimental departments had an obvious priority. Although histology is traditionally a "qualitative" approach, I felt very strongly in favor of making quantitative evaluations whenever possible. We thus hit on the method of studying nuclear size spectra, a procedure that had become popular in the German literature in

---

* A question most elegantly solved since with the methods of autoradiography. Flerkó and I knew the answer earlier but never really came to grips with this problem because of the change of our interest.

the late thirties, as a means to study the changes in functional activity in various tissues and organs. I did not succumb to the generally held unsophisticated view of the time that increased activity of the tissue goes hand in hand with increased cell nuclear volume and vice versa, because I understood that nuclear or nucleolar volume can only be a reflection of the actual balance between the uptake and discharge of various substances (in many cases probably simply of water). Nevertheless a change in nuclear or nucleolar volume could be considered as an indicator of some change in the functional equilibrium. In our group it was B. Mess who became most proficient in this type of research. He developed a number of workable biological assays—based on nuclear size spectrum changes—for various hormones, well before the modern bioassays became available (Mess, 1954). Another sign of our continuous struggle for making our histological observations quantitative, was the attempt (Mess, 1952) to evaluate the intensity of spermatogenesis after hypothalamic injuries by means of a counting procedure of seminiferous duct profiles in different cycle stages of the spermatogenetic wave.

Trying in retrospect to analyze my own attitude during this period, I have to realize that I had a negative bias against differential stainings. This was probably irrational, or had its roots in the depths of my unconscious (perhaps in connection with my early breaking away from the "dye-centered" technology of histology towards an almost exclusively silver impregnation centered approach in my neurohistological work), and I tell this only to show how the scientific activity of a whole group can be influenced by the irrational feelings or biases of their members. These characteristic traits of our work during the early and mid-fifties were still quite predominant in the first edition of our monograph (J. Szentágothai, B. Flerkó, B. Mess, and B. Halász, 1962), where most of our earlier papers were quoted in detail. Today, when there are different methods to trace the uptake and location of various general metabolites or other more specific substances, down to the level of the cell organelles, by electron microscopic autoradiography, and procedures to measure the contents of matter and of specific substances in single cells, most of this seems obsolete and hardly even of historical interest. And yet the old methods had the advantage of offering quick bird's-eye glimpses of an immensely complex pattern which in turn were leading to general concepts and theories. However unsophisticated and even false these may be, we were then less in danger of losing ourselves in an uncontrollable welter of detail than we probably are today.

Our strategy in hypothalamic research gained shape gradually during the mid-fifties. From the amorphous mass of often queer experiments and approaches, it was B. Flerkó's work that emerged first as a clear line of realistic investigation into the control mechanism of female gonadotrophic function. Particularly, his elegant experiment of parabiotically joined pairs of rats—one bearing the hypothalamic lesions and receiving the estrogen treatment, while the other served as test animal—was the first experimental model in which the hypothalamic action of estrogen could be unequivocally demonstrated. This paper was published in French (Flerkó, 1957) with the generous help of the group of Prof. J. Benoit in Paris, particularly of I. Assenmacher. It was some disappointment to realize that this crucial step in the development of this field passed virtually unnoticed until after Flerkó (1963) could tell the story again in English in a review type of paper, or after the appearance of our monograph. Dr. Flerkó became the first true neuroendocrinologist of our group who grasped the real spirit and got hold of the basic mental strategy of this new field of research.

My own role in this community remained that of some kind of "random generator" of often nonrealistic (if not mad) ideas, most of which led nowhere. Some of this may have had its origin in the character of "improvisation" of the early experimental morphology, still prevalent in the early thirties, when I received my introduction to scientific research. But I should not, perhaps, lay the blame for my basically romantic attitude upon the environment from which I received my first and most deeply ingrained impressions, because I most certainly grossly overplayed this game of improvisation. It was my idea to implant various endocrine organ fragments into the hypothalamus. If the idea of hypothalamic feedback was true, "why not implant the target organs and even the anterior pituitary into the hypothalamus and watch the result?" It would never have occurred to me, nor would I have had the patience to play around with—as has been done later by others—implanting or injecting the purified substances. Most of these experiments did not yield conclusive results, as could be justly expected if the many factors of uncertainty inherent to the method were considered. I positively had to force Flerkó, by using my prerogative as head of the department, to try this trick with ovarian tissue. This was some time around 1955 and the experiments were ready and evaluated (the actual work being done by Vera Flerkó-Bárdos) many months before Dr. Flerkó was prepared even to look at the results of "such an absurd experiment." The results were quite conclusive and were eventually published (Flerkó and Szentágothai, 1957). Trial and error, after all, is not always bad tactics.

The inside story of our pituitary transplants is even more amusing. Because of some observations of a young co-worker (Török, 1954) on pituitary circulation, we gained the impression that a fraction of the blood passing the anteriormost part of anterior pituitary tissue might be drained through veins at the posterior surface (adjoining the cleft) towards the median eminence. Being then completely immersed in the idea of feedback, I thought that this might be the anatomical basis of a short circuit feedback of anterior pituitary substances on the hypothalamus. An experimental study of this with B. Halász—still very young at that time and more under my influence than Flerkó, who was rapidly establishing his scientific independence—gave some semiconclusive results for the adrenal cortex (Halász and Szentágothai, 1960). (As a youngster Halász had the touching aura of a well-bred boy of an early Victorian family, for whom raising objections against the orders of a tyrannical "father" was out of the question.) In spite of this he was already then a keen observer and an astute thinker who understood the real implications of the anterior pituitary implants. The observation of intact basophilic cells in parts of the implant having immediate contact with a certain region of the mediobasal hypothalamus led to the definition and delineation of the so called hypophysiotrophic area of the hypothalamus (Halász, Pupp, and Uhlarik, 1962), one of the most elegant findings in the neuroendocrinological literature of the time. So, however unrealistic our implantation experiments may have been initially, they were turned into an important line of evidence by my excellent coworkers.

Our preoccupation with hypothalamic feedback had led us somewhat earlier to an interesting idea, the concept of neural feedback from endocrine organs. The assumption of neural channels, by which information from the periphery can reach the control centers of endocrine mechanisms, is not new. Such mechanisms of neural feedback were very generally believed to be at work in gonadotrophic mechanisms, where the significance of sensory information from the genital canal seems to be obvious. Similarly, information about peripheral tissue damage reaches the central mechanisms of corticotrophin control at least partly over neural routes. What we found, however, was quite different. The observation of an increase of cell nuclear volume in the ventromedial nucleus of the hypothalamus both after adrenalectomy and in adrenal atrophy induced by cortisone administration, and a decrease in nuclear size in adrenal hypertrophy, irrespective of whether caused by stress or by ACTH administration, induced us to study this effect more carefully. Astonishingly, unilateral adrenalectomy revealed this effect as being crossed: On the side contralateral to the removed adrenal the nuclear volume of cells in the ventromedial nucleus was increased, while on the ipsilateral side—i.e. contralateral to the remaining hypertrophic adrenal—the nuclei were shrunken (Halász and Szentágothai, 1959). Since such a crossed effect cannot be explained otherwise than by the assumption of a neural pathway, we hypothesized that an ascending neural path has to exist from the adrenal—probably from the capsule, which is rich in sensory endings—feeding rather directly into the contralateral ventromedial nucleus.

The mechanism is still rather obscure and has not, so far, aroused much interest, although apparently diencephalic effects after unilateral damage to the gonads were known long ago. The effect itself has been recently substantiated by modern methods using uptake by the cells of the ventromedial nucleus of tritiated amino acids (Gerendai, Kiss, Molnár, and Halász, 1974). These were the things that always fascinated me most, but I am a hopeless romantic.

Neurohistology proper of the hypothalamus remained my own domain, at least in the beginning. It is only relatively recently that the emerging new generation of neuroanatomists begin to see the great promise of this field: notably G. Raisman in Great Britain, Sousa-Pinto in Portugal, I. Akmayev from the USSR, and some of our own people in the two anatomy departments of Budapest. Research in this territory remained exceedingly frustrating throughout the fifties. Most of the classical neurohistological techniques for light microscopy were simply not suited for this region of the brain. I tried for many years to unravel the internal neuron connectivity of the hypothalamus by making small lesions in one part and by looking for degeneration of preterminal axons and synaptic terminals in another. The yield of such experiments remained discouragingly low even after the so-called suppressive silver stains for degenerating axons became available (Nauta and Gygax, 1954). Although I included some of our findings in our monograph (1962), I was never able to get this material off the ground, it remained a lame duck. The only reason I did not throw the whole material overboard was my almost fanatic conviction that this line of research has eventually to succeed one way or the other. One solution came through still another step in the development of the specific stains for degenerated axons and terminals: the method of Fink and Heimer (1967), which has since been joined by a score of similar other formulas. This new development came too late for me, too deeply engaged now in other fields of the nervous system. But this is, of course, irrelevant, because excellent work is being done in neuroanatomy laboratories all over the world both on the limbic system in its widest sense and on the hypothalamus proper, which will soon change our earlier naïve concepts beyond recognition. Another important step forward was to realize that secondary degeneration of axons and synaptic terminals could be used at great advantage by the application of the electron microscope. The pioneers in this field were Raisman (1969a,b); Raisman and Field (1971); Halász, Réthelyi, and Syentágothai (1968); Réthelyi and Halász (1970); and Sousa-Pinto (1970). It is not difficult to foresee that this line of research will gain momentum and great significance in the near future. I shall return to this briefly at the end of this paper.

There was, however, at least one line of research in hypothalamic neurohistology which not only gave satisfactory results but also contributed very much to my approach to and understanding of neural organization in general. The classical Golgi method, to which we owe practically everything we knew up to very recently about the fundamental architecture of the nervous system, was neglected for almost 50 years after the turn of the century. It is difficult to understand now the objective or more probably the psychological roots of this attitude of the neuroanatomists. There are, of course, fashions in research, as there are in social patterns or clothing, which may have many roots, from conscious manipulation by specific economic interests up to the irrational or the deep spheres of the subconscious. One should think, however, that fashions in biological research should be under the influence of more rational forces. It would be an interesting objective of a probably still nonexistent "sociopsychology of scientific research" to analyze the forces that are in the background of these shifts in attention, appreciation, and priority given to different modes of approach, beyond and above the obvious and not too glamorous motives that scientists also move in the direction of the least resistance and in the hope of harvesting the richest yields in the shortest time. Probably most neuroscientists felt after the appearance of the two magnificent volumes of Ramón y Cajal (1909, 1911) that little could be added to what has been described there, and if they wanted to discover something new they had to resort to other techniques. Additionally, neuroanatomy has vastly outrun the development of neurophysiology and it was quite logical that physiology had first to catch up—which it did with the emergence of the modern electrophysiology and unit level techniques from the early forties onwards—before neuroanatomy could resume its progress on the neuronal or neuron network level. It was, indeed, about during the mid-fifties that general interest in the Golgi procedures reappeared: in the studies of M. E. and A. B. Scheibel, of C. A. Fox, D. A. Sholl,* and others, soon followed by an increasing number of papers almost flooding the periodicals of today. Interestingly, this renaissance of the Golgi method preceded the development of electron microscopy of the central nervous system and hence anticipated the impressive demonstration by this new tool of the fact that from all the classical neurohistological methods the Golgi procedure gave the most realistic and most (if not only) useful picture of the real structure of neural tissue elements.

It was also in the mid-fifties that I started to work on the Golgi architectonics of the hypothalamus. The real pioneer, however, in this field was W. S. Krieg (1932), who gave an excellent general survey type description of the hypothalamus of the rat, including a very clear account of the Golgi architectonics. This paper was the main starting point of my own studies, which have yet to reach a stage at which I could summarize them in more than very preliminary form. Of course, our standards in requirements for an architectural study of any part of the gray matter have so radically risen in

---

* I do not quote the several publications because they have no immediate relevance to hypothalamus and neuroendocrinology.

recent years that it is unreasonable to expect an allover architectural description of the whole hypothalamus by any research group, let alone by a single author. Such a study would require a complete cross-identification and correlation of the Golgi and the EM architecture. This is now obviously beyond the reach of any single group, and we have to wait now for the gradual assembly of the whole picture of the hypothalamus from the bits and pieces on the architecture of single nuclei or parts thereof, now under way in many laboratories all over the world. I could, therefore, summarize my own Golgi observations only in a rather offhand fashion in the first edition (1962) of our monograph, and later with some improvements and bits of EM observations in the later edition (1968). My own understanding of the neuronal interconnections in the hypothalamus underwent a considerable change after the first summary in 1962. Although I earlier observed and illustrated types of axon terminals, mainly in the anterior hypothalamic and in the arcuate nucleus, which would be indicative of a specific termination of a single axon on a single or few neighboring cells (by means of grapelike clusters of terminal bulbs, Figures 23 and 29 in the 1962 edition), I was inclined to visualize the neuron network of the hypothalamus as some kind of diffuse connectivity system. More recent Golgi material (mostly unpublished, or Szentágothai 1969) has made me realize that there may be much more specific connectivity in the hypothalamus. Very unfortunately, the lack in regularity of orientation of dendritic processes and axonal arborizations makes it extremely difficult to disentangle the apparently diffuse neuropil into separate units. The only way of progress that I can visualize along these lines are three-dimensional reconstructions of whole parts of the neuropil from EM section series, as is being done with success in many other parts of the CNS. This type of fine-grain analysis of hypothalamic structures will probably be one of the most promising lines of the future and I would certainly encourage young scientists interested in the hypothalamus to take this route.

A result of major significance of my Golgi studies was the anatomical demonstration of the so-called parvicellular tuberoinfundibular neurosecretory system of the hypothalamus (Szentágothai, Flerkó, Mess, and Halász, 1962; Szentágothai, 1964). It was in these observations that the earlier assumed but still somewhat hypothetical system of neurons and nerve terminals that produced and discharged the hypothalamic releasing hormones into the pituitary portal system could be seen directly. Although the anatomical finding was clear enough (see Figure 49 of the 1962 edition of our monograph, or Figure 10 of my 1964 paper), they received little attention initially. When I presented the results first at an international meeting in 1962 (Szentágothai, 1964), they were received with incredulity and criticism—to say the least—by the "neurosecretologists" who had understandably little faith in the applicability of the Golgi procedure to these problems. (I hasten to add that the Scharrers were not among these; they immediately understood the implications of my observation.) This shows also how low in anatomical esteem the Golgi procedure stood in the beginning of the sixties. Only after the terminals in the superficial zone of the median eminence were demonstrated by the electron microscope (Szentágothai and Halász, 1964; Röhlich, Vigh, and Teichmann, 1965; Monroe, 1967) did the negativistic attitude subside very gradually, although many authors working on this system still do not seem either to realize or want to acknowledge that this system could be clearly demonstrated by the Golgi procedure. It is gratifying to see that the pictures yielded by the most advanced methods based on the immunohistological demonstration of releasing hormones (for example LH-RH; Barry, Dubois, and Poulain, 1973; Sétáló *et al.*, 1975) match the earlier Golgi pictures to the finest details.

My own direct involvement with the neuroendocrine studies largely ended with the publication of our monograph in 1962 and particularly with 1963, when I had to take over the chair of anatomy at Budapest Medical School, and my neuroendocrinologist co-workers stayed at Pécs. I had to confine myself to the role of an interested and benevolent spectator of the continuing work of my earlier pupils under the chairmanship of my successor at Pécs, Béla Flerkó. To my intense satisfaction they did much better on their own than under my romantic impetus. Quite understandably, because their grasp of the endocrine mechanisms was better and they received the benefits, from the late fifties onwards, of getting into fruitful communication with the international community of the neuroendocrinologists. Their methodology gained in scope and sophistication by adopting many of the internationally used techniques. The studies of B. Flerkó and co-workers on androgen sterilization and on estrogen uptake can illustrate what I mean. But I am also glad to see that the daring and romantic spirit of improvisation of our early efforts has not suffered from the use of more "legitimate" means and the new respectability gained by the international recognition of this group. The best example of this is the ingenious technique developed by B. Halász to produce isolated hypothalamic islands with the so-called Halász knife (Halász and Pupp, 1965) and the studies of this elegant experimental model are still far from having exhausted its potentialities.

For almost 10 years, since 1963, my interests have been absorbed by other problems of the CNS, notably the cerebellum, the subcortical relay nuclei, and the cerebral cortex, and until recently I had no intention of investing significant further efforts into the hypothalamus. However, this attitude has changed since B. Halász has been appointed to the second chair of anatomy of the Semmelweis University Medical School at Budapest, and we are again together in the same building. We have now several younger collaborators, or in fact whole research units, engaged in the type of fine-grain structural analysis of hypothalamic nuclei with continued Golgi and EM studies of the type hinted at earlier. Of course, such studies have to include experimental degeneration, both on the light microscope and EM level, the new methods of tracing nerve elements by uptake and axoplasmic transport of radioactive and other substances (procion yellow, cobalt, horseradish peroxidase), the fluorescence and microchemical methods for monoamines, and, last but not least, stereological methods to unravel the quantitative aspects of neural networks.

It is not difficult to realize that the study of the hypothalamus as a neural apparatus is still in its very beginnings. At my age it would be unreasonable to make ambitious plans of long duration, but I am thoroughly convinced that this type of analysis is one of the most promising lines in future neuroendocrinological research. What I would envision for the hypothalamus is the gradual emergence of neuron circuits or more probably of neuron network modules of known and tractable operational properties—as we begin to understand them in some other centers, notably the cerebellar and cerebral cortex. However, I am afraid this is still a distant promised land that I shall not be able to enter.

REFERENCES

Barry, J. M., P. Dubois, and P. Poulain (1973). LRF producing cells of the mammalian hypothalamus. *Z. Zellforsch.* **146:** 351.

Dey, F. L. (1941). Changes in ovaries and uteri in guinea-pigs with hypothalamic lesions. *Am. J. Anat.,* **69:** 61.

Dey, F. L. (1943). Evidence of hypothalamic control of hypophyseal gonadotrophic function in the female guinea-pig. *Endocrinology* **33:** 75.

Endröczi, E., K. Lissák, and M. Tekeres (1961). Hormonal "feedback" regulation of pituitary-adrenocortical activity. *Acta Physiol. Acad. Sci. Hung.* **18:** 291.

Fink, R. P., and L. Heimer (1967). Two methods for selective impregnation of degenerating axons and their synaptic endings in the central nervous system. *Brain Res.* **4:** 369.

Flerkó, B. (1951). Einfluss experimenteller Hypothalamuslaesionen auf das Eileiterepithel. *Acta Morphol. Acad. Sci. Hung.* **1:** 5.

Flerkó, B. (1954). Zur hypothalamischen Steuerung der gonadotrophen Funktion der Hypophyse. *Acta Morphol. Acad. Sci. Hung.* **4:** 475.

Flerkó, B. (1957). Le rôle des structures hypothalamiques dans l'action inhibitrice de la folliculine sur la sécrétion de l'hormone folliculo-stimulante. *Arch. Anat. Microsc. Morphol. Exp.* **46:** 159.

Flerkó, B. (1963). The central nervous system and the secretion and release of luteinizing hormone and follicle stimulating hormone. Pages 221–224 *in* A. V. Nalbandov, ed., *Advances of Neuroendocrinology.* University of Illinois Press, Urbana.

Flerkó, B., and J. Szentágothai (1957). Oestrogen sensitive nervous structures in the hypothalamus. *Acta Endocrinol.* (Kbh.) **26:** 121.

Gerendai, I., J. Kiss, J. Molnár, and B. Halász (1974). Further data about the existence of the neural pathway from the adrenal gland to the hypothalamus. Cell and Tissue Res. 153: 559.

Halász, B., and L. Pupp (1965). Hormone secretion of the anterior pituitary gland after physical interruption of all nervous pathways to the hypophysiotrophic area. Endocrinology 77: 553.

Halász, B., L. Pupp, and S. Uhlarik (1962). Hypophysiotrophic area in the hypothalamus. J. Endocrinol. 25: 147.

Halász, B., M. Réthelyi, and J. Szentágothai (1968). Examen électromicroscopique sur l'éminence médiane isolée (désafferentée neuralement). Arch. Anat. (Strasbourg) 51: 289.

Halász, B. and J. Szentágothai (1959). Histologischer Beweis einer nervösen Signalübermittlung von der Nebennierenrinde zum Hypothalamus. Z. Zellforsch. 50: 297.

Halász, B., and J. Szentágothai (1960). Control of adrenocorticotrophic function by direct influence of pituitary substance on the hypothalamus. Acta Morphol. Acad. Sci. Hung. 9: 251.

Hillarp, N. Å. (1949). Studies on the localization of hypothalamic centres controlling the gonadotrophic function of the hypophysis. Acta Endocrinol. (Kbh.) 2: 11.

Hohlweg, W., and K. Junkmann (1932). Die hormonal-nervöse Regulierung der Funktion des Hypophysenvorderlappens. Klin. Wochenschr. 11: 321.

Krieg, W. S. (1932). The hypothalamus of the albino rat. J. Comp. Neurol. 55: 19.

Laruelle, L. (1936). Contribution à l'étude du névraxe végétatif. C. R. Assoc. Anat. 31: 210.

Lenhossék, M. von (1898). Über Flimmerzellen. Verh. Anat. Ges. 14: 106.

Mess, B. (1952). Influence of hypothalamic injury on spermatogenesis in albino rats. Acta Morphol. Acad. Sci. Hung. 2: 275.

Mess, B. (1954). Kernvolumnia der Schilddrüse als Mastab für die thyreotrope Aktivität des Hypophysenvorderlappens. Acta Morphol. Acad. Sci. Hung. 4: 515.

Mihálik, P. von (1934–35). Über die Bildung des Flimmerapparates im Eileiterepithel. Anat. Anz. 79: 259.

Monroe, B. G. (1967). A comparative study of the ultrastructure of the median eminence, infundibular stem and neural lobe of the hypophysis of the rat. Z. Zellforsch. 76: 405.

Nauta, W. J., and P. A. Gygax (1954). Silver impregnation of degenerating axons in the central nervous system: A modified technique. Stain Technol. 29: 91.

Raisman, G. (1969a). A comparison of the mode of termination of the hippocampal and hypothalamic afferents to the septal nuclei as revealed by electron microscopy of degeneration. Exp. Brain Res. 7: 317.

Raisman, G. (1969b). Neuronal plasticity in the septal nuclei of the adult rat. Brain Res. 14: 25.

Raisman, G., and P. M. Field (1971). Sexual dimorphism in the preoptic area of the rat. Science 173: 731.

Ramón y Cajal, S. (1909). Histologie du Systeme Nerveux de l'homme et des vertébrés. I. Maloine, Paris.

Ramón y Cajal, S. (1911). Histologie du Systeme Nerveux de l'homme et des vertébrés. II. Maloine, Paris.

Réthelyi, M., and B. Halász (1970). Origin of the nerve endings in the surface zone of the median eminence of the rat hypothalamus. Exp. Brain Res. 11: 145.

Röhlich, P., B. Vigh, and I. Teichmann (1965). Electron microscopy of the median eminence of the rat. Acta Biol. Acad. Sci. Hung. 15: 431.

Sétáló, G., S. Vigh, A. V. Shally, A. Arimura, and B. Flerkó LH-RH-Containing neural elements in the rat hypothalamus. Endocrinology 96: 135–142, 1975.

Sousa-Pinto, A. (1970). Electron microscopic observations on the possible retinohypothalamic projection in the rat. *Exp. Brain Res.* **11**: 528.

Szentágothai, J. (1942a). Die innere Gliederung des Oculomotoriuskernes. *Arch. Psychiatr. Nervenkr.* **115**: 127.

Szentágothai, J. (1942b). Die zentrale Leitungsbahn des Lichtreflexes der Pupillen. *Arch. Psychiatr. Nervenkr.* **115**: 136.

Szentágothai, J. (1951). Short propriospinal neurons and intrinsic connections of the spinal grey matter. *Acta Morphol. Acad. Sci. Hung.* **1**: 81.

Szentágothai, J. (1952). The general visceral efferent column of the brain stem. *Acta Morphol. Acad. Sci. Hung.* **2**: 314.

Szentágothai, J. (1964). The parvicellular neurosecretory system. Pages 135–146 in W. Bargmann and J. P. Schadé, eds., *Lectures on the Diencephalon. Prog. Brain Res.* **5**. Elsevier, Amsterdam.

Szentágothai, J. (1969). The synaptic architecture of the hypothalamo-hypophyseal neuron system. *Acta Neurol. Belg.* **69**: 453.

Szentágothai, J., B. Flerkó, B. Mess, and B. Halász (1962). *The hypothalamic control of the anterior pituitary.* Akadémiai Kiadó, Budapest.

Szentágothai, J., B. Flerkó, B. Mess, and B. Halász (1968). *The hypothalamic control of the anterior pituitary.* 3rd rev. enlarged ed. Akadémiai Kiadoó, Budapest.

Szentágothai, J., and B. Halász (1964). Regulation des endokrinen Systems über Hypothalamus. Pages 227–248 *in* R. Zaunick, Hrsg. *Die Nervenphysiologie in gegenwärtiger Sicht. Nova Acta Leopoldina N. F.* **28**, Leipzig.

Török, B. (1954). Lebendbeobachtung des Hypophysenkreislaufes an Hunden. *Acta Morphol. Acad. Sci. Hung.* **4**: 83.

21

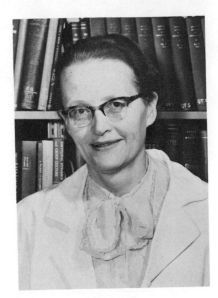

Marthe Vogt

Marthe Vogt, born and educated in Berlin, graduated in medicine in 1928 and gained a Ph.D. in Chemistry at the Kaiser Wilhelm Institut für Biochemie in the following year. She was then (1929–30) Research Assistant in the pharmacology department of Berlin University (Professor P. Trendelenburg), and Research Assistant and later a Department Head at the Kaiser Wilhelm Institut fur Hirnforschung, Berlin-Buch. As a Rockefeller Traveling Fellow, Marthe Vogt worked at the National Institute for Medical Research in Hampstead with Sir Henry Dale and at the Department of Pharmacology, Cambridge, with Prof. E. B. Verney before her appointment as Alfred Yarrow Research Fellow at Girton College, Cambridge, from 1937 to 1940. During this period she earned a Ph.D. in Pharmacology in the University of Cambridge.

The years 1941–1946 were spent on the staff of the pharmacology department of the Pharmaceutical Society of Great Britain, before she joined the pharmacology department of Edinburgh University, where she stayed as Lecturer and later Reader from 1947 to 1960. In 1960 Marthe Vogt was appointed to the headship of the Pharmacology Unit, Agricultural Research Council Institute of Animal Physiology, Babraham, Cambridge, until her retirement in 1968.

Marthe Vogt has enjoyed visiting appointments at Columbia University in New York, University of California at Los Angeles, University of Sydney in New South Wales, and McGill University in Montreal, and is currently still engaged in research at the Institute of Animal Physiology, Babraham, Cambridge.

Nervous Influences in Endocrine Activity

MARTHE VOGT

My first reaction on being asked to contribute personal reminiscences to the subject of neuroendocrinology was one of disbelief that I had ever worked in this field. I was then reminded by one of the editors that the subject covered every aspect of the relation between the nervous system and endocrine glands, and I suddenly realized that my very first efforts in the field of endocrinology were about nervous influences on endocrine activity. In 1929, Paul Trendelenburg had taken the chair of pharmacology in Berlin, and attracted to his institute a group of recently qualified medical graduates. These flocked to his laboratory to work without pay as "apprentices" in research, a custom now unknown and forgotten the world over. This happy state of affairs was cruelly interrupted by Trendelenburg's premature death early in 1931. During 1930, Trendelenburg was writing a monograph on the endocrine glands, and suggested that I should work on two *neuroendocrine* problems. The first was the nervous control of thyroid activity. This gland has a sympathetic innervation and the question was whether the nerves could act by enabling the gland to adapt its secretion to the varying needs of the body as determined by food intake. The answer was a clear-cut no. After sympathectomy, and even after cervical cord transection, the secretory state of the gland (assessed histologically) varied with the nutritional state, showing colloid storage during fasting and colloid discharge after feeding. A recent paper on the mouse (Melander, Ericson, Sundler, and Ingbar, 1974) nevertheless suggests that sympathetic nerves may serve to effect prompt, short-term alterations in the rate of thyroid hormone secretion.

The second problem proved to be far more involved. Trendelenburg had wondered whether a hormonal substance in the uterus was responsible

MARTHE VOGT • Institute of Animal Physiology, Babraham, Cambridge, England CB2 4AT.

for eliciting secretion of gonadotrophins, in conditions when mechanical stimulation of the cervix caused pseudopregnancy in the rat, or copulation with vasectomized males produced ovulation in the rabbit. No humoral factor was found. Yet the impression of nervous sympathetic control created by a statistically highly significant reduction in the occurrence of pseudopregnancy in the rat after cervical sympathectomy was fallacious. It did not mean that the sympathetic nerves were essential for the production of pseudopregnancy, but indicated a loss of cervical sensitivity in rats from which daily vaginal smears had been taken for prolonged periods of time. However, a nervous element was involved, since local anesthesia of the cervix was found to prevent pseudopregnancy, and the convulsive drug picrotoxin caused ovulation in the rabbit (Marshall, Verney, and Vogt, 1939); the search for this nervous pathway was resumed several years later (Vogt, 1942). Parasympathetic fibers running in the greater superficial petrosal nerve enter the carotid plexus and might reach the pituitary together with the blood vessels. Bilateral destruction of the greater superficial petrosal nerves was performed, but did not prevent ovulation in the rabbit. We now know that gonadotrophin release is produced by releasing factors elaborated in short hypothalamic neurones, but the pathway from the uterus to the hypothalamus has not been traced.

INTERACTION BETWEEN CORTEX AND MEDULLA OF THE ADRENAL GLAND

During the 4½ years I spent in England before the outbreak of war, foreigners (later "enemy aliens") like myself were not allowed to take up employment and they worked exclusively on research grants. Prof. E. B. Verney, with whom I spent most of the time, was interested in the kidney, and renal hypertension became my field of activity till 1940. I was then offered, and allowed to take up, the first post I had in Britain. It was in the pharmacology department of the Pharmaceutical Society. Its head was Prof. J. H. Gaddum, who, however, was away on war work and, in 1942, took up the chair of pharmacology in Edinburgh. My duties at the Pharmaceutical Society were the standardization, usually by bioassay, of certain medicinal products before they reached the market. Half of my time was my own, the problems were of my own choosing, and I decided to resume work in endocrinology. I concentrated on the adrenal cortex, which was a new and little explored field. I was fortunate in finding that the hormone concentration in adrenal blood was much higher than that in the gland and lent itself to rather inaccurate, but feasible bioassays.

The problem of the control of adrenocortical secretion led to the next episode in neuroendocrinological work. It was mostly done in Edinburgh where I had joined Gaddum in 1947, having ascertained that I would be allowed to pursue work on the adrenal cortex. It was concerned with the release of ACTH and the relation between medullary and adrenal cortical secretion. Circulating adrenaline is a stimulant of ACTH release at least in some species, the rat in particular, and indirectly leads to accelerated cortical activity whenever the splanchnic nerves are stimulated. How essential is medullary secretion in stress-elicited ACTH release? Cannon's and Elliott's work in the first decades of this century had shown the many conditions leading to splanchnic stimulation and thus secretion of medullary hormones; they could all be classified as *stresses*. In the 1940s *stress* was established as the accelerator of adrenocortical secretion, via release of ACTH. However, not all forms of stress activate the adrenal medulla, and the question arose whether in some forms of stress circulating adrenaline was indispensable for cortical activation, or whether it only reinforced an independent cortical response. In other words, how important for survival was the neural part of the response? Before discussing the experiments, it should perhaps be emphasized that this work (Vogt, 1947; 1951*a,b*; 1952) was carried out before chemical micromethods for the estimation of cortical hormones had been developed; the state and secretion of the adrenal cortex had to be assessed by histological means or by chemical estimation of loss of ascorbic acid from the adrenal gland.

It was shown (Vogt, 1947) that hemorrhage, as well as exposure to low or high environmental temperature, produced, in the rat, a loss of cortical lipids indicative of hypersecretion, whether or not the nerves to the adrenals had been cut. In a study in which the method of ascorbic acid depletion was used to obtain more quantitative information, it was then found that denervation of the adrenals did not prevent the ascorbic acid loss produced by insulin; the same held for demedullated rats in which there could be no doubt about the complete inactivation of the adrenal medulla. It was further ascertained that the effect of insulin was entirely caused by the hypoglycemia produced, as it could be prevented by offering glucose to drink. The hypoglycemia produced in demedullated rats is much more severe than in rats which can release adrenaline; this probably explains why the ascorbic acid loss after insulin is not appreciably reduced by denervation. In the demedullated rat, release of ACTH is due to hypoglycemia alone, and in the normal rat, to the combined effect of circulating adrenaline and a much milder hypoglycemia.

The question remained open whether there are forms of stress which depend entirely on the release of adrenaline for activation of ACTH secretion. Two conditions in which the role of adrenaline might have been expected to be decisive were emotion and the administration of β-tetrahydronaphthylamine, a substance which is now called 2-aminotetraline, and which causes vigorous sympathetic discharge through a central action. The result was clear-cut: No difference in the response of the adrenal cortex to 2-aminotetraline was found between demedullated and normal rats. However, after a very mild emotional stress (introduction of a rectal thermometer in the untrained animal), rats without adrenal medullae continued to show a fall in adrenal ascorbic acid, but the fall was less than in the normal rat. Thus, even mild emotional stress is not wholly dependent on medullary activity for causing release of ACTH.

Finally (Vogt, 1952), direct estimations were carried out of circulating adrenaline in stressed normal and demedullated rats. After a few minutes' operative stress under ether, arterial plasma of normal rats contained between 1 and 6 ng adrenaline per ml, whereas none (< 0.5 ng/ml) was found in demedullated rats. When doses of adrenaline were administered intramuscularly which were too small to produce an adrenal cortical response, they nevertheless raised the circulating adrenaline to values detectable by the methods used. Thus the response to stress in the demedullated rat was not due to residual traces of circulating adrenaline. After demedullation, the speed of cortical response in stress involving stimulation of sensory nerves during ether anesthesia was rapid, significant falls in ascorbic acid developing within a few minutes of ether administration.

These experiments define the role of the adrenal medulla in eliciting an adrenocortical response to stress as one of accelerating and supporting the response. They also show that afferent stimuli cause ACTH release within a few minutes of the stress even without the aid of medullary secretion. Irreplaceable, however, are the peripheral actions of the medullary hormone, such as effects on circulation or blood sugar, so that certain forms of stress are poorly tolerated in the absence of medullary activity.

NORADRENALINE IN THE BRAIN

Adrenaline played a central role in the work described in the previous section. With the discovery of noradrenaline as transmitter at peripheral postganglionic sympathetic neurones, work crowned by the first experiments demonstrating release of noradrenaline on stimulation of the splenic nerves (Peart, 1949), my interest grew in exploring the possibility that noradrenaline might play an important role in brain function, perhaps as a transmitter. There was a second reason for looking for potential transmitters in the brain. This was the fact which had become very obvious from work on the distribution of choline acetyl transferase in the brain (Feldberg and Vogt, 1948) that acetylcholine could only be a cerebral transmitter at a limited number of synapses; how did all the other terminals transmit their impulses? This is hardly a topic which merits classification as neuroendocrinology, though its early findings could have been so defined, and I therefore follow the advice of one of the editors to dwell a little on the origin of this work.

The occurrence of noradrenaline in the brain was shown by v. Euler in 1946. It was assumed to be present in cerebral vasomotor nerves. This was undoubtedly correct, but the question was whether it also occurred in the cerebral tissue proper. A detailed study of the distribution of noradrenaline (and adrenaline) in different parts of the brain left little doubt that much of the cerebral noradrenaline was not situated in blood vessels (Vogt, 1954). There was no correlation between vascularity of a region and its noradrenaline content: Thus there were only traces of noradrenaline in the highly vascularized cerebellum, and the concentration in the hypothalamus was too large to be accounted for by its vasomotor nerves. Another possibility was uppermost in my mind during the initial phases of the work: Catecholamines had been shown to be involved in release of gonadotrophins (Sawyer, Markee, and Everett, 1950). The finding that the highest concentration of cerebral noradrenaline was in the hypothalamus suggested a physiological mechanism controlling activity of the anterior lobe involving locally produced catecholamines. Such a view has now been put on a firm basis by many observations, such as the demonstration that selective destruction of cerebral adrenergic neurons (dopaminergic neurons remaining intact) does interfere with gonadotrophin secretion (Zolovick, 1972). Yet the overall distribution of noradrenaline in the brain was incompatible with such a restricted view of its role in brain function. In 1952, when the work on the distribution of noradrenaline had been completed (the delay in publication till 1954 was due to a temporary loss of the manuscript in the office of the editors of the *Journal of Physiology*), it would have been rash to state with any degree of confidence that cerebral noradrenaline was a transmitter at adrenergic neurons. The neuronal localization of the amine had not been demonstrated, and the occurrence of noradrenaline in gliomas was a warning not to take anything for granted. However, some conclusions could be confidently drawn: Hypothalamus, midbrain, and medulla contained so much noradrenaline that vasomotor nerves could not be its only site of occurrence; secondly, the capacity of a variety of drugs to reduce the noradrenaline content of hypothalamus and midbrain, provided the drug produced a centrally initiated sympathetic discharge, left no doubt that noradrenaline took part in brain function. At the time of writing, 13 years after the demonstration, by fluorescence microscopy, that cerebral noradrenaline was indeed situated in neurones (Carlsson, Falck, and Hillarp, 1962), the pendulum has swung from underestimating the functional role of this brain constituent to, perhaps, overestimating it. Psychiatrists, psychologists, pathologists, and pharmacologists vie with each other in finding new and exclusive functional roles for what is, after all, only one of the transmitters of impulses within the brain.

ACKNOWLEDGMENT

The work published after 1950 was supported by Edinburgh University and the Medical Research Council.

REFERENCES

Cannon, W. B. (1932). *The Wisdom of the Body*. Kegan Paul, London.

Carlsson, A., B. Falck, and N.-Å. Hillarp (1962). Cellular localization of brain monoamines. *Acta Physiol. Scand.* **56**(Suppl. 196): 1.

Elliott, T. R. (1912). The control of the suprarenal glands by the splanchnic nerves. *J. Physiol.* **44**: 374.

Euler, U. S. v. (1946). A specific sympathomimetic ergone in adrenergic nerve fibres (sympathin) and its relations to adrenaline and noradrenaline. *Acta Physiol. Scand.* **12**: 73.

Feldberg, W., and Vogt, M. (1948). Acetylcholine synthesis in different regions of the central nervous system. *J. Physiol.* **107**: 372.

Marshall, F. H. A., E. B. Verney, and M. Vogt (1939). The occurrence of ovulation in the rabbit as a result of stimulation of the central nervous system by drugs. *J. Physiol.* **97**: 128.

Melander, A., L. E. Ericson, F. Sundler, and S. H. Ingbar (1974). Sympathetic innervation of the mouse thyroid and its significance in thyroid hormone secretion. *Endocrinology* **94**: 959.

Peart, W. S. (1949). The nature of splenic sympathin. *J. Physiol.* **108**: 491.

Sawyer, C. H., J. E. Markee, and J. W. Everett (1950). Activation of the adenohypophysis by intravenous injections of epinephrine in the atropinized rabbit. *Endocrinology* **46**: 536.

Vogt, M. (1931). Zur Frage der nervösen Regulation der Schilddrüsentatigkeit. *Arch. Exp. Pathol. Pharmakol.* **162**: 129.

Vogt, M. (1931). Über den Mechanismus der Auslösung der Gravidität und Pseudogravidität, zugleich ein physiologischer Beweis für die sympathische Innervation des Hypophysenvorderlappens. I. Mitteilung. *Arch Exp. Pathol. Pharmakol.* **162**: 197.

Vogt, M. (1933). Über den Mechanismus der Auslösung der Gravidität und Pseudogravidität. II. Mitteilung. *Arch Exp. Pathol. Pharmakol.* **170**: 72.

Vogt, M. (1942). Ovulation in the rabbit after destruction of the greater superficial petrosal nerves. *J. Physiol.* **100**: 410.

Vogt, M. (1947). Cortical lipids of the normal and denervated suprarenal gland under conditions of stress. *J. Physiol.* **106**: 394.

Vogt, M. (1951*a*). The role of hypoglycaemia and of adrenaline in the response of the adrenal cortex to insulin. *J. Physiol.* **114**: 222.

Vogt, M. (1951*b*). The effect of emotion and of β-tetrahydronaphthylamine on the adrenal cortex of the rat. *J. Physiol.* **114**: 465.

Vogt, M. (1952). Plasma adrenaline and release of adreno-corticotrophic hormone in normal and demedullated rats. *J. Physiol.* **118**: 588.

Vogt, M. (1954). The concentration of sympathin in different parts of the central nervous system under normal conditions and after the administration of drugs. *J. Physiol.* **123**: 451.

Zolovick, A. J. (1972). Role of central sympathetic neurones in the release of gonadotrophin after hemiovariectomy. *J. Endocrinol.* **52**: 201.

Index